Educating Adolescents with Learning and Behavior Problems

Bruno J. D'Alonzo

Arizona State University

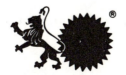

AN ASPEN PUBLICATION®
Aspen Systems Corporation
Rockville, Maryland
London
1983

Library of Congress Cataloging in Publication Data
Main entry under title:

Educating adolescents with learning and behavior
problems.

Bibliography: p. 491
1. Mentally handicapped children—Education (Second-
ary)—Addresses, essays, lectures.   I. D'Alonzo,
Bruno J.
LC4604.E34   1983   371.92′82   82-16363
ISBN: 0-89443-847-6

Publisher: John Marozsan
Editorial Director: R. Curtis Whitesel
Managing Editor: Margot Raphael
Editorial Services: Eileen Higgins
Printing and Manufacturing: Debbie Collins

Library of Congress Catalog Card Number: 82-16363
ISBN: 0-89443-847-6

Printed in the United States of America

1   2   3   4   5

IN MEMORIAM

To *R. Curtis Whitesel,* whose encouragement provided
direction and foresight. Curt brought to his profession
a unique blend of vigor, enthusiasm, and knowledge.
To his memory, I dedicate this work.

Table of Contents

Preface xiii

Acknowledgments xv

Contributors xvii

PART I—OVERVIEW AND ORIENTATION 1

Chapter 1—Introduction to Secondary School Programming for
LBP Students 3
Bruno J. D'Alonzo

Introduction 3
Adolescents and Secondary Schools 4
Causes of Organizational Problems 6
High School Curriculum: Trends and Issues 8
Problems in Programming for LBP Youths 15
Broad Range of Teacher Roles 22
Crisis-Resource Teacher/Room 27
Itinerant Interventionists 28
Teacher Consultants 29
Peer Tutoring/Support 30
Learning Specialists 31
Learning Assistance Centers 31
Summary 33

PART II—THE STUDENT AND FAMILY IN THE SCHOOL
ENVIRONMENT 35

Chapter 2—Adolescents with Learning and Behavior Problems 37
    Harold J. McGrady

        Introduction 37
        Perspective 37
        Common Characteristics 43
        Identification 49
        Curriculum and Instructional Objectives 50
        Mainstream Education 55
        Summary 65

Chapter 3—LBP Adolescent Offenders 67
    Jeffrey Schilit

        Introduction 67
        Identification, Incidence, and Legal Rights 68
        The LBP and the Psychology of Crime 72
        Criminal Behavior in LBP Adolescents 78
        Myths and Misconceptions 79
        Advocacy: Helping Adolescent Offenders 80
        Prevention Through Education 82
        Summary 89

Chapter 4—Communicating with Parents of LBP Adolescents 91
    L. Kay Hartwell, Roger L. Kroth, and Douglas E. Wiseman

        Introduction 91
        Parent Rights, Responsibilities, and Advocacy 93
        Conferencing Strategies 97
        Model for Increasing Parent Involvement 101
        Ways to Involve Parents 107
        Three Model Parent Involvement Programs 112
        Strategies for Parent Involvement 115
        Summary 120

**PART III—CURRICULA, CLASSROOM, STRATEGIES,
    AND VALIDATION 121**

Chapter 5—Classroom Organization and Synthesization 123
    Michael J. Fimian, Mark S. Zoback, and Bruno J. D'Alonzo

Introduction 123
Organizing and Synthesizing 124
Organizing the Physical Environment 124
Organizing the Learning Environment 131
Synthesizing the Instructional Environment 145
Pulling It All Together 149
Summary 151

Chapter 6—IEPs for LBP Adolescents **153**
    Bruno J. D'Alonzo and Michael J. Fimian

Introduction 153
The IEP Defined 153
Assumptions Underlying the IEP 155
Principal Concepts of P.L. 94-142 157
Developing the IEP Process and Product 163
Minimum Credits for Graduation 194
Summary 195

**Chapter 7—Instructional Approaches and Curricula for
       LBP Adolescents** **197**
    *Suzanne Lanning-Ventura, Maribeth Montgomery-Kasik,
       and David A. Sabatino*

Introduction 197
Remediation and Tutoring 198
Academic Achievement and Remediation 199
Auditory, Auditory Sequential Memory 206
Auditory Closure 207
Auditory Discrimination 209
Auditory Association 210
Auditory Comprehension 211
Visual Memory 213
Visual Discrimination 215
Fine Motor Skills 216
Time Orientation Disability 218
A Review of Remediation 220
Tutoring 220
Exemplary Lesson 1 224
Exemplary Lesson 2 228
Exemplary Lesson 3 229
Exemplary Lesson 4 229

Exemplary Lesson 5 230
A Review of Tutoring 232
Summary 232

**Chapter 8—Methods of Instruction: A Process-Task Approach for
LBP Adolescents 233**
Kathleen M. McCoy and Nancy Ralph Watson

Introduction 233
Evaluation Model 233
Organizing/Analyzing Content Material 236
Evaluating the Student 237
Application of the Evaluation Model 242
Mathematics Instruction 251
Summary 259

**Chapter 9—Formative Evaluation and Data Management Systems
for LBP Adolescents 261**
Michael J. Fimian and Stuart A. Goldstein

Introduction .... ` 261
Evaluation and Exceptional Learners . ` 262
Formative Evaluation 265
The Instructionally Based Model 271
Norm- and Criterion-Referenced Evaluation 281
Direct Observation Methods of Evaluation 284
Choosing an Observation System 299
A Procedural Analysis 300
Summary 312

Chapter 10—Applied Research Techniques for LBP Adolescents 315
David A. Sabatino and Patrick J. Schloss

Introduction 315
Traditional Research Application 317
A Simplified Classroom Evaluation Model 322
Behavioral Assessment 327
Applied Research with Mildly Handicapped 345
Summary 350

**PART IV—ALTERNATIVE MODELS TO TRADITIONAL
SECONDARY PROGRAMMING 351**

Chapter 11—Mainstreaming LBP Adolescents **353**
     Harold Wm. Heller

     Introduction 353
     The Concept 353
     Definitions 354
     Legal Basis 357
     Moral and Ethical Basis 358
     Placement Considerations 360
     Structural Aspects 367
     Role Interactions 374
     Trends and Issues 378
     Summary 380

Chapter 12—Parallel Alternative Curriculum for LBP Adolescents .. **381**
     L. Kay Hartwell, Douglas E. Wiseman,
          and Anthony Van Reusen

     Introduction 381
     Rationale for a PAC 382
     Trends in Providing Alternative Programs 384
     Parallel Alternate Curriculum (PAC) 389
     Specific Procedures for PAC Development 390
     Content Presentation 397
     Testing Options 398
     Student Assessment 399
     Other Instructional Considerations 405
     Monitoring Student Progress, Performance 407
     Evaluation Considerations 412
     Summary 418

Chapter 13—Career and Vocational Education for
          LBP Adolescents **421**
     Bruno J. D'Alonzo and William S. Svoboda

     Introduction 421
     Definitions of Career Education 422
     Theories on Career Education Delivery 425
     Categories of Career Development 429
     Career Developmental Tasks in School 430
     Principles of Career Development Program 432
     Student Goals and Competencies 432

Career Education Components 433
Decision Making 434
Vocational Education 439
Career and Vocational Service Models 446
Career Education Models 448
Other Options 453
State of the Art 459
Summary 460

Chapter 14—Alternate Educational Service Models for
                LBP Adolescents 461
                Janice M. Schnorr, Bruno J. D'Alonzo, and
                   David A. Sabatino

Introduction 461
Alternative Schools 461
Selected Alternative School Programs 463
Private School Programs 467
Characteristics of Private Schools 468
Evaluation Criteria for Private Schools 472
Directory of Private Schools 481
Summary 489

Index 513

Preface

The major purpose of this text is to provide an individualized approach to the education of adolescents with learning and/or behavior problems (LBPs). Such adolescents traditionally have been labeled as either educable mentally retarded, behavioral disordered, or learning disabled. Instructionally, the label has been virtually useless in singling out those classified as mildly handicapped. Therefore, the editor seeks in developing this book to focus on the specific learning characteristics these adolescents display, their more typical responses to educational tasks, and the environment in which they traditionally perform. The interaction resulting from examining student, task, and environment may provide special educators with a broader range of curricular options and alternatives to work effectively with these students while developing meaningful learning environments.

An eclectic approach leading to reasonable program choice is recommended for the education of these students. The contributing authors have selected from among the best of existing principles, practices, and theories and have incorporated them into their respective chapters. These approaches should assist educators in removing the barriers created by the use of traditional secondary school environments and the historic attitude of neglect experienced by youths who fail that system. The categories tend to limit rather than broaden the development of the technology, methodology, strategies, and program options needed to provide a free appropriate public education for these students.

The editor believes this book to be a pioneering effort in the field of special education and much needed in bringing adolescents with learning and behavior problems to center stage in the secondary schools. LBP students have been too long neglected in special education by those charged with the responsibility for the teaching and care of these adolescents.

This text is designed for students being prepared by the nation's colleges and universities and for their professors. However, it also is developed for use by experienced regular and special education teachers, program specialists, and supervisors and administrators in public educational institutions responsible for the delivery of services to adolescents with learning and/or behavioral problems. The content provides a modern-day synthesis of the critical educational issues and practices for these teenagers who fail and are failed by the system.

The book is divided into four discrete but interrelated sections. In Part I, the single chapter provides an overview and orientation of the field. In Part II, the learning and behavioral characteristics of the students are reviewed and juvenile adolescent offenders are studied. The final chapter in the section looks at the problem of bringing parents and professionals together.

Parts III and IV provide a theoretical and process orientation to curriculum content and program delivery. Together, a conceptual-to-operational phase-in program development for LBP adolescents is offered in a single source. Several chapters deal with the current issues of mainstreaming, resource rooms, and alternative and private school services for adolescents. Others focus on individualized education plans, methods of instruction, observational and management systems, and classroom research and evaluation techniques. Still others provide information on critical areas such as alternate curricula and career and vocational education.

It is the editor's intent to contribute a textbook to the field of special education that will serve as a launching pad from which future missions in scholarly contributions for LBP adolescents will embark.

Bruno J. D'Alonzo, Ph.D.
December 1982

Acknowledgments

Once committed to the development of this textbook, it became obvious that I was not one of those few experts who has such an encyclopedic acquaintance with our field as to permit him to outline chapters required in the subspecialty areas of special education. Indeed, it was a bit of a task to choose the chapter headings and the chapter authors who would carry the ball. I was fortunate to recruit a group of dedicated professionals who were willing to serve as members of a team to develop this unique book.

Any multiauthored text has inborn problems. Not everyone uses the same style, and I have made a few contributors less than happy by the delays caused through intensive editing. The chapter authors have been most patient and cooperative. In any event, it has been a challenge—and a stimulating one at that. I personally thank each chapter author for the final product. If there are any imperfections, inconsistencies, and annoying variations in style in this book, I assume full blame. The individual authors have done what was asked of them.

An editor incurs many debts. Besides the chapter authors I want to especially thank Dr. David A. Sabatino and Dr. Allen A. Mori for their encouragement and support and Dr. Harold Wm. Heller for permission to use portions of his original mainstream chapter in Chapters 1 and 2. I am grateful to the staff at Aspen Systems Corporation: John Marozsan, Margot Raphael, Eileen Higgins, Jane Coyle, Scott Ballotin, Dorothy Okoroji, Ruth Judy, Ruth Bloom, Martha Sasser, Anne Hill and the late Curt Whitesel.

These individuals have been responsible for the respect Aspen has achieved among special educators for its excellent contributions and publications to this field.

Special thanks to Anne Cantor, who provided valuable typing support that is necessary for the success of any writing effort.

I also want to acknowledge the administration, faculty, staff, and students at Arizona State University, who provide me with a scholarly, supportive, and stimulating environment from which to serve others.

Contributors

BRUNO J. D'ALONZO, PH.D.
Associate Professor
Department of Special Education
Arizona State University
Tempe, Arizona 85287

MICHAEL J. FIMIAN, PH.D.
Educational Consultant
Seaside Education Associates
Lincoln Center, Massachusetts
01773

STUART A. GOLDSTEIN, M.S.
Reading Specialist
Kenai Peninsula Borough Schools
Soldotna, Alaska 99669

L. KAY HARTWELL, PH.D.
Associate Professor
Department of Special Education
Arizona State University
Tempe, Arizona 85287

HAROLD WM. HELLER, ED.D.
Professor and Dean
College of Human Development
and Learning

University of North Carolina at
Charlotte
Charlotte, North Carolina 28223

ROGER L. KROTH, ED.D.
Professor
Department of Special Education
University of New Mexico
Albuquerque, New Mexico 87106

SUZANNE LANNING-VENTURA, PH.D.
Visiting Instructor
Department of Special Education
Southern Illinois University
Carbondale, Illinois 62901

KATHLEEN M. MCCOY, PH.D.
Associate Professor
Department of Special Education
Arizona State University
Tempe, Arizona 85287

HAROLD J. MCGRADY, PH.D.
Director
Special Education
Mesa Public Schools
Mesa, Arizona 85203

MARIBETH MONTGOMERY-KASIK, M.ED.
Research Assistant
Department of Special Education
Southern Illinois University
Carbondale, Illinois 62901

DAVID A. SABATINO, PH.D.
Professor and Dean
School of Education and Human
  Services
University of Wisconsin-Stout
Menomonie, Wisconsin 54751

JEFFREY SCHILIT, PH.D.
Professor and Chairperson
Department of Exceptional Student
  Education
Florida Atlantic University
Boca Raton, Florida 33431

PATRICK J. SCHLOSS, PH.D.
Assistant Professor
Department of Special Education
The Pennsylvania State University
University Park, Pennsylvania
  16802

JANICE M. SCHNORR, PH.D.
Associate Professor
Department of Curriculum and
  Instruction
Northern Arizona University
Flagstaff, Arizona 86011

WILLIAM S. SVOBODA, ED.D.
Professor
Department of Secondary
  Education
Arizona State University
Tempe, Arizona 85287

ANTHONY VAN REUSEN, M.ED.
Doctoral Candidate
Department of Special Education
University of Kansas
Lawrence, Kansas 66045

NANCY RALPH WATSON, M.ED.
Research Associate
Department of Elementary
  Education
Arizona State University
Tempe, Arizona 85287

DOUGLAS E. WISEMAN, ED.D.
Associate Professor
Department of Special Education
Arizona State University
Tempe, Arizona 85287

MARK S. ZOBACK, M.S.
Doctoral Candidate
Department of Educational
  Psychology
University of Connecticut
Storrs, Connecticut 06268

Part I

Overview and Orientation

This section serves as an overview and orientation to adolescents with learning and/or behavioral problems, the traditional secondary school environment, and special educational alternatives. The section can serve as a review for inservce special education teachers. It also can present introductory information to regular educator inservice audiences new to alternative programming and current special education delivery service modes in secondary schools. It may be useful to school psychologists, administrators, guidance counselors, and even interested and informed parents as a single reading source that reviews the current state of the art.

However, it is written as an introduction to preservice college students beginning a course in characteristics, methods, or program delivery that focuses on secondary high-incidence handicapped (learning disabilities, behavioral disorders, and mild mental retardation).

Chapter 1

Introduction to Secondary School Programming for LBP Students

Bruno J. D'Alonzo

INTRODUCTION

Perhaps the most populous category of underserved handicapped youths, in response to Public Law 94-142 (the Education for All Handicapped Children Act of 1975), are the learning and/or behavior problem (LBP) adolescents in today's secondary schools. The LBP acronym is used throughout this text in place of the traditional terminology that describes mildly handicapped adolescents who may be mentally retarded, learning disabled, and/or behaviorally disordered.

Only one-fifth of all secondary handicapped students receive the required special education services, while elementary pupils receive almost four-fifths (Metz, 1973). Malouf and Halpern (1976) advance a strong argument that few handicapped students of high school age are served by special education programs—they are either encouraged to drop out or are excluded from general school activities.

There is evidence that many secondary school adolescents who have records of nonattendance and whose reading levels are below those necessary to be functionally competent in course work should properly be considered handicapped. According to Byrne (1982), based on data collected from State agency reports submitted to the Department of Education, Special Education Programs (as required under P.L. 94-142), the number of mentally retarded (MR), emotionally disturbed (ED), and learning disabled (LD) children and adolescents receiving special education and related services during academic year 1981-82 was:

		Classification		
Ages	MR	LD	ED	Total
		Actual Figures		
6-17	610,185	1,538,284	284,541	2,433,010
18-21	71,096	49,965	13,125	134,186
Approximate figures averaged from ages 6-17 and added to actual ages 18-21 figure.				
14-21	292,980	609,341	116,594	1,018,915

These estimates are probably more than the actual number of MR, LD, and ED students classified at the 14-21 age level, because allowances were not made for the attrition rate at the high school level. For 1977 the Census Bureau (United States Bureau of the Census, 1978) reported 3,442,000 adolescents between 14 and 21 years dropping out of school.

It is apparent from these data that a need exists for programs and qualified teachers for these adolescents. Despite the need, special education programs exist for only 85 percent of the mentally retarded, 54.8 percent of the learning disabled, and 44.1 percent of the behaviorally disordered youths in the United States (Miller, Sabatino, & Larsen, 1980).

In recent years an emerging special education trend has emphasized the necessity for service and program delivery to handicapped adolescents. One of the major reasons for this is the increased number of LBP students who have been identified and provided with special education intervention at the elementary school level and now have advanced to the secondary school. The incidence of students in this group has created a demand for service that the educational community cannot continue to ignore.

This chapter presents an overview of special education for the LBP student at the secondary level. Several of the issues analyzed have an impact on the education of handicapped students in today's schools. The rest of the chapter introduces trends and issues in secondary schools in general, and specifically current principles and practices as they relate to special education for LBP adolescents; causes of organizational problems; and high school curricula, including trends, issues, and problems in programming.

ADOLESCENTS AND SECONDARY SCHOOLS

The growth of secondary schools in the United States has been unprecedented in comparison to other nations. In 1900, secondary schools accommodated approximately 10 percent of the adolescent population; today they serve more than 90 percent of such students, with about 75 percent of them graduating. But that upsurge developed only in the last 30 years, when they passed the 50 percent level. This phenomenal growth can be appreciated better when it is compared to Western Europe, where even the most educationally sophisticated nations provide formal schooling for only 4 to 20 percent of their adolescents (Martin, 1976).

The sole reason for the expansion in the number of students served in the United States is the compulsory school attendance law. First initiated in Massachusetts, compulsory attendance requires students to stay in school until legal age (generally 18) or earlier (usually 16) if they request a permit to work, or are expelled.

Youths who experience difficulty with their academic and social response to school present four major, overlapping characteristics: (1) truancy, (2) being dropped or stopped from school attendance, (3) histories of school failure (primarily academic), and (4) mild handicap.

Besant (1969) describes an occupational training program at the Rodman Job Corps Center in New Bedford, Mass., where nearly 85 percent of the youths who attended two levels of study completed a high school equivalency exam and qualified for a diploma. The Rodman Center sought to benefit from observations on teaching dropout youths. Dropouts have a deep sense of school inadequacy that is partially supported by their prior record of failure. The center hypothesized that if the dropouts were to succeed in any preventive or remedial program they must experience early success. Failure was quickly identified and checked by recycling students through the units they did not master.

Initial instruction was verbal, with a gradual shift to written material as student reading ability increased. Individual and job-related counseling was intensive, highly personal, and realistic. Besant reports that "six to nine months of classwork and concurrent on-the-job training were sufficient to qualify the average 17-to-22-year-old trainee for an entry level job in a range of office skills" (p. 52).

Douglass (1969) developed a junior high school dropout prevention program based on the premise that youths quit because of their inability to learn to read and their consequent failure in other subjects. Douglass recommends these major approaches in preventing dropouts:

- improve pupil-teacher interpersonal relations
- increase junior high school remedial work
- offer special study habits and skill-building guidance center prevention classes
- improve counseling relationships with an eye toward dropout prevention systems
- increase the number of work study programs

Millions of dollars and more than half a century of program efforts have been expended; yet the dropout problem remains. Proposed solutions include abolishing compulsory schooling laws and providing on-the-job training, career education, and more relevant curricula. As educators confront the issue today it would benefit them to keep in mind the fact that school is not a panacea. In fact, as the evidence suggests, it has been anything but that for lower socioeconomic class youths.

Accordingly, while attempting to improve the quality of schooling for all children, educators should refrain from making misleading promises and inaccurate statements. Furthermore, they should consider the possibility that, at least for pupils of high school age, school might not be the best place. Above all, they never should engage in a campaign against dropouts that results in social stigmatization.

Dropping out of school may be said to be a symptom of preexisting problems rather than a problem itself. In the opinion of many authorities, the source of that problem may well be in the fiber of society, of which the schools are an integral part. Programs that work must focus on attitude; if the school reinforces feelings of inadequacy and continues to deny success, youths' options dwindle to but one. A few concerned teachers and an overworked counselor can make only a small difference. If leaving school is viewed as a community problem that must be addressed by all parties—courts, employers, service agencies, and schools—effective measures for dropout prevention as well as for returning to class those who have left can commence.

CAUSES OF ORGANIZATIONAL PROBLEMS

The growth of secondary schools has created organizational problems of increasing complexity. Primarily, these have occurred because of (1) consolidation and centralization of school districts; (2) parental, governmental, and community demands that schools provide diverse curricula to better serve heterogeneous populations; (3) the perception that school personnel are to serve in loco parentis in the supervision of students; (4) the adolescents' transition from smaller elementary, self-contained classes to departmentalized classes in larger junior and senior high schools designed to be economically and logistically justifiable; and (5) the view that schools are capable of solving all of society's problems promptly before graduation (Martin, 1976).

Reactions to such stresses vary among adolescents, but those who do not follow the commonalities in music, fads, dress, and vocabulary create an illusion of deviation from the norm, some of which is expectable adolescent rebellion and some of which results in willful norm-violating behavior.

Adolescents have provided researchers, philosophers, and educators with much to say. Adolescence is marked by a divergent break from childhood at puberty, theoretically culminating in psychological maturity—for some in their late teens and for others, much later. The biological beginning and the psychological ending make adolescence a unique period during which a balance of independence and dependence within selected social and personal relationships stabilizes. It is in this struggle between independence and dependence, in the context of the social agency known as the schools, that adolescence appears to many educators—and to students themselves—as a period of storm and stress.

Rapid physical growth, newfound concerns for a place in an enlarged world, the establishment of sex role relationships, and intense pressures from without to accept the adult world and declare an earned place in it, all interact to create tremendous internal needs with which the middle and secondary schools must cope. If to those normal developmental dimensions is added a combination of school and societal failure overlaid by a handicapping condition, it is little wonder that the secondary schools remain academically oriented, functionally denying the existence of "problem youths."

In this country, literature from the 1950s onward described adolescents who became aggressive toward the system or withdrawn from traditional social structures as alienated (Bailey, 1969; Havighurst, 1970). The term alienation is troublesome because it creates one more label for youths who already may feel different and who may react to such labeling by in fact behaving differently. The concern with being different is doubly heightened for youths who fail to meet their own expectancies or those of society. In essence, the schools tend to amplify the uniqueness of adolescence, especially when youths do not succeed within the system.

Research by Reckless (1967), substantiated by a number of other studies (Jones, 1972; Rosenthal & Jacobson, 1968), points out the dangerous influence of labels on students and teachers alike. Reckless essentially reports that all adolescents experiment with limits, values, and relationships. Those who become chronic disruptives or norm violators tend to hear the expression *bad* associated with their behavior much more often. It could be that disruptive behavior is initiated as a reinforcement of specific behavioral incidents.

Of more critical importance to educators is the fact that once chronic-disruptive, norm-violating behaviors begin, the schools may not have the means of stopping them. What alternative treatment forms do secondary schools use for youths in trouble?

Such individuals may be removed from the normal flow or mainstream. The system thus punishes students for troublesome behavior by removing them from the setting. Secondary school youths are suspended and expelled from school daily at an alarming rate (Splaine, 1975). The public schools appear to have the attitude that education is a privilege, and it therefore can be denied. The result is that the street or some agency now must provide for youths who are well under 21. The mean age at which most youths either drop out or stop attending school remains around 14 (Schreiber, 1968).

Another element in the behavioral continuum are violent or vandalistic youths who display norm-violating and chronic disruptive behavior through overt aggression, placing a low priority both on other people and on their property. Aggressive youths cannot be submitted to the care of the streets. The public values property, the ability to control, and the capability to establish viable norms for its future citizens. Therefore, incarceration is the most common practice for dealing with aggressive youths who intimidate persons or destroy property. Society naively believes that incarceration is a form of treatment. Incarceration may include treatment, but in itself it is not treatment. There are those in fact who believe that incarceration only begets incarceration (Shore & Massimo, 1969), pointing to the recidivism (parole violations and recommitment) rate, which remains at 75 percent to 80 percent (Moore, 1962).

The rate of recidivism among previously institutionalized juvenile delinquents appears to remain the same today. However, reduction in recidivism among previously incarcerated adolescents has been reported through a systems behavioral family therapy approach (Alexander & Parsons, 1973) and an employment related program approach (Mills & Walter, 1977).

A study by Ganzer and Sarason (1973) identified several variables common to recidivists. Their findings indicate that female delinquents in general come from more disorganized and socially less adequate families than do males, and that the most promising potential predictors of recidivism were associated with (a) family background factors, (b) age at first offense and commitment, and (c) diagnostic classification of the adolescent.

The traditional professional response to chronic disruptive, norm-violating adolescents is disappointing. There are no simple solutions to complex problems. Yet there are no solutions to any problems if they are not first sought. These two principles hang in the balance, suspended there by regular, vocational, and special educators who must select an integrated professional posture. Currently, that posture is that the secondary schools teach subject matter, such as mathematics, chemistry, political science, metal or wood shop. The subject matter is important, and the student who does not respond to it must make the decision to make an effort to master it or drop it. That attitude places the secondary public schools in direct conflict with the letter and intent of P.L. 94-142.

There is another contributing factor. By the end of the first 70 years of the 20th century, while the high schools were experiencing their extraordinary growth, the onset of puberty for males and females was occurring at a younger age—in fact two years earlier for today's adolescents than for their grandparents. While this earlier physical maturation is universal in the technologically advanced countries representing Western civilization and generally is credited to improved diet, a parallel growth in intellectual potential can logically be assumed. Nevertheless, the high schools retained authoritarian controls and supervisory practices, teaching democracy while practicing minority rule. These practices impede self-realization, deny the self-regulation potential of adolescents, and increase dependence on direction from adults. Thus, during the day, the schools baby-sit (at a very high cost) the adolescents who become the nation's nighttime baby sitters.

HIGH SCHOOL CURRICULUM: TRENDS AND ISSUES

Concern has been expressed throughout the literature about the relevance and structure of the high school curriculum not only in general education but also in special education. Gearhart (1980) states that:

Much of our knowledge in providing programs for handicapped students is based on successful experience with elementary-age children. When we attempt to plan for handicapped adolescents, we find that both the structure and goals of the school and the characteristics and drives of the students are different. (p. 419)

In regard to services to mildly handicapped students, data collected by the National Center for Educational Statistics (NCES) from 1970-1971 to 1978-1979 produce two findings. First, at least 50 percent more elementary than secondary students received special education services each year. Second, from 1973 to 1978 (the last part under P.L. 94-142) the percentage of mildly handicapped secondary students receiving services increased by nearly 25 percent each year. The rapid increase in services to that population does not mean that the gap between those needing and those receiving help has been closed. NCES data for 1978-79 place the percentage of handicapped aged 5 to 17 receiving services at 7.9 percent of the general population. Slightly more than 10 percent of that group is in the elementary grades, with less than 6 percent (or half of the estimated total handicapped secondary group) still not served.

Data on the incidence of handicapped secondary students and the increasing percentage who are receiving services lead to two assumptions:

1. Special education efforts in the secondary schools may be a new phenomenon to many regular educators.
2. Special education service delivery modes may be a new phenomenon to many special educators whose training and experience were at the elementary school level.

It may be that secondary special education for the mildly handicapped, and especially the learning disabled, is a new experience for educators, and one that requires new approaches.

Research on the focus of secondary learning disabilities programs (Lerner, Evans, & Meyers, 1977) clearly indicates that the most prevalent role played by secondary resource teachers is that of academic remedial educators. In this role, resource room teachers attempt to support the classroom teacher's required academic subject learning by strengthening the youths' basic skills. The preliminary data reported by Miller, Sabatino, and Larsen (1980) suggest a third assumption: the most prevalent practice among secondary special education resource teachers is the elementary remedial model used in support of mainstreaming.

Further, data collected in 1977-78 and reported by Miller, Sabatino, and Larsen in 1980, show sharp disagreement between university and local special education directors as to what constitutes a training program for secondary special teachers. Statistically significant differences between the two groups involve (1) the need for secondary resource teachers to work in a liaison function, especially with vocational educators (one of the highest priorities named by local educational agency directors); and (2) the continued need for remedial training (the highest priority by universities and the lowest for local educational directors). Thus, three further assumptions:

1. Colleges and universities are continuing to prepare elementary and secondary learning disability resource teachers in the same mode.
2. Local education agencies see an urgent necessity for secondary resource teachers who can perform a liaison or brokerage function for students.
3. Colleges and universities are not paying attention to the needs of the users of a major group of their products (secondary teachers) and are not preparing these individuals properly.

The major postulate drawn from these assumptions is that there should be a sharp distinction between the special education program delivery modes of resource teachers in elementary as opposed to secondary schools. The principal point of differentiation is the means by which the two groups support mainstreaming of students as a major program goal.

In summary, elementary school is designed to teach developmental skills and remediate their shortfall. High school is designed to teach the academic, vocational, social, and personal skills needed for work, future education, the maintenance of successful sound relationships, and harmonious interpersonal adjustment. These objectives call into question the secondary school's traditional role with the mildly handicapped. On the basis of all the new evidence, rather than perpetuating that role, mainstreaming in secondary schools now requires:

- assisting the youths in establishing a career or goals in the four objective areas: academic, vocational, social, and personal
- integrating the secondary school curriculum to capture the students' career life plans during their remaining years of school and under self-monitoring conditions
- projecting an attitude of willingness to forego the teaching of academic subjects
- accepting the students' educational handicap as the teachers' problem, not the youths'

Secondary school personnel must make a humane, goal-directed response toward these young adults as decision makers. Recognizing that these students fear failure, secondary educators need to present them with realistic information, help them restructure their expectations, and assist them in the search for incentives that provide life values.

Clark (1980) believes that the major curricular domains for the mildly handicapped adolescent are (1) occupational development, (2) daily living skills, and (3) personal-social skills. These areas are described in the following section.

Occupational Development

As part of the National Assessment of Educational Progress (1978a, 1978b), data were provided on occupational development. A sample of 34,000 17-year-olds in school and 1,000 who had graduated or dropped out comprised the study. Of particular interest was the finding that only about 2 percent of the students considered school or academic areas as useful preparation for a job. Only 25 percent rated the high school counselor among their top five sources of job information. Furthermore, these adolescents achieved only 50 percent accuracy in such personally useful skills as measurement, conversions, cost computations, writing job application letters, and critical thinking. Finally, the attitudes they expressed toward work revealed a dislike for repetitive jobs, a high degree of stereotyping in female aspirations for occupations, and a desire for prestige and status without a willingness to accept the accompanying responsibility.

If these data raise questions about the appropriateness of the regular high school curriculum for large numbers of nonhandicapped adolescents, then what are the implications for its effect on the handicapped?

The Carnegie Council of Policy Studies in Higher Education sponsored a study conducted by Clark Kerr (1979) that revealed that about one-third of today's youth are ill educated, ill employed, and ill equipped to make their way in society. The Council's report boldly states that high schools are an alienating experience for thousands of young people. In some schools, dropout rates soar to 23 percent for Caucasians, 35 percent for blacks, and 45 percent for Hispanics. The dropout rate for low-income whites is even higher than for low-income blacks. The Council warns that the nation is in danger of developing a permanent underclass—a self-perpetuating culture of poverty.

Some of the Council's recommendations reveal alarm over high schools' miserable rate of success in career preparation—the very environment held by many to be least restrictive. The Council's recommendations include the following structural and administrative changes: making high schools smaller and more specialized, moving skills training into business and industry or community colleges, and establishing federal and state work-study programs for 16- to 19-year-olds modeled on the present college level work-study system. The Council also recommended that literacy, numeracy, and good work habits become the basic vocational and academic skills taught at the secondary level.

Although this study focuses more on educational opportunity for minority group populations and school- and work-alienated youths than on exceptional students, special educators and advocates for the handicapped cannot ignore the Council's indictment of today's high schools. The implication of the study strikes at the heart of what constitutes "appropriate education" under P.L. 94-142 and the least-restrictive environment concept in high schools.

Daily Living Skills

In three separate reports on health practices and skills in accident prevention and emergency care, social studies and citizenship, and consumer skills, the National Assessment of Educational Progress (1978a, 1978b, 1979) provides interesting data on selected skills of daily living. The results indicate many 17-year-olds lack knowledge or understanding of such topics as first aid, contraception, energy resources, purposes of various branches of government, consumer protection, and personal finance. This can be remedied by functional teaching.

Functional teaching assumes that goals and objectives of the traditional developmental curriculum are not within the students' reach. Therefore, the developmental curricular goals of achieving academic success in a traditional sense are replaced with aims of attaining functional literacy for vocational entry. Students are taught exactly what they need to know in order to function at a basic level academically. One functional teaching goal—driving—is provided as an example. A partial list of objectives is included to illustrate actual functional teaching strategies.

Driving is a major objective of the majority of high school age youths. Therefore, key functional words related to driving and the ultimate obtaining of a driver's license are important objectives that carry great motivation. The goals might be set up as follows.

Driving and Driving Safety Objectives

The teacher helps students identify color cues appropriate to the safety signs:

Red: danger, stop
Yellow: caution, yield
Green: go, clear, safe zone

The teacher and the class discuss where signs are most likely to be found and where they can be observed, e.g., railroad crossings, school crossings, and pedestrian crossings.

The teacher obtains a state driver's license manual for each student. Students identify the section on signs and name each sign and its use.

The teacher uses the sentences or paragraphs involving signs in the manual to assist the students to read the context of that paragraph based on the meaning of a particular sign.

Familiarity with Driving Manual Objective

The student should be able to read and memorize key words related to common driving signs and signals in the manual. The key words involve freeways, exits, intersections, entering town, city streets, secondary roads, country roads, and county roads.

Personal-Social Skills

The broad area of personal-social skills generally includes knowledge and abilities in values and attitudes, self-esteem, personal habits, and human relationships. Certainly, from the perspective of how the adult handicapped have fared in the past, a significant body of literature supports the importance of personal-social skills (Butler & Browning, 1974; Cobb, 1972; Henrick & Kriegel, 1961; Zigmond & Brownlee, 1980). However, the more immediate concern is for current high school programs in this field. The following research findings are important:

- Leming (1978) reports that knowledge of moral conduct (i.e., moral judgment) and actual behavior in certain situations differ in high school students, who rationalize these differences in a "get-it-when-you-can" philosophy.
- The U.S. Bureau of the Census (1978) shows a steady increase in juvenile delinquency between 1969 and 1977, with a 44 percent rise for individuals under 18 years of age.
- The violent crime arrest rates increased 283 percent between 1960 and 1978. The Federal Bureau of Investigation Uniform Report for 1979 indicated that 34 percent of all reported arrests involved 11- to 19-year-old youths.
- Bachman, O'Malley, and Johnston (1978) report that senior boys admitted to the following behaviors one or more times during the two-year period immediately preceding their senior survey:

Participated in a group fight	21%
Involved in a serious fight at school	32%
Damaged school property on purpose	19%
Involved in shoplifting	36%
Involved in theft under $50	37%

- Steinitz (1976) says high school seniors find it difficult to reconcile personal ambition and personal achievement goals with social responsibility. Today's culture, and schools that reflect it, teach a basic message that self-reliance is a measure of an individual's worth and that people are to be judged on the basis of how hard they try and how much they accomplish. The conflict arises in students' ambivalent attitudes toward and treatment of others who appear not to be trying and who have not achieved material success.
- The high estimated rates of sexual intercourse (52 percent) of those between the ages of 15 and 19, along with American teenage childbearing rates that rank among the highest in the world (Planned Parenthood Federation of America, 1977), may be as related to current personal-social values and attitudes as to knowledge of contraception noted in the National Assessment of Educational Progress (1978a).

These studies reflect a growing awareness that high school curricula are either ignoring the issues of personal-social skills through direct instructional efforts or that the incidental learning approach through discussion, counseling and guidance, and related curriculum materials is inadequate. Given that personal-social values and attitudes require instruction that may be highly verbal, handicapped students might find it difficult to achieve desired goals in current high school programs, even if instruction were available.[1]

PROBLEMS IN PROGRAMMING FOR LBP YOUTHS

Secondary level special educators frequently perceive LBP students from far too narrow a base. They attempt to isolate the learning and/or behavioral problem without considering the context of the ecological system in which the students function. Even though these teachers are deeply concerned for the total person and espouse their commitment to the individual student in all aspects of their profession, quite often their approach to education is limited to the youth's learning or behavior problems, which generally pertain to academic learning experiences. Special educators should have a broader focus when instructing handicapped adolescents. One of the major differences between elementary and secondary students involves the circumstances adolescents encounter while growing up in a complex society, which places great stress on them to define their purpose in life.

Grinder (1980) explains the development of the individual during the adolescent period:

Growing up is an intricate process. During adolescence, as the body grows, cognitive capacity develops for achieving high levels of awareness of both self and society. Adolescents, in contrast to children, acquire the potential to cope with risks to physical and mental health, experiment with new forms of social interaction, explore career prospects, and develop perspectives on social and moral issues. Adolescence, thus, is represented . . . as the most consequential period in the life span for attaining the attributes that underlie future personal and social growth. (p. 1)

In addition to developmental concerns, there are many other problem areas that recur to professionals in their quest to provide a free and appropriate education to LBP adolescents. These areas of concern are discussed in the remaining sections of this chapter.

Methodological Concerns

Several methodological or curricular concerns should be mentioned. Secondary teachers usually employ methods that rely heavily on the students' listening skills. Taylor (1973) reports that more than 50 percent of a student's time in the elementary classroom is spent in the act of listening. It therefore can be postulated that this percentage of student time would be even higher in secondary schools. Although listening is one of the most continuously needed educational skills, it probably is the most neglected of those taught in the schools.

This fact becomes even more important for LBP adolescents. Listening skills for students of average intelligence and scholastic ability generally are more advanced than reading abilities. For students who encounter reading problems, the reliance upon listening becomes even more marked. For example, Taylor (1973) concludes:

In general, less competent students, those judged to be less intelligent and scholastically below average, show a marked preference for listening over reading in most learning situations, and do retain more from listening. The slower student depends on the special attributes of listening for much of his understanding. In listening, he is assisted in interpreting content by the phrasing and expression of the speaker, while in reading he must construct his own linguistic units in order to realize meaning. (p. 3)

Although the auditory channel of communication is heavily relied upon as the primary information receptor for many adolescents, research and material developments in the area lag far behind efforts in reading. Similarly, the development of reading material outdistances that of auditory material. For example, Kass and

Lewis (1973) surveyed 382 members of the Council for Exceptional Children's Division on Children with Learning Disabilities to identify materials and techniques used with learning disabled children. They report that by far the greatest number of identified materials and techniques involve remedial reading and visual perception (44 percent). Only 5 percent related to the auditory area, and they were defined as "auditory perception" materials. Although the vast majority of learning disabled youths suffer reading problems, it appears that few auditory materials are available for their instruction, essentially because professionals lack the interest to develop them.

As these disabled readers, many of whom have LBPs, move through the various grade levels, their inability to meet their schools' reading standards often becomes obvious. These discrepancies between actual and expected performance place the students in a precarious position academically as they enter various learning environments, especially at the high school level, where they are manifested in many ways. Students' frustration levels increase and boredom and anxiety become common behaviors that often result in increased failure and dropout rates.

Lack of Instructional Materials

Teachers commonly give a brief lecture or demonstration, then rely heavily on such materials as textbooks, workbooks, programmed instruction, task sheets, and cassette or video recordings to supplement their direct instruction. This method makes both students and teachers dependent on instructional materials. The validity of these materials then becomes an important consideration, especially since there is such widespread use of instructional materials. A data base is needed to better document whether such materials are effective and produce learning in these students.

Stowitschek, Gable, and Hendricksen (1980) state that "after more than sixty years of research in education, there is very little that we can unequivocally say is a critical variable affecting instruction. The one factor that is quite clear is instruction time—specifically, the time that students spend working at educationally relevant tasks" (p. 2). This involves also how much time is permitted for practice and its intensity. Popham and Baker (1970) call this "the principle of appropriate practice." Given that practice time-at-task is so critical, it is important to analyze how materials play a part.

Programming for Individual Differences

The basic philosophy that prevails in special education is that of individualization of instruction, with a considerable body of literature focusing on this concept. Some educators indicate that materials play an important part in instruction and that this is the single, most conclusive finding in research on individual differences (Stowitschek, Gable, & Hendricksen, 1980).

However, a growing number of educators view individualized instruction differently. Instead of a singular focus on learners and their inherent characteristics, or on the materials and their basic concepts, many believe it is the interaction among teacher, materials, and learners that is critical to individualized instruction. Poor materials and failing learners can be offset by good teaching practices. Likewise, a lack of teacher time to devote to individual students can be compensated for by carefully sequenced interactive materials and motivated youths. For this reason, the techniques of a materials technology do not focus only on materials and their characteristics, the types of learners to be dealt with, or particular teacher attributes. Instead, these techniques are intended to assist in increasing or improving the interactions (Exhibit 1-1). This diagram demonstrates the type of interactions within and between variables that takes place.

Adolescents in the Ecological System

Surprisingly little has been written about adolescents within the ecological system; most research assesses learning disabled children. Parents, for example, describe their learning disabled children as more impulsive, anxious, and dependent than their typical nonhandicapped siblings or matched controls (Owen, Adams, Forrest, Stolz, & Fisher, 1971). The effect of the LBP adolescent on the family system, meanwhile, includes parental feelings of guilt and self-blame for contributing or causing the youth's learning and/or emotional disability; frustra-

---

Exhibit 1-1 Three-Way Interaction Relationships

Teacher _____ and _____ Materials
(selecting, adapting)

Teacher _____ and _____ Learner
(integrating direct instruction with materials)

Learner _____ and _____ Materials
(evaluating materials)

Source: Reprinted with permission from *Instructional Materials for Exceptional Children: Selection, Management, and Adaptation* by J.J. Stowitschek, R.A. Gable, and J.M. Hendricksen, Aspen Systems Corporation, © 1980, p. 9.

tion because of a lack of practical information and understanding about the disability; increased anxiety, fear, and/or depression among siblings; a greater potential for parental separation and/or divorce, and resistance by the family in acknowledging any of these effects on its members (Briard, 1976; Bryant, 1978; Kaslow and Cooper, 1978; McWhirter, 1976).

Longitudinal studies should be conducted to examine the relationship among self-concept, family interactions, and nonacademic adjustment in community activities and organizations. Adaptive behavior scales can evaluate chronological changes in peer relationships, independent living and survival skills, and generalization of academic training into practical community applications such as utilizing money and math concepts for shopping, budgeting, and planning.

Finally, the effects of the LBP on vocational choices and success, marriage and family attitudes and practices, and subsequent attitudes toward schools and education must be investigated. A great deal of attention has been concentrated on these youths in the lower levels of the school system. Now they are grown up, and it is time to assess the long-term success of educational interventions and identify the students' continuing needs.

Ecological assessment requires ecological programming and intervention. To program effectively for high school LBP students, and to prevent their maladaptive behaviors from emerging, the most critical intervening variable—self-concept—must be controlled. Continuous evidence of adolescents' positive self-concept will confirm effective programming in the education, social skills and counseling, peer, family, and community systems. Thus, a comprehensive program for high school LBP adolescents must address these systems interdependently (Beare, 1975; Cook, 1979; Greenlee & Hare, 1978; Jacks & Keller, 1978; Philage, Kuna, & Becerril, 1975; West, Carlin, Baserman, & Milstein, 1978).

Planning must include identification and definition of student participants; determination of long-term and short-term program goals; designation of primary and support personnel; coordination of specific orientations, methodologies, and interventions; and a predetermined procedure for formative evaluations and program assessments.

Periodic reports from the students' program planning team to the principal, teachers, and parents will maintain and encourage communication and commitment. Information and orientation sessions with all of these individuals prior to the program's start should nurture positive attitudes and expectations. These sessions may include information and films about learning/behavior disabilities, affective education activities and modeling exercises, and initial counseling or therapy where appropriate (Briard, 1976; Marandola & Imber, 1979; Nielson, 1979; Robinson & Brosh, 1980; Shelton, 1977).

Eventually, the program should include interventions with the LBP students, their parents, and the educational staff. Continuous attention also should reinforce the positive attitudes of others in the school (principal, teacher, nondisabled students) to allow as much mainstreaming as possible. Interventions with the LBP adolescents should include:

1. Educational training that integrates remediation into coping or compensatory techniques. Typically adolescents have experienced and failed the structured remediation procedures. Now, it is easier to answer a math problem successfully with a calculator than to demonstrate a step-by-step understanding of the operation. Compensatory strategies, such as the use of a calculator, should minimize the effects of the specific learning disability while maximizing success and accomplishment.

2. Challenging activities outside of the pure academic domains should allow students to discover self-confidence, self-reliance, and a group of new skills and talents. The LBP adolescents must learn that success in a job is not completely dependent upon information taught in school. Further, the disability may not even interfere with some activities, or it can be circumvented successfully.

3. The adolescents should receive training in problem-solving strategies. They should be able to analyze a problem; identify its goals; determine, test, and evaluate potential solutions; and experience the satisfaction of resolving it correctly. This training can be applied academically, vocationally, or socially. For example, conflict-producing situations can be analyzed, appropriate solutions generated, and successful resolutions practiced with problem-solving strategies. This constitutes an excellent application of greater student self-control.

4. Individual, peer, and group counseling, directed by the school social worker or psychologist, should be an integral part of the class day. Affective education units, values clarification, and reality therapy techniques adapted from Glasser (1976) all can be used to improve student self-understanding, self-acceptance, and positive self-concept. Activities also could teach better social perception and interpretation. Non-LBP students can be included in these groups where appropriate.

5. Students should receive prevocational instruction, career exploration and counseling, and vocational skill analysis and training. Junior high school is not too early to begin vocational planning. This should explore a wide assortment of possibilities and should not discourage consideration of jobs that require college or postsecondary education (Cook, 1979; Freeman & Thompson, 1975; Jacks & Keller, 1978; Shelton, 1977).

Interventions with parents of LBP adolescents should include individual counseling, and sessions both with the youths and with the entire family. Parents may need assistance in working through feelings of guilt and anger, in developing more appropriate communications and realistic expectations of their youngster, and in recognizing the effects of the disability on their daily lives. Group sessions with all parents in the program may provide specific information on learning and/or behavior disabilities or group counseling and/or sharing times (Abrams & Kaslow, 1976; Kaslow & Cooper, 1978; McManman & Cohn, 1978; McWhirter, 1976).

Finally, program coordinators must continually analyze staff morale, staff-student interactions and patterns, decision-making procedures and results, and specific conflicts that may arise between staff members and/or adolescents. These group process issues must be discussed and resolved before they interfere with program effectiveness, efficiency, and success. Addressing the group process may necessitate weekly sensitivity sessions or outside consultants or facilitators. Clearly, a coordinated, communicating staff will ensure the most positive effects on these adolescents and their futures.

Lack of Basic Skills at Secondary Level

Another important area is the teaching of basic skills. There is a consensus among educators that the content of arithmetic and reading at the basic level follows a sequence and that the methods used in instruction should be those in which the teachers have competence. It also has been recommended that the teachers use an eclectric approach and utilize cross-age or peer tutors to assist in direct instruction. Unfortunately, secondary schools have a two-fold problem.

First, many secondary teachers have not taught reading or arithmetic under supervision (i.e., during their student teaching), even though they have university course work in those areas. Many secondary teachers originally were certified in secondary subject areas and, for one reason or another, have changed to special education. Many may have majored in elementary and/or special education, have done their student teaching in an elementary classroom with no previous experience at the secondary level, and have found their first position to be in a secondary school. This is not to imply that such teachers are any less competent, but they could very well be deficient in direct or vicarious arithmetic and/or reading instructional experiences. However, this does identify a discrepancy in education practices that has and will continue to create instructional problems for some secondary teachers if something is not done.

Second, the attitude exists that since many of these adolescents are nearing completion of formal schooling, the priorities should shift from basic skill acquisition (if they have not reached mastery at that level) to functional skills. From a developmental point of view, this would not be educationally sound, simply because many of these students who manifest developmental or educational lags now are more than ever ready for intense systematic instruction in the basic skill areas of reading and arithmetic. Instead of decreasing the qualitative and quantitative aspects of instruction in these areas, it should be increased. This, unfortunately, is seldom done.

Lack of Secondary Level Teacher Preparation

Secondary programs for LBP students, as noted earlier, have proliferated at a rapid rate in recent years. However, the preparation of secondary level special education instructors in teacher education programs has not kept pace with this program growth (Clark & Oliverson, 1973; Little, 1977; Miller, 1975; Miller, Sabatino, & Larsen, 1980). Training for secondary special educators in traditional roles (e.g., self-contained programs) or new roles (e.g., cross-categorical resource teachers) has not emerged quantitatively or qualitatively to meet needs in the field.

There are several possible reasons for the lag in secondary level teacher education preparation:

- the increased emphasis on behaviorism as a catch-all method purportedly applicable to all levels of special education
- the increased emphasis on mainstreaming LBP adolescents because of the belief that most can be educated in general education programs
- the limited number of practitioners with direct or vicarious experience and/or interest in secondary special education
- the limited number of preservice students expressing an interest in, or being encouraged to pursue, secondary school teaching careers
- the K-12 certification practice in existence in all but 12 states that makes possible the employment of teachers without a special core of secondary school LBP adolescent courses.

BROAD RANGE OF TEACHER ROLES

A range of roles has emerged for secondary special education teachers, possibly as a result of the variety of programs in secondary schools. Marsh and Price (1980) believe that because of this variety, the special educator's role in a secondary school could be substantially different from the traditional concept of that teacher. This range of roles has been noted by several authors: D'Alonzo (1974); D'Alonzo and Wiseman (1978); Evans (1980); Marsh and Price (1980); Safran (1980); Younie and Clark (1969). An example of the range the role of one type of secondary teacher encompasses is described by D'Alonzo and Wiseman (1978). They believe that this person is:

1. a teacher who must be among the best
2. a curriculum specialist with a comprehensive understanding of a variety of subject areas
3. an expert in methods of working with students who are difficult to instruct and reach
4. a technician competent in the use of the "tools of the trade," both hardware and software
5. an administrator who keeps reports and records and arranges schedules of others
6. a counselor who deals firsthand with educational, social, occupational, and personal problems
7. a public and human relations expert in working and communicating with administrators, colleagues, students, and parents
8. a diagnostician whose competence plays a major part in adolescent learning

It is not always a simple process to identify which duties, tasks, and responsibilities will encompass any particular special education teacher's role. The behaviors associated with a particular position will be determined by the role expectations as perceived by the incumbent as well as by parents, general and special education administrators and teachers, state department of education representatives, and, of course, the local school board.

An institution such as a school probably can be measured best in terms of the degree to which it successfully fulfills its purposes, tasks, and goals. The efforts of secondary special education teachers therefore should be directed toward the facilitation of those purposes, tasks, and goals and be reflected in the administration of their program, thereby justifying their position. Role clarification thus becomes imperative. With knowledge of their role, high school teachers may be more effective in the selection of the problems to be overcome, the ranking of these issues in order of priority, and the making of decisions concerning alternative solutions.

Several teacher roles have been identified and exist in secondary schools:

- the self-contained teacher
- the single category resource teacher
- the itinerant resource teacher
- the cross-categorical resource teacher
- the crisis intervention teacher
- the work-study or prevocational coordinator
- the alternative class teacher
- the teacher consultant
- the learning specialist

The following section examines several roles of the special education teacher and programming settings at the secondary level.

The Resource Room

The resource room represents one of the most used and abused program alternatives in education today. The idea is a viable one, but its conceptual base has been stretched considerably as school systems seek a means to place students in the mainstream. School administrators have seen it as part of a system that enables them to remove from academic situations those who do not learn or behave well. Therefore, handicapped learners may be moved out of the regular class for reading, arithmetic, and science and placed in a special education setting, taught by a special educator, in essentially a self-contained room for one or more periods a day. Conversely, it is indeed interesting that the emphasis on academics to a large extent is why students are moved from the special class to the regular classroom for instruction.

Organized and operated properly, the resource room has great potential as an alternative (short-term) support placement for LBP adolescents. For students with learning problems, the resource room should be designed to focus on the areas where such deficits are most severe. This focus is not merely the teaching of academic subjects (in lieu of the regular class) but rather is an addition to instruction in academics by the regular classroom teacher. For example, if students are having difficulty in performing math functions, they should not be assigned to math only in a resource room. Not at all. To do so causes the resource room to become a replacement for academics in the regular classroom.

Unfortunately, this is not the rationale for the resource room. As the name implies, it should serve in a "resource" capacity as a complement to the regular classroom. This requires that the regular and resource room teachers work closely in planning how to intervene effectively in the amelioration of a given learning or behavior problem. The resource room educator under this approach would not be presenting academics but teaching strategies to the adolescents for use in academic situations. The difference is one of content vs. strategy. The students may acquire the content (even in a regular class) if they have developed the proper strategies.

Similarly, a resource room for adolescents with behavior problems must not emphasize academics but instead should help the students to improve their behavior so they can be retained maximally in an academic setting for learning purposes. To the extent necessary, the resource room becomes a center for counseling, redeveloping self-confidence, stimulating improved motivation, and building in the students a capability to understand their own behavior as a means of learning to control it. If students who have behavior problems reject reading in the regular classroom, it is not likely that they will accept it any better in a resource room. What needs to be determined is why they do not perform in the academic setting (why they reject reading) and, if they have learning problems, what occurred first, the problem or the behavior?

Once that has been resolved, the possibilities for delineating effective intervention strategies are greatly enhanced. The interaction between problems in learning and in behavior often are closely intertwined. Cause-and-effect relationships must be assessed adequately and accurately before implementing a strategy to deal with the behavior problem. Then, and only then, is a solution to the learners' problems plausible.

The success or failure of the resource room as a facilitator of mainstreaming rests with the maintenance of its integrity as a resource and the degree to which the teachers in both the regular and resource rooms communicate with each other. Without this communication it is impossible for the students to receive maximal assistance as learners in either placement. Accountability rests jointly on both teachers; therefore, they are mutually responsible for the degree of success the students ultimately realize.

The Role of the Resource Teacher

The role of the special education resource teacher varies greatly according to the presenting problems of the students. However, most resource rooms work from a general role model. The most common role of the secondary resource teacher is that of academic remedial educator (Lerner, Evans, & Meyers, 1977). In this role, resource room teachers attempt to support classroom teachers in academic or subject learning by strengthening the youths' basic skills, comprehension, or understanding of the information necessary to demonstrate success in a subject area.

The Remedial Model

The remedial model is built on the philosophy that once basic academic achievement skill (developmental learning) occurs, the youths will be able to progress without additional academic support services. Academic remediation in secondary schools obviously is differentiated from academic skill development at the elementary level. Both remedial efforts are undertaken primarily to support the successful mainstreaming of the handicapped in the regular curriculum. Certainly, all the support that can be given to academic skill development in elementary school, especially in the first three grades, should be provided. But if the youths have not developed at grade level proficiency in tool subjects (reading, math, handwriting, spelling) by ages 12 to 14, then resource teachers may wish to consider another option. Beginning in the fourth grade, pupils may need compensatory help through tutoring to overcome basic skill deficits. Tutoring in the middle school years, sometimes in combination with remediation, may provide the students with the information and comprehension necessary to demonstrate success in required subjects.

The difficulty with the basic skills approach is that by junior high school, the student has become so deficient that constant remediation cannot close the gap in written expression, listening, speaking, and thinking needed to cope with secondary school work. In short, remediation of basic skills at the secondary level frequently is a no-win situation because it cannot provide the abilities necessary for students to meet the subject demands being presented. Slow readers, nonreaders, poor spellers, and students who fail to write well because of all these problems simply cannot catch up with daily assignments that consider these skills as given.

The Functional Model

When academic remediation or direct tutoring of basic skills fails, many resource educators initiate a functional role model, teaching so-called survival skills. The functional teaching model assumes that the youths have pressing needs in preparation for a specific vocational career. Survival teaching may include learning a very specific functional word list needed to pass a driver test or a technical vocabulary to understand career information or enter a specific vocational-technical training pattern. Functional teaching may cover making change, a basic sight word vocabulary, a technical vocabulary, and social skills necessary to receive positive peer acceptance.

Functional Skills/Vocational Approaches

Various approaches emphasize survival and/or vocational-career skills. These require a separate curriculum for teaching LBP students how to function in society. Development and delivery of the curriculum are the primary responsibilities of special education teachers, who often have little or no training in this area and who may duplicate the efforts of vocational educators. This model is sound if the students receiving instruction are indeed nonfunctional. This determination must be made by comparing performance of LBP adolescents on functional or vocational skills to that of normal peers. Many LBP students have at least average intelligence and, for the most part, are clearly capable of benefiting from the regular classroom curriculum. Limiting instruction for these students to a basic survival skills curriculum would be denying the significant potential that most of them possess.

Tutorial Approach

In programs using primarily the tutorial approach, special education teachers help students with their academic classwork. The adolescents are tutored in specific subjects and may attend a resource room for English or math credit. The emphasis, then, is on course work, not on the underlying inability to learn efficiently that is causing the youths' problems in regular classes. They may be unwilling to do general remedial work knowing that they are supposed to be dealing with a specific content area. Also, the tutorial model assumes that special education teachers, with little background in content instruction, can effectively present a variety of high school subjects.

Using a tutorial approach, even under the best of circumstances, teachers might be able to meet only one of a student's lifetime learning needs. Other seriously damaging effects of the tutorial model include classroom teachers' decreased tolerance for student differences, increases in inappropriate referrals, and the youths' dependence on the special education program. A growing number of educators and agencies (i.e., state departments of education) view the tutorial model as the least desirable of all available options.

CRISIS-RESOURCE TEACHER/ROOM[2]

As the name implies, the crisis factor must be considered when applying this alternative to LBP students. Generally, this model will be of greatest value to those with behavior problems, but students with learning problems who suffer stress also may benefit.

This alternative has the advantage of being need related and is therefore in congruity with the students. The students have the option of being responsible for their behavior to the maximum extent possible but, should it become necessary, therapeutic assistance is available. In many instances this alternative is internalized by the students and not by the system, which is even more advantageous for the adolescents. Few intervention strategies have this desirable characteristic from the learners' point of view.

The key person in this intervention strategy is the crisis-resource teacher. This individual must be able to quickly read situational and personal behavior cues to be maximally effective. This means the teacher must know the LBP adolescents both as students and as individuals and must have a clear understanding of the instructional environment and climate in which they participate as learners and peer members.

Crisis-resource teachers must work hard to ensure that they do not become viewed as disciplinarians in the school setting. Too often, students with behavior problems are considered to be a "discipline crisis" and crisis-resource teachers are called in to administer discipline. This is not the role such educators should play. The real concern, however, should be what precipitated the need for discipline, not the administration of the corrective measures themselves. It is hard for any students, adolescents or otherwise, to seek assistance from someone they view as an enforcer.

Crisis teachers may function on an itinerant basis or from a resource room. If itinerant (the preferred approach), they should not be housed in conjunction with the principal's office or other perceived authority figures within the school for two basic reasons. The first is that the students will view them as an arm of the principal's office or as authoritative figures. The latter image is one that is not well received by adolescents with behavior problems who are seeking to establish their own parameters of self-control and/or autonomy. The second is that the classroom teachers with whom the crisis educators must relate will not view these individuals much differently from the way the students do because they do not want perceived disciples of the principal in their rooms. It always is quite difficult to function out of an office of authority and not have some residual association attached to it.

If crisis-resource teachers work out of a room, every effort should be made to keep it strictly a place of service and contact rather than for classwork. One of the distinct advantages to the crisis educators is that they then are not viewed as teachers by the youths they serve. To many students with problems, the classroom teacher is the problem. Should a room assignment occur, the crisis teachers must work to keep it in operation half a day at the most and the ratio with students as close to a one-to-one as possible. The value of crisis-resource teachers is diminished if they must be confined to a room and required to work with adolescents on a group, rather than on an individual, basis. The confinement to a room also may preclude the crisis teachers from having an opportunity to view the students functioning in the classroom and in the process identify possible antecedents for their learning or behavioral problems.

The crisis-resource teacher alternative has not been widely adopted, but there is every reason to believe it will become more common in the future. The role is difficult and not everyone has the characteristics necessary to fulfill it effectively. The problem of being an advocate for both students and teachers is difficult to resolve, especially when a side must be taken. Yet, given the right kind of person, such dilemmas will occur infrequently and few of them will go unresolved.

ITINERANT INTERVENTIONISTS

This alternative is highly analogous to the crisis teacher strategy except that the practitioners are totally itinerant and therefore are not based at any one school on a permanent basis. Itinerant interventionists work on a regular basis primarily with students who have various kinds of problems involving learning or behavior. They are scheduled across the schools and follow an established routine. However, while they are not primarily used to deal with crises, they are skilled in dealing with those that might occur while they are at a given school or in a particular classroom.

As interventionists, teachers are concerned about developing programs for the students that will seek to reduce problems almost along the lines of a preventive model. Once developed, these programs are left with the regular teachers so they can utilize the strategies once the itinerant interventionists leave the school.

This alternative has advantages for the rural or small school system because it gets help to the learners and does provide a plan for the teachers. However, it lacks the intensity of the crisis-resource teacher and does not provide for close analysis of the students and their learning situations. For students with very mild problems, this alternative can be most effective by supporting them in the mainstream as well as preventing the further deterioration of their performance in the classroom. Through this procedure everyone benefits some, but for some youths it just may not be enough.

TEACHER CONSULTANTS

Whereas the itinerant interventionists work primarily with students, teacher consultants deal mainly with regular classroom teachers. This alternative places an emphasis on teaching the regular educator how to deal with LBP students. Teacher consultants may be itinerant or school based, depending on the size of the schools in the system or the size of the system itself.

Teacher consultants are first of all excellent teachers in their own right. They have been in regular classes and have been well trained in instruction and classroom management. They are skilled at diagnosis, prescription, and evaluation. In short, they are learning or instructional strategists in the purest sense.

Probably the single most important trait of teacher consultants is their ability to communicate effectively with regular classroom teachers. This communication is essential if the students are to benefit from the knowledge and skill of the consulting teachers. The regular classroom teachers must respect the ability of these consultants and, at the same time, the latter must respect the quality and rights of the classroom teachers. The use of the word "rights" is of particular significance because the regular classroom is the responsibility of the regular teachers. Teacher consultants must recognize this right as well as the classroom teachers' accountability for the students' progress, or lack of it.

Teamwork and shared responsibility are bywords in the success of the teacher consultant alternative. Referrals to teacher consultants result in initiation of a systematic process of observation, diagnosis, and interaction among students, teachers, and parents regarding the perceived problem. Once this has occurred, then—and only then—a plan of action (prescription) is suggested to the regular teacher for implementation. The effectiveness of the prescriptive action plan is a joint responsibility between teacher consultants and regular educators. Continuous evaluation is essential to ensure that the plan either is working, needs revision, or should be discarded.

The teacher consultant approach is one in considerable use in various forms across the nation. Like the other alternatives that require a strong instructional specialization, much is dependent upon the person selected to serve as the teacher consultant. More than mere skill is required since personal interactions are so much a part of the planned application and implementation of the prescriptive strategy.

If the elements of quality are met, however, this alternative is highly viable and effective. It is effective because the regular classroom teacher learns to deal effectively with the students without direct intervention from a special educator. This means one less adjustment for the adolescents and removes one more point where accountability may be delineated. The approach is appropriate for both large and small systems and does provide a means of effectively using master teachers for the good of all students rather than for just a lucky few.

PEER TUTORING/SUPPORT

A major strategy for adolescent students is the use of peers for tutoring and support. The need to belong is of paramount importance to adolescents and they generally will accept more structure and direction from peers than from adult authority figures, especially those identified as representing the school establishment. The use of peers for tutoring is not new in education. The old one-room country school relied heavily on the older students' working with the younger ones as teacher assistants. Their general effectiveness was quite good, as attested by the success of many who were educated in such settings. Present-day literature includes numerous references to this activity, citing various arguments for and against the practice.

Special educators have used nonhandicapped peers as tutors for years with reasonable success. While there are problems with the strategy, these are not of any major consequence if peer utilization is well planned and supervised. The advantages of peer utilization are many but the most obvious include the following:

- the peers' ability to communicate on the same terms and from a common base of interest
- the absence of a generation gap, which otherwise places an artificial barrier between students and tutors
- the peers' familiarity with classroom routine, procedures, goals, and rules
- the peers' knowledge of the material to be taught as well as practice in its acquisition
- the peers' ability to follow up on a supportive basis beyond the confines of the school
- the resulting mutually rewarding activity for both tutors and students

Often the tutor provides an entree to the school's social structure that previously was not available to the students on their own. This "buddy" or "friend" relationship has tremendous benefit to adolescents who need to belong and feel wanted by their peers. For adolescents with behavior problems, the peer tutor also may serve as a role model for them to view and possibly emulate.

But peer tutoring requires careful planning and structure. Not every fellow adolescent may be qualified to serve as a peer tutor. The selection process must be sensitive to the kinds of characteristics that are necessary for an effective tutor-pupil relationship. Once identified and selected, the peer tutor should receive training in the basics of how to reward, the value of repetition, how to maintain consistency, and rudiments of what it is to teach.

Classroom teachers must be willing to delegate but not forget that they still are responsible for the results of the peer tutoring, whether positive or negative. Likewise, the teachers must seek to establish the best match between the LBP adolescents and their tutors. By no means is the use of peer tutors easy, but the potential results make it well worth the effort.

One final comment and caution regarding the use of peer tutors: Teachers never should place one peer in the role of disciplining another. Peer tutoring does not embrace the practice of peer discipline.

LEARNING SPECIALISTS

An emerging support service model is that of the learning specialist who operates in a learning or educational services center. The center provides teachers with a diagnostic-prescriptive intervention service that emphasizes retention of the students in the regular classroom.

The learning specialists who function in the center are skilled in the analysis of diagnostic data, intervention and remedial strategies, evaluation, prescription development, and instruction. These specialists work to help regular class teachers develop a better understanding of what constitutes learning and/or behavior problems and the derivation of a given problem. The learning specialists are highly skilled and oriented to a systematic approach toward instruction, based on the diagnostic data collected through evaluation of the student's present levels of educational and behavioral functioning.

LEARNING ASSISTANCE CENTERS

A number of learning and educational center models have been developed by school systems. They vary as might be suspected in both design and program. An example of one such program is that operated by the Palo Alto Unified School District, Palo Alto, Calif. Titled *The Learning Assistance Program for Education-*

ally Handicapped Pupils, this is described by Gearhart (1973) as one of the more acceptable and effective models. The goals of the Palo Alto program, which serves the educationally handicapped (including both learning disabilities and behavior problems) are:

1. To assist educationally handicapped students to function more adequately in the regular classroom.
2. To establish an educational guidance committee in each school for the purpose of early identification of the educationally handicapped student. The committee will usually include the principal, the classroom or subject area teacher, the learning assistance teacher, the speech therapist, the school nurse, the counselor, and the guidance consultant.
3. To utilize diagnostic findings from the fields of psychology, education, and medicine in developing a realistic individualized education program for each educationally handicapped student.
4. To coordinate the special services provided for each educationally handicapped student with the student's basic educational program.
5. To provide continuous evaluation of each educationally handicapped student's progress in both the special program and the regular class, modifying his program when indicated.
6. To arrange for parent conferences, both individual and group, to facilitate understanding of their child's educational problems.
7. To provide a careful and systematic program of in-service study for professional growth.
8. To research the total program and utilize the findings of this research to develop a preventive, as well as remedial, program for educationally handicapped students.
9. To be knowledgeable of all available community resources for the educationally handicapped student.
10. To convey to the community the goals, organization, and philosophy of the program. (Gearhart, 1973, p. 160)

Basic to the Palo Alto program is the formulation of learning centers. These are designed and developed to facilitate handicapped students' being returned to or retained in the regular classroom through a coordinated process of interchange between the learning assistance practitioner and the regular classroom teacher. The major role of secondary level learning assistance teachers, according to Gearhart, is that of liaison among teachers, counseling staff members, and administrators in the school. The learning assistance teachers utilize a variety of techniques, all intended to mainstream educationally handicapped students.

The major responsibility of learning specialists or learning assistance teachers often is one of interpretation of what the various diagnostic findings mean in relation to a given student's performance or behavior in the regular classroom. The learning assistance specialist may then transpose the information into a viable instructional prescription for the regular teacher to utilize in the classroom.

The learning assistance center is not a resource room. Students receive intensive instruction there for a very short time. The type of instruction is focused on the students' specific learning or behavior problems that precipitated their referral to the center by the teacher. The learning specialists apply to the students a particular type of program that they feel will be effective based on the information the regular teacher has provided as well as on data they have obtained from their own diagnostic analysis.

Once applied, the prescriptive programs are evaluated by the learning specialists to determine whether or not they are appropriate and, if not, what modifications should be made. Once the evaluation indicates that the instructional models or prescriptions are effective, the learning assistance specialists provide them to the regular teachers for their classroom use. Thus, the learning specialists not only develop a prescription but also apply it in a controlled situation—the learning center—and then transmit it to the regular teacher for its ultimate implementation.

The value of a learning or educational center to a school is high. The center not only provides the locus for learning specialists to operate but also offers classroom teachers an easily accessible place to obtain technical assistance. The opportunities for follow-up and monitoring of the applied prescription facilitate and support the mainstreaming of LBP adolescents.

As a concept, the learning assistance center also has tremendous potential for acceptance in high schools because it can be operated under the auspices of the guidance program. Such an operation may serve to reduce its negative image from the viewpoint of the adolescents while at the same time accord to it the positive aspects that association with the guidance program might provide. Without question, the learning assistance or educational center concept has great potential value as a means of facilitating the retention and/or placement of handicapped learners at the junior high and secondary school level.

SUMMARY

This chapter has made possible a better understanding of the complexity of secondary level special education. This area of special education has experienced enormous change in recent years and will continue to do so in the future. The differences between elementary and secondary programs, particularly the instructional strategies, teacher roles, intervention systems, problems encountered in the schools, and adolescent behavior, now should be better comprehended.

NOTES

1. Gary M. Clark. "Career preparation for handicapped adolescents: A matter of appropriate education." *Exceptional Education Quarterly,* 1980, *1*(2), 11-17. Portions of this article were used with permission in this section.

2. The author expresses his appreciation to Dr. Harold Wm. Heller for his contributions to the crisis resource teacher/room and learning specialist sections.

Part II

The Student and Family in the School Environment

There are no simple descriptions of secondary students with learning and/or behavioral problems. These youths provide a complex mosaic of learner characteristics that have a profound impact on the teaching task in the educational environment. Chapter 2 reviews the common characteristics used to describe the handicapping categories constituting secondary mild or high incidence handicapped groups. It focuses on learning and behavioral problems as generic terminology because the LBP definition makes sense educationally. That fact is explained in the identification section. How LBP students may be managed in the most general sense, from both an instructional and behavioral point of view, also is discussed.

Logically, if LBP youths remain without proper interventions, the result may be tardiness, truancy, vandalism, and violent behaviors. Chapter 3 looks at adjudicated youths and the correctional efforts of the juvenile justice system. It presents the harsh reality of one type of alternative when public school intervention is not provided in time, or at all. It speaks to the role the streets play in attempting to restructure a quality of life aspect for youths who have failed, and were failed by, the system.

Chapter 4 examines the communication process with parents, including the role students and their families can play in providing self-determination in the educational decision-making process.

Chapter 2

Adolescents with Learning and Behavior Problems

Harold J. McGrady

INTRODUCTION

This chapter is an overview of the educational characteristics and instructional approaches for adolescents who have learning and behavioral problems (LBPs).[1] The purpose is to point out their unique characteristics and highlight ways in which these factors dictate the need for special education. In essence, this chapter responds to the questions: What are the unique features of adolescents with LBPs, and how should these elements be accommodated in special education programs?

The discussion covers important aspects of special education for LBP adolescents: (1) identification, assessment, and diagnosis; (2) design of overall curriculum programs and individual instructional objectives; (3) use of various intervention strategies such as behavior modification, prescriptive teaching, and mainstreaming strategies; and (4) the broader aspects of programming and delivery systems.

As an overview, this chapter may have some overlap with later ones on assessment or specific instructional programs and methodologies. The purpose here is to touch on each of these areas, providing perspective, issues, and guidelines, while leaving fuller details to those chapters.

PERSPECTIVE

The problems and issues involving the treatment of LBP adolescents are a microcosm of the questions faced by the entire field of special education. Professionals express varied opinions in regard to definition, identification, assessment techniques, diagnosis, remedial approaches, and the nature of service delivery systems. Many opinions are reported in subsequent chapters, substantiated in varying degrees by research data.

Although professionals seem to be in agreement that something ought to be done about LBP students beyond elementary school, there are few proved treatment models to emulate, essentially because extensive and comprehensive programming for LBP adolescents is an emerging and developing trend in special and general education. Secondary schools often attempt to carry elementary level models of special education treatment. There are distinct differences and similarities between elementary aged and adolescent LBP students. These are discussed in the following sections.

Differences

There are valid reasons why models of treatment that have been shown to be useful with younger children have not been productive when applied to adolescents. The primary reason is deceivingly simple: The two groups *are* different.

Adolescents with learning and behavior problems are different, according to several perspectives. They share the same differences from younger and older age groups as are experienced by normal adolescent youths. The total physical, psychological, and social changes that affect normal adolescents also occur for disabled youths. These are the normal differences described in Chapter 1. But the passage from childhood to adulthood, characterized by dramatic behavior shifts, is compounded by the presence of special learning or behavor problems such as socio-sexual relations, cognitive learning at the formal operations level in academic subjects, and delinquency.

The second difference is that LBP adolescents do not have the normal base of learning and social behavior to cope with this particularly challenging period of life. Thus, they come into adolescence ill prepared to deal with the sudden changes and demands placed upon them. Their academic skills usually are well below expectancy, their social behavior is inferior, and attempts to rectify either of these circumstances tend to meet with failure.

A third major difference, which sometimes is overlooked, is the cumulative effect of the many attempts to help these youngsters prior to their adolescent years. They reach this stage of life with a characteristic history of failure. They have lived with their learning and/or behavior problems and the resulting academic and social failures for a decade or so. Thus, these students whose problems persist (or begin) beyond the elementary school years may manifest a variety of difficulties quite different from those of their elementary counterparts. As a result, they may require more age-appropriate materials and strategies to counteract the various internal and external stimuli affecting them as they progress through the adolescent years. The practical fact is that practitioners must examine how each student has been treated educationally in the past.

Some educators reason that if opportunity is provided to adjust handicapping conditions in elementary school, then youths who do not appear to be different physically or mentally should outgrow the problems and respond favorably at the secondary level without the need for additional program adjustments. The inability of secondary teachers to see youths positively when they fail to learn or evidence other negative experiences in social and extracurricular activity indicates the students do not take advantage of the privilege of learning. In that case, prejudicial views concerning their indifference and overt measures to stop them (stop out as opposed to drop out) from attending school continue. To be realistic, many secondary handicapped youths must face the subject-matter-centered attitude of educators that excludes from teacher consciousness those who fail to achieve in the secondary academic setting. Students fall roughly into three classes:

1. They have never been treated. The prevalence of this circumstance should diminish as nationwide mandatory programs are developed.
2. They have been treated for a long time. The amount of continuing treatment may become a significant problem in the field of learning and behavior disorders. What can be done when, after years of treatment, students display minimal or decreasing effects? Do educators continue treating students in the same way indefinitely?
3. They have been mistreated. This is more difficult to deal with, but students have been misclassified and/or treated inappropriately.

The truth is that eventually children with learning and behavior problems reach physical maturity but, as they progress through various phases of development, their disorders manifest themselves in ways that affect them in their adult lives in varying degrees.

Academic, Social, and Behavioral Difficulties

These aspects attracted the attention of this author during a longitudinal study of students with language learning disabilities during the 1960s (McGrady, 1969). It was startlingly clear upon interviewing parents of aphasic boys aged 7 to 9 in the early 1960s that the pupils' learning disabilities were manifested in behaviors such as severe academic difficulties starting with elementary school and disruptive social-emotional or affective problems during adolescence and beyond.

The progression was mirrored by the concerns of parents. The students studied had been identified as having significant language/learning problems during their preschool years. At that time the parents were concerned about factors such as: Will they be able to talk normally? Will they be able to go to school? Are they retarded? Will they be able to go to college? The parents' primary questions concerned academics: How will these youngsters be taught to read and do arithmetic? Will they have to be in special classes? How can they pass various academic tests? These same students were tested at ages 13 to 15, and the parents reinterviewed. Their perspectives and concerns had shifted. College was seen as a less prominent goal; merely getting through various grade levels, subjects, or courses was more important than excelling. But, very dramatically, these parents were expressing great anxiety over the social/emotional behavior and well-being of their children. The adolescents frequently were reported to be loners; they were viewed as "different" by their peers; they often had few friends; they did not participate heavily in social activities such as school clubs, extracurricular activities, and the like. The families began to question their vocational potential and their probabilities for marriage and family success.

The clear conclusion from this is that the affective, social, and emotional behavior problems manifested by adolescents with long-standing learning disabilities transcend the basic academic/learning problems after a period of time. It is an axiom among personnel workers that few adults lose their jobs as a result of poor skills or aptitudes. These can be taught. They usually leave jobs because of an inability to manage the communication and interpersonal relationships required of their employment. Similarly, it is not academic failure, per se, that is most detrimental to adolescents' future success—it is the accompanying personal social factors. For that reason alone, the treatment of LBP adolescents is different from that of preteen youths.

It is not safe to assume that LBP elementary students pass tranquilly into junior high school and adolescence. During this transition, numerous variables impact significantly upon them. For example, educational systems (Johnson, Blalock, & Nesbitt, 1978; Kokoszka & Drye, 1981; Zigmond, 1978) and families (Beare, 1975; Bryant, 1978; Klein, Altman, Dreizen, Friedman, & Powers, 1981a, 1981b) are ill prepared to analyze, adapt to, and address these students' academic and social-emotional needs. Peers misunderstand, devalue, and reject these "different" individuals (Bryan, 1976, 1978; Bruininks, 1978; Siperstein, Bopp, & Bak, 1978); and nature creates a temporary, physiological chaos (Cook, 1979; Hurlock, 1973; Jacks & Keller, 1978).

Without systematic attention and intervention to all of these variables, the LBP junior high school student often begins (or continues) a pattern of frustration, poor self-concept, social withdrawal, and depression (Bryant, 1978; Siegel, 1974). Ultimately, this may lead to anger, overt aggression and frustration, crime, and delinquency. The learning disabled elementary student now presents behaviors more characteristic of an emotionally (behaviorally) disturbed junior high school age student (Shea, 1978; Stephens, 1977).

Following are two capsule case studies from the author's personal observation:

CASE 1: ALLEN

Allen, a young adult, came to us as a college freshman. He had just been dismissed from an excellent school of music because he had threatened to kill another student with a knife after a trivial incident in the dormitory hall. Although this young man had had serious learning problems since early childhood, he had managed to navigate all of the academic obstacles and eventually be admitted to this program of higher education. He had an extraordinary talent for music and somehow had survived all of the academic hurdles through intensive work on his part and that of his parents.

His undoing was his inability to control his behavior. The incident was one in which he simply became annoyed over some noise in the corridor. His anger became uncontrollable, and he threatened to kill the offending student. This was a sudden outburst of emotion and never had occurred to that degree before. Eventually he was readmitted to the conservatory and, with intensive counseling and guidance, succeeded in graduating. He since has developed into a successful musician and teacher and is enjoying a happy marriage.

CASE 2: ANNE
(Also described in another textbook, Van Hattum, 1980.)

In 1976, Anne was 18 years old. Although she had experienced learning and behavior problems throughout her school years, she never had been retained at any grade level. Her behavior always had been erratic. She was impulsive and seemed to respond unevenly to various circumstances. Her memory was very bad, particularly for spoken information, but she appeared to learn when tasks were organized carefully. Her parents, teachers, and friends referred to her as immature. She always had had difficulty in planning ahead or seeing the consequences of her actions.

At the completion of high school, she faced two problems. She never had been able to keep even the simplest job and was having trouble gaining employment. She had no salable skills. She also had just become pregnant, although she was not married.

Anne always had been a puzzle to her parents. Furthermore, dozens of specialists over the years had not been able to pinpoint her learning disability. Her school system never provided a comprehensive program for children with learning disabilities until recent legislation forced the establishment of such activities. Anne was about to enter the adult world, still trying to cope with an unknown, and essentially untreated, learning disability.

This case has an even more dramatic and compelling epilogue. The author was in contact with Anne's parents in 1982. Anne was 26. Kathy, the girl born of Anne's teen-age pregnancy, was 7 and had completed the first grade. However, Kathy was manifesting the same pattern of behavior and learning problems seen years before in her mother. The similarities were remarkable.

The question is whether these problems are genetically based or whether Anne's own personal failures have contributed to poor parenting skills in adulthood. This writer's opinion is that the truth is somewhere in between. Evidence points to dramatic similarities that probably result from heredity, although Anne's adult life has been characterized by poor social-emotional behaviors. Her marriage ended in divorce, her vocational success was sporadic, and her social life deficient. These factors logically would have an effect on the mother-child relationship. Anne's impulsiveness, forgetfulness, and inconsistent behavior can only serve to diminish her parenting skills.

Thus, there is a vicious cycle of cause and effect that appears to be transmitted across generations. This alone should give educators pause to realize the importance of dealing forthrightly with every child with learning and behavior problems. Otherwise, simply by their omission or lack of assistance, educators may be contributing inadvertently to the perpetuation of such problems in society.

These cases exemplify the intricate intertwining that occurs between learning/academic problems and the accompanying behavioral difficulties. Planning for appropriate special intervention must take into account the following factors:

1. the residuals of the basic learning and behavior problems (and the associated reductions in levels of academic and social skills)
2. the adolescents' reactions and responses to their consequent successes/failures in attempting to cope
3. the current and cumulative effects of reactions from others in the environment to past failures and low current levels of functioning

In summary, LBP adolescents are different primarily in three ways:

1. they are different from other age group children because they are adolescent
2. they are different from their adolescent peers because they have learning and behavior problems
3. each individual is different from other adolescents with learning and behavior problems because of the cumulative effect of their problems and their life history of failure.

Each of these elements of the problem must be considered in establishing a program for LBP students in secondary schools. Perhaps the key factor in all treatment of these adolescents is whether such differences are given proper consideration in the design and implementation of intervention techniques, methods, approaches, or total programs.

COMMON CHARACTERISTICS

Definition/Description

In traditional categorical terms, special education students include those who are referred to as learning disabled (LD), educable mentally handicapped/retarded (EMR), or emotionally/behaviorally handicapped (EH). In more generic terms, this group might be assigned the rubric of mildly educationally handicapped. Although this amalgamation of categories may give some teachers concern, these special students share common characteristics: they enter adolescence with below normal academic and/or social behavior skills and their functional levels of performance exist in direct proportion to those skills. Thus, symptomatically they are similar. Although they require individual treatment, there are generic principles of teaching for behavioral and academic learning skills that apply to all.

Attempts to develop an operational definition and classification system for LBP adolescents have stirred controversy among special educators in recent years. This is most evident in attempts to define students who fall in the traditional LD and EH categories.

Problems of Classification

The dilemma in attempting to describe the characteristics of students with learning and behavior problems is that there exists no set of common behaviors that constitute a universal syndrome of characteristics. For example, at an international exposition in Montreal, a medical display showed a large mock-up of a human cell, with appropriate flashing lights and accompanying audio description. This allowed observers to identify parts of a typical human cell. The accompanying commentary said every human cell was different from every other specific human cell, even if they were of the same type in one human being. The concluding remark capsulized the problem: "There is no such thing as a typical cell; you have just seen a typical cell."

It is traditional to state in academic texts and university courses that a certain type of problem, such as learning disabilities or emotional handicap, is characterized by a group of certain specified behaviors. Thus, many college level courses are devoted to the characteristics of learning disabilities, or mental retardation, or behavior disorders, or whatever.

This approach is unproductive and often misleading. If educators were to follow that line of reasoning and provide a list of universal behavior characteristics for adolescents with learning and behavior problems, they would have to conclude by paraphrasing from the Montreal exhibit: "There is no such thing as a typical student with learning and behavior difficulties; let us now describe the typical student with learning and behavior problems." This predicament is demonstrated by authors who have attempted to stereotype learning disabilities among adolescents. The following section looks at efforts to isolate the characteristics of LD adolescents.

Learning Disabilities

Goodman and Mann (1976) discuss the problems inherent in the procedure of diagnosis by exclusion. They describe what adolescents with learning disabilities are *not*:

> In summary, secondary level learning disabled pupils are not sensorially or physically handicapped, mentally retarded or slow learners, or pupils whose general intellectual levels are insufficient to master the more complex demands of secondary education. Neither are they victims of severe behavioral disturbances caused by brain injury, neurological disturbance, or emotional pathology. They do not suffer from pathologically impoverishing social-cultural histories; nor do they represent the many dismotivated, disinterested, turned-off constituents, and products of modern society and its educational systems. (p. 10)

What are the characteristics of adolescent students with learning disabilities? A subsequent attempt by Mann, Goodman, and Wiederholt (1978) met with similar frustration for anyone attempting to clarify a taxonomic scheme. In that volume, Deshler concludes that it is improper to use terms and concepts from studies of characteristics of younger children with learning disabilities. This results "in the inappropriate and eventually meaningless application of terms such as *hyperactivity, perceptual deficit, distractibility*, and *disorders of thinking*" (p. 49). Deshler adds: "The presence of any given characteristic is neither conclusive nor required in determining if a youngster has a learning disability. Conversely, all characteristics commonly associated with learning disabilities need not be present in order to cause a reduction in a student's educational and social adjustments" (p. 49).

Consequently, Deshler settles on a descriptive, rather than a diagnostic-categorical, approach to defining learning disabilities among adolescents. The approach essentially is to categorize (and therefore treat) behaviors, rather than pupils. Thus, he categorizes behavioral characteristics according to whether they are academic-cognitive, personality-social, or perceptual-motor. He concludes that each of these factors must be included in any strategy for studying the characteristics of learning disabled adolescents. The assumption is that a thorough cataloguing and understanding of significant characteristics of a given student are essential to serving the psychoeducational needs of that particular individual, regardless of any system of diagnostic classification.

Deshler continues this approach in a more recent book coauthored with Gordon Alley (Alley & Deshler, 1979). They make no effort to recapitulate the characteristics of adolescents with learning disabilities. Instead, they categorize the learning strategies needed to overcome such problems. They call this the "learning strategies approach" and define it as follows: *"Learning strategies are defined as techniques, principles, or rules that will facilitate the acquisition, manipulation, integration, storage, and retrieval of information across situations and settings.* A learning strategies model of instruction for LD adolescents is designed to teach students how to learn rather than to teach students specific content" (p. 13). They include seven skill areas; "reading, writing, mathematics, thinking, social interaction, speaking, and listening" (p. 22).

The preceding discussion highlights the problems of trying to categorize students with learning disabilities. The LD hallmark is the presence of severe intraindividual differences in learning in the absence of other significant factors such as low general mental ability, sensory or motor problems, cultural, economic, or environmental factors. These factors and how they are represented in the federal definition of learning disabilities are discussed in McGrady (1980).

Emotional Disturbance/Behavioral Disorders

This discussion so far has utilized primarily examples of characteristics from the field of learning disabilities. However, the same circumstances prevail in the attempt to describe or characterize adolescents with behavioral or emotional problems. Taxonomic systems based on diagnostic categories from the field of psychiatry and mental health such as psychoses, neuroses, schizophrenia, autism, and others have proved to be unproductive in solving individual problems or designing treatment programs, especially in educational settings. Interventions based primarily on dealing directly with observable behaviors have been more successful, as is discussed in the final section of this chapter. Reality therapy, assertive discipline, and various behavior modification programs have been the product of this shift in thinking.

Of the major categories that purport to classify exceptional children and youths, few appear to have such inconsistency as does the area of study known as emotional disturbance or behavioral disorders (Kanner, 1962). The basic difficulty in describing emotional disturbance is that it requires a definition of normality, a most difficult task (Laing, 1967; Szasz, 1969). Unlike mental retardation, which by definition is fixed in the developmental period, emotional development not only is influenced by the growth of the nervous system and the opportunity to learn but also may be threatened by the events of unpredictable human relationships. To obtain a fixed position in time and space, as is true with mental retardation, is impossible with emotional disturbance: there are those who function normally in all but one situation, where fears of that condition alone trigger abnormal reactions. Unlike deafness or blindness, it is impossible to determine the degree of deviance in precise psychological or physical measures.

Manual of Mental Disorders (DSM-III)

The *Diagnostic and Statistical Manual of Mental Disorders, DSM-III* (American Psychiatric Association, 1980, 3d ed.) improved upon the previous ones—DSM-I (1952) and DSM-II (1968)—by specifying more precise criteria for clinical judgment. It increased the list of psychological disturbances significantly to 230 separate categories, named the disorders, and described them precisely. This change resulted in a better system of clinical classification.

According to McDowell (1982):

A second important change in DSM-III over previous editions is that it requires much more information about the person being diagnosed. DSM-III instructs the diagnostician to evaluate the person on five different axes or areas of functioning [Exhibit 2-1]. This multiaxial classification system means that instead of simply placing a person in one category, each case is evaluated in terms of a number of important factors.

Axis I describes abnormal behavior patterns such as anxiety or depression. Axis 2 covers two areas: personality disorders in adults or specific developmental disorders in children and adolescents. Axis 3 refers to any medical or physical disorders that may be relevant to the psychological problem. Axis 4 assesses psychosocial factors such as divorce that may have been causing the person stress. Examples for both adults and children are included. Axis 5 is the highest level of adaptive functioning attained by the person during the previous year. A rating of the person's adjustment in such areas as occupation or social relationships is used.

Axes 4 and 5 are especially significant. Knowing what demands the person has been trying to meet is necessary to understand the problem behavior that has developed. Moreover, knowing the person's general level of success in meeting the demands of adjustment can help in formulating an appropriate, realistic treatment plan. (p. 7)

Exhibit 2-1 DSM-III Classification: Axes I and II Categories and Codes

The long dashes indicate the need for a fifth-digit subtype or other qualifying term.

Disorders Usually First Evident in Infancy, Childhood, or Adolescence

Mental retardation
(Code in fifth digit: 1 = with other behavioral symptoms [requiring attention or treatment and that are not part of another disorder], 0 = without other behavioral symptoms.)
317.0(x) Mild mental retardation, _____
318.0(x) Moderate mental retardation, _____
318.1(x) Severe mental retardation, _____
318.2(x) Profound mental retardation, _____
319.0(x) Unspecified mental retardation, _____

Attention deficit disorder
314.01 With hyperactivity
314.00 Without hyperactivity
314.80 Residual type

Conduct disorder
312.00 Undersocialized, aggressive
312.10 Undersocialized, nonaggressive
312.23 Socialized, aggressive
312.21 Socialized, nonaggressive
312.90 Atypical

Anxiety disorders of childhood or adolescence
309.21 Separation anxiety disorder
313.21 Avoidant disorder of childhood or adolescence
313.00 Overanxious disorder

Other disorders of infancy, childhood, or adolescence
313.89 Reactive attachment disorder of infancy
313.22 Schizoid disorder of childhood or adolescence
313.23 Elective mutism
313.81 Oppositional disorder
313.82 Identity disorder

Eating disorders
307.10 Anorexia nervosa
307.51 Bulimia
307.52 Pica
307.53 Rumination disorder of infancy
307.50 Atypical eating disorder

Stereotyped movement disorders
307.21 Transient tic disorder
307.22 Chronic motor tic disorder
307.23 Tourette's disorder
307.20 Atypical tic disorder
307.30 Atypical stereotyped movement disorder

Other disorders with physical manifestations
307.00 Stuttering
307.60 Functional enuresis
307.70 Functional encopresis
307.46 Sleepwalking disorder
307.46 Sleep terror disorder (307.49)

Pervasive developmental disorders
Code in fifth digit: 0 = full syndrome present, 1 = residual state.
299.0x Infantile autism, _____
299.9x Childhood onset pervasive developmental disorder, _____
299.8x Atypical, _____

Specific developmental disorders
Note: These are coded on Axis II.
315.00 Developmental reading disorder
315.10 Developmental arithmetic disorder
315.31 Developmental language disorder
315.39 Developmental articulation disorder
315.50 Mixed specific developmental disorder
315.90 Atypical specific developmental disorder

Source: Reprinted with permission from *Diagnostic and Statistical Manual of Mental Disorders* (3d ed.). American Psychiatric Association. © 1980. p. 15.

Although the DSM-III classification system is the most prevalent used among professionals, it does not have unanimous support. Many professionals make modifications of these postures or, depending upon orientation, others totally eschew them. McDowell (1982) also indicates that acceptance of DSM-III by professionals "implies acceptance of the medical model for explaining abnormal behavior, which states that, like physical diseases, emotional disorders have their underlying causes, etiology, and resultant observable symptoms" (pp. 8-9).

Mental Retardation

Appropriate definition and cataloguing of characteristics for mildly retarded students have not been any easier. In fact, the American Association on Mental Deficiency (AAMD) dramatically changed the definition of mental retardation (Grossman, 1977) simply by describing it as follows: "Mental Retardation refers to significantly subaverage general intellectual functioning existing concurrently with deficits in adaptive behavior, and manifested during the developmental period" (p. 11).

Using this definition, professionals consider persons to be mentally retarded if their general intellectual functioning, as measured by an individualized intelligence test such as forms L-M of the Stanford-Binet or the three Wechsler scales, is identified as being significantly subaverage. Significantly subaverage refers to an IQ of two or more standard deviations below the mean. The mean, according to Grossman (1977), is "usually (IQ) 100 of a standardized general intelligence test" (p. 12). Mental retardation is "represented by an IQ of 67 or below on the Stanford-Binet and an IQ of 69 or below on the Wechsler Scales" (p. 12). In addition, an individual must exhibit deficits in adaptive behavior, "the degree with which an individual meets the standards of personal independence and social responsibility expected for their age and cultural group" (p. 11). These deficits in adaptive behavior must exist concurrently with significantly subaverage general intellectual functioning.

Previously the cutoff point for mental retardation was subaverage general intellectual functioning reflected in an IQ score of below one standard deviation from the mean. By virtue of that one "stroke of the pen," 13.59 percent of the population of the United States who theoretically would be classified as mentally retarded no longer were considered as such. What a miraculous cure. The fact is that whether a person is labeled as mentally retarded, emotionally disturbed, or learning disabled depends entirely on a set of arbitrary characteristics and cutoff points.

This is illustrated beautifully by the following passage from Lewis Carroll's *Alice in Wonderland*. When Humpty Dumpty says to Alice, "There's glory for you!", the following repartee ensues:

"I don't know what you mean by 'glory'," Alice said. Humpty Dumpty smiled contemptuously. "Of course you don't—till I tell you. I meant 'there's a nice knock-down argument for you'!"

"But 'glory' doesn't mean 'a nice knock-down argument'," Alice objected.

"When *I* use a word," Humpty Dumpty said, in a rather scornful tone, "it means just what I choose it to mean—neither more nor less." (Gardner, 1960, pp. 268-269)

Words are arbitrary symbols. Labels and definitions for LBP adolescents are arbitrary designations. They are meaningful only to their users. Any use of these terms is subject to misuse and miscommunication. Thus, it seems best not to try to define a syndrome or precise diagnostic category for these youths. Rather, it would be best to merely state and describe in objective terms the exact behaviors that need to be developed or corrected/eliminated.

IDENTIFICATION

The problems of identification stem from the dilemma posed above, viz., that there are no clear-cut syndromes for a taxonomy of LBPs. If practitioners cannot clearly and precisely outline a list of characteristics for specified types of learning and behavior problems, how can they hope to devise systems to identify them? The answer begs for simplicity.

It is similar to the attempts to define pornography (McGrady, 1980): "Jokingly, one colleague has said that the definition of learning disabilities is like the definition of pornography: 'No one seems to be able to agree on a definition, but everyone knows it when they see it' " (p. 510).

Similarly, everyone knows LBP adolescents when they see them. These students have failed consistently in school and/or they misbehave. It is as simple as that. Ask any classroom teacher; ask any parent; ask any student. Identifying youngsters with problems is simple. Knowing and understanding the precise nature of their problems and discerning exactly what treatment is required are more difficult.

One dictionary definition of identify is: "to show to be a certain person or thing." It is easy for individuals to show that they are persons with learning or behavior problems—that they are that thing: a learning/behavior problem. The concrete evidence is readily available: scholastic grades are lower than expected, either in total or in specific courses/subjects; social failures abound; aptitude and achievement tests yield low scores; teachers complain of misbehavior in the classroom; attendance patterns are erratic; other students even complain about adolescents who are "different."

Thus, the identification process is simple. To screen for possible LBP, practitioners need only ask those who know: the classroom teachers, the parents, and the students themselves.

Screening checklists can be given to classroom teachers; they should be simple and objective. Exhibit 2-2 is an example of a checklist used in the Mesa Public Schools, Mesa, Ariz. Teachers can be asked to refer any students for whom they have concern, accompanied by this referral checklist. Parents can be screened in a similar vein, or informed of normal referral processes. Students can be made aware of remedial services available to them; thus, self-referrals can occur. Someone can be given the responsibility to check student achievement test results and periodic grade report cards to identify potential problem individuals.

Too often professionals confuse identification with diagnosis. They expect a screening test to tell the entire story. They anticipate that the identification process will provide the answers as to what needs to be done to help. This is not so. The identification of learning and behavior problems is only a preliminary step to the actual evaluation, assessment, or diagnosis of the adolescent. The use of informal techniques often is suitable for this stage of the process.

Which system, which tests, and which checklists are to be used is almost immaterial. What is important is that every school should have a designated, systematic process for identifying students with problems. In fact, it is best for a school or system to develop its own process and its own checklists. Then, it is to be hoped that the identification will be consistent with available programs for intervention. Furthermore, the teachers, counselors, and others will feel an "ownership" of the process. Once identification of students with LBPs has been accomplished, the process of assessment and diagnosis can begin.

CURRICULUM AND INSTRUCTIONAL OBJECTIVES

The curriculum objectives and the specific instructional techniques will depend entirely on the major philosophy or approach that professionals might assume toward LBP adolescents. For example, there are four major types of approaches that shape the goals that practitioners might choose for youngsters with learning problems:

1. The remedial-clinical approach: The goal is to change the students' constituent learning patterns. It often is stated that professionals will teach persons to "learn how to learn." The term expresses it: the students will learn to remediate; they will change their thinking, perception, language, reading attack, or whatever. Whether teachers concentrate on psychological processes or academic tasks, the goal still is the same: to change the students' mode of thinking.

Exhibit 2-2 Behavior Problems Checklist, Mesa Public Schools, Mesa, Arizona

Name of Student _____ School_____ Teacher_____

Please indicate which of the following constitute problems, as far as this student is concerned. If an item does *not* constitute a problem, encircle the zero; if an item constitutes a *mild* problem, encircle the one; if an item constitutes a *severe* problem, encircle the two. Please complete every item. Additional comments would be appreciated.

Date _____

No Problem	Mild	Severe	
0	1	2	1. Restlessness, inability to sit still
0	1	2	2. Attention-seeking, "show-off" behavior
0	1	2	3. Stays out late at night
0	1	2	4. Doesn't know how to have fun, behaves like a little adult
0	1	2	5. Self-consciousness, easily embarrassed
0	1	2	6. Fixed expression, lack of emotional reactivity
0	1	2	7. Disruptiveness, tendency to annoy and bother others
0	1	2	8. Feelings of inferiority
0	1	2	9. Steals in company of others
0	1	2	10. Boisterousness, rowdiness
0	1	2	11. Crying over minor annoyances and hurts
0	1	2	12. Preoccupation, "in a world of his own"
0	1	2	13. Shyness, bashfulness
0	1	2	14. Social withdrawal, preference for solitary activities
0	1	2	15. Dislike for school
0	1	2	16. Jealousy over attention paid other children
0	1	2	17. Belongs to a gang
0	1	2	18. Repetitive speech
0	1	2	19. Short attention span
0	1	2	20. Lack of self-confidence
0	1	2	21. Inattentiveness to what others say
0	1	2	22. Easily flustered and confused
0	1	2	23. Incoherent speech
0	1	2	24. Fighting
0	1	2	25. Loyal to delinquent friends
0	1	2	26. Temper tantrums
0	1	2	27. Reticence, secretiveness
0	1	2	28. Truancy from school
0	1	2	29. Hypersensitivity, feelings easily hurt
0	1	2	30. Laziness in school and in performance of other tasks
0	1	2	31. Anxiety, chronic general fearfulness
0	1	2	32. Irresponsibility, undependability
0	1	2	33. Excessive daydreaming
0	1	2	34. Has bad companions
0	1	2	35. Tension, inability to relax

Exhibit 2-2 continued

0	1	2	36. Disobedience, difficulty in disciplinary control
0	1	2	37. Depression, chronic sadness
0	1	2	38. Uncooperativeness in group situations
0	1	2	39. Aloofness, social reserve
0	1	2	40. Passivity, suggestibility, easily led by others
0	1	2	41. Clumsiness, awkwardness, poor muscular coordination
0	1	2	42. Hyperactivity, "always on the go"
0	1	2	43. Distractibility
0	1	2	44. Destructiveness in regard to own and/or others' property
0	1	2	45. Negativism, tendency to do the opposite of what is required
0	1	2	46. Impertinence, sauciness
0	1	2	47. Sluggishness, lethargy
0	1	2	48. Drowsiness
0	1	2	49. Profane language, swearing, cursing
0	1	2	50. Nervousness, jitteriness, jumpiness, easily startled
0	1	2	51. Irritability, hot-tempered, easily aroused to anger
0	1	2	52. Often has physical complaints, e.g., headaches, stomach aches

Source: Harold J. McGrady, Department of Special Education, Mesa Public Schools, Mesa, Ariz.

2. The compensatory approach: In this mode, educators essentially decide they cannot teach students to learn "normally." The practitioners may decide that the adolescents never will learn to read any better, or develop better memory, or do certain levels of mathematics. Thus, they teach these students how to learn a subject through their intact learning processes. They might try a nonreading curriculum, or take all examinations orally, or provide the pupils with whatever learning aids are available. The educators teach the students to circumvent their problems.

3. The tutoring approach: In this method, practitioners simply try to teach a particular subject or content matter that is being learned by the students' peers. By whatever techniques possible or available, they try to teach the problem students English, or algebra, or American government, or whatever. The goal is merely to teach subject matter or content of current relevance in the educational program. This approach might be used while attempting the remedial or compensatory goals above.

4. The counseling approach: The educators eventually may decide that the students have reached an impasse or have achieved to the upper limits of their learning abilities. The goal then is to teach them to learn to live with their problem. The students must accept others' reactions to them yet have a positive self-concept, emphasizing the things they can do. They must learn

to avoid situations that require them to perform in their weak areas and strive to put themselves in situations in which they can utilize their strengths. Vocational and life counseling are primary elements in this approach.

Thus, these four approaches set differing goals:

1. learn how to learn (remedial)
2. learn through alternative systems (compensatory)
3. learn specific content (tutorial)
4. learn to live with the problem (counseling)

For each LBP youth, a decision must be made about which of these goals to stress. The goals usually proceed in the order discussed and are determined on an individual basis. They will change over time as the students mature, gain mastery, and develop new needs.

Similarly, paradigms could be envisaged for dealing with behavior problems, depending on whether the primary goal is to teach the adolescents how to behave, how not be behave, or how to adjust their behavior. A schemata for viewing this is presented later in Figure 2-1.

Another way of viewing instructional objectives for adolescent LBPs is to determine which aspects of the regular curriculum will receive the greatest emphasis. As these students move from elementary to junior high or middle school, remediation of basic skills should be only part of the total curriculum. Emphasis must be placed on preparation for the students' eventual graduation to a job and a self-sufficient life within the community. This adjustment requires preparation for the change from a protected school environment to one where individuals are expected to be independent and fend for themselves. LBP students can quickly become lost in high school where this shift of environments and demands occurs. Many of the academic and social gains from past educational experiences may show regression. This may cause the students to fail, drop out, or just "disappear into the woodwork," as many low achievers do at the high school level, especially in large or academically stringent schools.

All students who receive services in a special education program must have a program to meet their individual needs. At the secondary level, the needs cover a wide range of curriculum areas. These include at least academic and vocational skills.

Academic

Specific instructional objectives must be in concert with the goals that have been written into the student's individualized education program (IEP). If practitioners select a remedial approach as opposed to a compensatory, tutorial, or counseling one, remediation procedures must be designed to reduce known deficits in academic areas. The most common areas of academic remediation are reading skills, language (i.e., penmanship, vocabulary, spelling, or English), and mathematics.

These areas are important to the students' success in the regular classroom if they are planning to earn the credits necessary for high school graduation or for possible entrance into a college, university, or technical school. Remedial work at the secondary level is only for students who still can benefit from such instruction.

As stated previously, the ultimate goal must be determined. The remedial approach will assist the students to learn in the future; the tutorial approach will only help them pass certain subjects or courses. At the high school level, educators often are encouraged by outside forces to merely "get the students through," i.e., to allow them to meet minimal course requirements so they can graduate. This often is shortsighted. Despite claims that there are reduced benefits from a remedial approach for older students, results still are being obtained.

If the students can "learn to learn," it is to their long-term benefit. There is an old proverb that states: "Give me a fish and I'll eat for a day; teach me to fish and I'll eat for a lifetime." Alternative learning approaches can be used to teach content while remedial efforts are continued. (See Chapter 12 for a discussion of a successful program of this type, the Parallel Alternative Curriculum in the Mesa Public Schools, Mesa, Ariz.)

Vocational

Vocational objectives are especially important to adolescent LBP students. Those experiencing difficulties with the decisions they confront when choosing and acquiring employment should have the opportunity to visit a career information center. Very few LBP students find their way into vocational classes during their high school years, and many of them are not employable when it is time for them to leave school. Those who are moderately or severely handicapped typically have vocational training included in their regular educational program. However, the mildly handicapped adolescents usually are offered minimal services in this area. If LBP students are to be successful in getting and holding jobs after high school, the appropriate skills must be taught as a part of their educational program.

Specific goals of a vocational program include:

- Attitudes: toward employers, fellow employees, and the job itself
- Work Habits: completion of forms, attendance, entry level skills
- Social Skills: communication skills, interviewing, grooming, acceptance of criticism from supervisors and peers to improve performance
- Use of Resources: where to go to find employment opportunities
- Skill Training: classroom-based, as well as on-the-job, training for specific careers or specialties

Simply put, many youths need vocational classes at the high school level but are not receiving them. Vocational, industrial arts, or home economics teachers often deny entry of such students into their classes, particularly at higher levels on the ground that these individuals lack necessary skills or their behavior poses a safety hazard to themselves or to the class. In truth, the situation often is that the vocational teachers do not understand the characteristics and capabilities of such youngsters. Vocational educators working with special needs learners may need to:

1. provide inservice training for vocational teachers
2. hire resource teachers or aides to assist the vocational teachers in their classes
3. convert vocational classes to the Parallel Alternative Curriculum (PAC) approach

By doing so, the LBP adolescents would have greater employability, an enhanced self-concept, and a higher probability of success in life.

MAINSTREAM EDUCATION

As stated earlier, academic, vocational, and life successes depend strongly on the development of adequate social skills. For social personal development to occur, students must participate as fully as possible in the mainstream of education.

The extent to which adolescent LBP students receive instruction in the regular classroom depends on a variety of factors. To receive a high school diploma, specific requirements must be completed, including specified course credit hours, some of which are content courses mandatory for all students. The LBP students should complete independently as many of these classes as they can manage successfully, with some assistance from the special education teachers and other support personnel. The degree of student success will depend on:

1. The students' capabilities: They must be able to handle the day-to-day demands of the class (e.g., homework assignments, taking notes, taking tests, etc.).
2. Academic standards: These will have a definite effect on the students' success because, if they are exceptionally stringent, there is less chance of survival in the regular classroom for such youths.
3. Grading requirements: A fair break for all students is important. They should be able to earn grades based on the material learned. Some teachers have been found to automatically assign LBP students an average or below-grade mark based on the fact that they are receiving support services. This type of

policy makes it less likely that special education counselors will place students in mainstream classes. It unfairly removes incentives from youngsters who could learn with assistance.

4. Degree of individualization: The structure of a classroom is important when making decisions as to when and how much time students will spend in the regular class. The special education teacher or counselor becomes very selective in choosing a classroom that will offer students the maximum opportunities for success. If a history teacher uses only a textbook and classroom lectures, LBP students usually will experience frustration and failure in that course. Many high school textbooks have a readability that is two or more years above the grade level for which they are intended. Very few LBP students are capable of reading these texts. Note taking is another problem they encounter; if notes are required, it may be very difficult for them to keep up.

All of these problems can be solved without sacrificing quality standards. It has been shown that students who are given appropriate assistance can learn at the same level of instruction as others. Only the methods of instruction need to be varied. This is a challenge to regular teachers who do not wish to modify their instructions, their lectures, their texts, or their course materials.

As stated by Sabatino and Mauser (1978): "The secondary public school is an achievement-oriented academic area of departmentalized curricula, where teachers tend to view pupils as good or bad, and sense their roles as behavioral change agents as minimal" (p. 17).

In reality, secondary teachers have a large role to play in the lives of adolescents with learning or behavior problems. To the degree they are willing to recognize this role, and to modify their instruction accordingly, students will continue to progress in the reduction of learning and behavior problems in succeeding years.

Intervention Strategies

As stated earlier, this chapter provides an overview of how LBP students are unique and how the field of education might accommodate such characteristics. The remaining sections present some schemata for looking at the intervention process for dealing with these adolescents.

Remedial Approach

One of the most logical plans for the classification of remediation is presented by Lerner (1978). She proposes, "A taxonomic model that divides remediation into three classes: analysis of the student, analysis of the subject matter to be learned, and analysis of the environmental conditions under which the student learns . . . each type of analysis is subdivided into specific categories of remediation" (p. 102).

To oversimplify her approach, the "analysis of the student" is typified by the diagnostic or clinical approach. The general procedure is to test the students in various psychological processes or stages of development and proceed according to subsequent knowledge of their abilities and disabilities along those chosen parameters. In contrast, in the "analysis of the curriculum content" approach, teaching techniques and materials are presented only in terms of the type and/or level of content to be taught, regardless of the students' profile of characteristics. The skills development approach, in which a hierarchy of subskills is established and the students are taught each one accordingly, is one logical route. This method is enhanced by the presence of criterion-referenced tests for various academic skill levels to be taught.

Lerner's final category, the "analysis of environmental conditions," is best exemplified by the behavioral approach, although any psychotherapeutic or pedagogical method might also fit. Behavior modification, contingency management, and other related techniques have been used most successfully to reduce, eliminate, or modify unsatisfactory classroom or school behaviors, rather than to teach academics per se.

In a previous review of the state of the art of remediation for learning disabilities, this author (McGrady, 1980) summarized:

> The essence of the learning disabilities approach is clinical teaching: that process through which the child's capabilities are thoroughly analyzed and whereby the child is guided through the necessary sequence in order to learn a projected task. What makes learning disabilities teaching different from regular teaching is that it attempts to design an individualized program for a specific child, based on the discernible characteristics of his or her unique learning system. (p. 555)

There has been considerable argument about which approach is preferred—child analysis or a learning task analysis. The simple answer is that both are needed; one is insufficient without the other. "The competent, well-trained learning disability professional knows how to modify the 'normal' instructional process to match the unique characteristics of the child with an aberrant learning system—the child with a specific learning disability "(McGrady, 1980, p. 556).

Because of the range of disabilities and learning styles within the LBP adolescent population, it is difficult to find a theoretical base from which most programs are designed. Goodman and Mann (1976) simply resort to a series of rationale statements that conclude that secondary LD programs (1) are basic—teach reading, math, and language arts; (2) utilize mastery learning; (3) emphasize curriculum, including academic and career education; and (4) may be fully self-contained or integrated. They do not recommend process training.

Later, Mann and Goodman, with the assistance of Wiederholt and a collection of other contributors (1978), produced another text on teaching adolescents with learning disabilities. Although they state no organized theory of intervention, they appear to continue the type of position summarized above. Their general approach appears to be to simply articulate assessment and intervention procedures, techniques, or materials according to what is to be taught (language, reading, math, occupational education, etc.). They add to this potpourri a survey of current practices as exemplified by various federal model projects funded throughout the United States.

Wiig and Semel (1976) have written an entire text on language disabilities in children, including adolescents. Their approach is simply to identify the deficits in language processing, auditory perception, and cognitive and linguistic processing, then remediate those areas. This is the classic diagnostic-clinical approach reported above.

It seems paradoxical, but regardless of the theoretical bias stated by various authors, they usually report similar interventions. They may preach the doctrine of assessment/diagnosis of students or they may support the use of mastery learning, stressing the teaching of skills in some orderly sequence. But the end result is the same when they discuss intervention: they name skills/subjects to be learned and they follow with presentations of materials, methods, and techniques for teaching them. Often they report the same techniques, regardless of their school of thought.

Thus, it is not uncommon to merely catalogue interventions that are being attempted. Sabatino and Mauser (1978) do just that in describing strategies for intervention among adolescents with LBPs. They simply describe programs that have been developed throughout the United States for troubled youths, including disruptive students and suicidal adolescents, and for other problems such as learning disabilities. Again, their approach is not so much to present a theoretical framework as to merely describe what techniques and programs have been successful.

This is why the learning strategies approach of Alley and Deshler (1979) makes sense. As discussed, it merely determines what is to be taught and considers a spectrum of techniques that might accomplish that goal. It is pragmatic, useful, and productive.

Thus, to oversimplify the obvious, it can be concluded that, in the area of learning problems, the need is to identify what the adolescents are not learning, then teach them that skill or skills. Just as it was said that it is easy to identify the LBP students, it seemingly is equally easy to know what to do: simply teach them what they have not learned.

There remains the notion that that teaching process should be "different." When polled about their basic philosophy for teaching adolescents with learning disabilities (Lerner, Evans, & Meyers, 1977), special teachers agreed on two philosophies: (1) remediate deficit learning processes and (2) teach basic academic skills using special education materials. This is in preference to teaching basic academic skills using regular classroom materials. The problem seems to be to identify just what those special education materials and techniques are.

Thus, when reviewing the learning problems dimension of LBP, the solutions are relatively simple and represent common sense. The goals are to teach the students what they have not learned by whatever means the competent teacher can devise. The approach is largely to deal with the behavior to be taught.

Behavior Management

There are parallels in dealing with problem behaviors. The current trend is to forsake complex theoretical frameworks based on psychodynamics and hit the behavior head on. Through whatever techniques are favored by the intervener, the approach usually is to eliminate undesirable behavior and build in new repertoires. This is accomplished most often by some form of behavior management.

It is recognized that management of individual behaviors is part of a total group program or environment. In schools, this total system usually is referred to as the discipline program. This entire program of behavior management and discipline can be presented as a range of alternatives. D'Alonzo (1980) in the staff development and special education departments of the Mesa, Ariz., public schools has diagrammed such alternatives (Figure 2-1).

This represents the range of behavior management and discipline programs in operation there. The schematic conceptualizes the total context and alternatives of available behavior management programs in a particular school system. The array of choices and interventions represents the type of options that should be made available through all schools.

These alternatives represent a range from structured group (usually classroom) management systems with external controls by the teacher, through flexible, personalized treatments with internal controls by the student, which typically are individualized. Thus, the Mesa programs range from assertive discipline (Canter & Canter, 1976), which is handled through staff development department in-service training, to individualized counseling, through the guidance department. Either the special education or psychological services department provides a range from the highly structured engineered classrooms (Hewett & Taylor, 1980) to behavior management of individuals in classrooms or use of reality therapy (Glasser, 1976).

The approaches, objectives, and implementations vary, but each is aimed at shaping individual or group behavior to conform to acceptable social standards in a school situation. "Normal" behavior deviations can be managed through the more global approaches or environmental manipulations represented on the chart. Stu-

Figure 2-1 Sample Method for Managing Behavior Problems

MESA PUBLIC SCHOOLS/MESA, ARIZONA
BEHAVIOR MANAGEMENT-DISCIPLINE PROGRAMS

Structured ← External Controls   Flexible → Internal Controls / Personalized

	Assertive Discipline	Engineered Classroom	Behavior Modification	Reality Therapy	Citizenship and Personal Development	Individual Counseling
Group						
Training or Service Provider	STAFF DEVELOPMENT	SPECIAL EDUCATION	SPECIAL EDUCATION PSYCHOLOGY	PSYCHOLOGICAL SERVICES	PREVENTION SERVICES	GUIDANCE DEPARTMENT

Characteristics						
Approach	Competency-Based	Environmental-Management System Objective-Based	Environmental Manipulation—Behavior Management Interventions	Concept of Facing Reality and Responsibilities	Curriculum & Management • self-concept • communication • stress management • critical thinking	Therapeutic and Behavior Management • education process • personal-social • occupational • leisure

	To establish a classroom environment conducive to optimal learning	To develop appropriate school-related behaviors	To change or modify inappropriate or deviant behavior	To develop social responsibilities necessary to solve behavioral and educational problems	To develop skills in making effective life decisions	To develop skills in exhibiting appropriate behaviors; in rational thinking; in interpersonal relationships
Objective						
Implementation	Systematic Discipline Plan (class-school) • Hierarchy of consequences • Positive reinforcers	Structured Environment • Specific instructional objectives • Specific behavioral objectives	Systematic Reinforcement Procedures • Behavior—Observed —Measured —Modified • Reinforcers-consequences	Ten-Step Approach • evaluation of behavior • problem-solving alternatives • peer group control • positive reinforcers	Teacher's Inservice • Instructional units • Instructional objectives and activities	Student Needs Assessment • Behavior modification • Transactional analysis • Role playing • Crisis intervention
Teacher Role	Total Group	Group (Max. size-12)	Group or Individual	Group or Individual	Group or Individual	Individual

Source: Rosemarie L. D'Alonzo, Mesa, Arizona, Public Schools, © 1980, reprinted by permission.

dents with behavior problems will require the more structured, specialized, or individualized interventions, usually administered through the special departments and their technically trained staffs. However, the presence of a consistent schoolwide discipline plan will serve as a deterrent or preventive program for the reduction or elimination of more serious behavior problems.

This latter statement is important. Too often the field of special education has attempted to take over the teaching of any student with learning or behavior problems. As certain specialized techniques appeared to work with moderately or severely handicapped students, the temptation and tendency was to try those methods on the less severely disabled. However, the implementation often was through special classes, thus removing the youngsters from the educational mainstream.

The pendulum has swung back. Now P.L. 94-142 dictates that each youngster must be taught in the "least restrictive environment." The trend is to leave the students in regular classes as much as possible. That requires adequate support services, together with some interventions with regular teachers. Providing such assistance will help those teachers in learning to modify their instruction and enhance their understanding of the needs of the mildly or moderately handicapped students. For example, Edwards (1980) presents a model for "Curriculum Modification as a Strategy for Helping Regular Classroom Behavior-Disordered Students." She concludes from a review of the literature that: "First, teachers can be trained to use behavior modification procedures effectively in their classrooms. Secondly, reduction of disruptive student behaviors results in an increase in attention to task and, conversely, increased attention results in decreased disruptive behaviors" (p. 2).

The Edwards study sought to identify the combination of factors that could lead to academic success and behavioral adjustment for LBP students in regular classrooms. Her conclusion supports "a modified curricular approach paired with a token reinforcement system in which academic percent correct is rewarded" (p. 10). Therefore, the student is rewarded for mastery of the stated criterion.

The conclusion here is that traditional special education techniques of behavior modification can be taught to regular classroom teachers and will be beneficial to secondary students with behavior disorders. Another approach is to request the assistance of ancillary personnel such as guidance counselors in order to help LBP students better understand themselves in relation to the variety of environments in which they must interact and survive. This approach is presented in the following section.

Guidance/Counseling

A guidance program provides for direct services to students, including: (1) appraisal of their personal, social, and psychological status; (2) provision of information about educational, vocational, and personal-social opportunities so they can make intelligent choices and decisions; (3) individual and group counseling designed to facilitate self-understanding and personal growth; and (4) planning, placement, and follow-up regarding available vocational opportunities.

While each of the services offered by a guidance program will be of value to teachers of LBP adolescents at one or more times during the youths' educational experience, nevertheless it is most likely that the educator will rely heaviest on the counseling service. Wrenn (1951) offers this definition: ". . . counseling is a dynamic and purposeful relationship between two people in which procedures vary with the nature of the student's need, but in which there is always mutual participation by the counselor and the student with the focus upon self-clarification and self-determination by the student" (p. 57).

Counseling thus focuses on individuals' problems and their needs and is designed to help them learn what is needed to solve those difficulties. The effort of the counselor, like the teacher, is designed to facilitate the student's capability to deal independently with their problems so they can handle future difficulties without external assistance.

While there are several theories of counseling, the ones practitioners use most often in dealing with LBP adolescents are those referred to as directive and nondirective counseling. In directive counseling, counselors assume an active role in directing the counselees in arriving at a solution to a problem. The directive counselors present their own understanding of the students' problems based upon input from the youths and from others with whom they come into contact. In nondirective counseling, the practitioner's role is essentially passive. There is a heavy emphasis on the counselor-counselee relationship that provides a climate in which the students are free to explore their problems, leading to increased understanding and resolution of them. Intervention by the counselor is very minimal.

The degree of effectiveness of either of these approaches depends largely on the capability of the counselors. While there may be cases where a given student may respond more favorably to directive as opposed to nondirective counseling, generally speaking such instances are infrequent. If the counselors are qualified and well prepared in the utilization of the theory they are practicing, their effectiveness with any particular student ought to be maximum.

Either approach may be used on an individual or group basis. For adolescents who place great significance on group membership or group participation, this enables them to increase their capacity to develop mutually satisfying interpersonal relationships. Group counseling also may facilitate a better understanding of the handicapped youths' needs in relation to those of the nonhandicapped. The handicapped can pick up much information about the interests and attitudes of the nonhandicapped through the group process. This information may assist them in better understanding their own behavior as well as providing them an understanding of why their behavior is appropriate, or inappropriate, from the viewpoint of others.

There is no intent here to offer group counseling as the most beneficial model for developing a relationship. While it may be much more efficient and may accommodate the needs of the total school more fully, the desirability of the individual counseling relationship cannot be overlooked. However, there are some real benefits in group counseling. Ohlsen (1964) suggests that an adolescent benefits particularly from group counseling by learning:

1. that his peers have problems too;
2. that despite his faults, which his peers want to help him correct, they accept him;
3. that at least one adult, the counselor, can understand and accept him;
4. that he is, himself, capable of understanding, accepting, and helping his peers;
5. that he can trust others;
6. that when he can express his own real feelings about himself and others, as well as about what he believes, it helps him to understand and accept himself. (p. 148)

In determining whether or not students may benefit more from individual or group counseling, teachers may be able to provide information to facilitate such a decision. Mahler (1969) sets forth eight statements that describe situations in which individual counseling should be used and eight for group counseling. Those for individual counseling are:

1. Crisis situation complicated by a quest for causes and possible solutions.
2. Situations in which confidentiality is needed to protect clients and others.
3. Interpretation of test data in respect to self-concept.
4. Individual who exhibits extreme fear of talking in a group.
5. Individual who is so grossly ineffective in relating to peers that he may not be accepted by group members.
6. Individual whose self-awareness is limited.
7. Situation in which sexual behavior, particularly of a deviant nature, is involved.
8. Individual who has compulsive need for attention and recognition. (pp. 18-19)

The following are the suggestions on including in group counseling an:

1. Individual who needs to learn to better understand a variety of people and how they perceive things.

2. Individual who needs to learn deeper respect for others, particularly those who are different.
3. Individual who needs to gain social skills (talking and relating to others).
4. Individual who needs to share with others (needs to experience belongingness).
5. Individual who is free to talk about concerns, problems, values.
6. Individual who needs others' reactions to his problems and concerns.
7. Individual who finds support from peers helpful.
8. Individual who prefers to involve himself slowly in counseling and who can withdraw if it becomes threatening. (pp. 18-19)

These suggestions indicate that teachers probably have more insight into whether or not youths can benefit from individual or group strategy than perhaps any other persons in the school. By providing this information up front to the counselor, teachers may eliminate a possible trial-and-error situation that could prove nonproductive to both student and counselor. Teachers of LBP adolescents should view counselors as resource persons and as those with whom they may consult for assistance and information.

SUMMARY

Any discussion of intervention for LBP adolescents must examine the total situation—student, task, and environment. As noted, the students' past life and treatment of their problems are important factors; the type and level of family involvement can be critical; the quality of training and expertise of any specialists are important. But the intervention must be within the total educational program context, and often that is what needs to be modified.

If special programs are to work for LBP students, they must exist within a context of a total educational program. There must be a plan that addresses for all students (1) systematic discipline and (2) systematic teaching of the basic subjects and the curriculum. If a school or a district has no plan, no direction, no student-oriented objectives, no organization, no guidelines, and so on, the system creates learning and behavior problems. It is only when that total system is corrected and functioning that practitioners can truly know which students have the real learning and behavior problems.

Thus, special educators need to work closely with general educators to treat the ills of the system, not by taking over the system but by providing resources, creative ideas, and energy to resolve the problems. Special educators should:

1. influence the administrators of regular education to develop consistent discipline plans for their schools

2. develop specific learning objectives for all levels, classes, and subjects
3. make sure that regular teachers are aware of simple behavior management or behavior modifications that they can implement early in their regular classrooms
4. show a positive attitude toward students with LBPs

It is not the geographic location or the demographic makeup of a school that produces successful learning and appropriate behavior in students—it is the overall institutional climate. The attitude that all students are good, regardless of their behavior, and that all students can learn, regardless of how much they have failed, is more important than all of the techniques, methods, and curricular changes that experts can devise. Students will grow and learn in a warm, supportive, but structured environment. Those advances will be stunted and distorted in a cold, nonsupportive, disorganized ecology.

NOTE

1. The author wishes to thank Dr. Harold Wm. Heller and Marilyn Prehm for their contributions to portions of this chapter.

Chapter 3

LBP Adolescent Offenders

Jeffrey Schilit

INTRODUCTION

Adolescents with learning and behavior problems (LBPs) and the criminal justice system come into contact with one another frequently. When this contact occurs, be it social or professional, most often what occurs is negative. Because of this, it is extremely important that those working with LBP adolescents be aware of the type of interaction that generally results when these individuals come into contact with law enforcement agencies. It also is imperative that the police, attorneys, and judges be more knowledgeable about these youths.

More LBP persons are being identified, recognized, and served in the community now than ever before. Much of this results from legislation that has provided all handicapped persons with their basic rights, which previously had been denied them. The concepts of deinstitutionalization, decentralization, and normalization also have caused special education professionals to scrutinize the administrative and programmatic aspects of services provided to the handicapped, who as a result have entered the community and are functioning as independent citizens.

Because of the new freedoms accorded to LBP individuals, they are more likely to come into contact with the criminal justice system than previously. This is not to imply that persons with these problems will have more contact with the system than any other population. However, they will not be exempt from such contact. A number of writers (Blackhurst, 1968; Brown & Courtless, 1971; Brown & Robbins, 1979; Haggerty, Kane, & Udall, 1972; Herman, Gelhausen, & Childress, 1980; Keilitz, Zaremba, & Broder, 1979; and Murray, 1976) are concerned about what happens to LBP individuals once they become involved with the legal system.

This chapter discusses (1) the identification, incidence, and legal rights of LBP adolescents; (2) the psychology of crime and these youths; (3) criminal behavior among such young people; (4) myths and misconceptions about LBP adolescents; (5) advocacy; and (6) prevention through the education of adolescents, police officers, attorneys, and judges.

IDENTIFICATION, INCIDENCE, AND LEGAL RIGHTS

Several critical areas need to be examined with respect to the treatment of LBP adolescents by persons in the criminal justice system, especially police officers, attorneys, and judges. The following three sections cover the identification, incidence, and legal rights of these adolescents.

Identification and Awareness

There appear to be a number of blocks in awareness, knowledge, and general understanding of LBP adolescents among individuals in the legal system. Questions frequently asked by special educators are: Do these persons know LBPs' identifying characteristics? Do they have the ability to recognize these adolescents when they come into contact with them? What are their attitudes toward them and their problems—positive or negative? Answers to these questions provide insight to those concerned about the education and general welfare of these young people.

The attitudes of the police, the lawyers, and the judges determine to a great extent how LBP adolescents who have broken the law are treated. It is important for those in the legal system to understand how these adolescents behave, function, and think, and be knowledgeable about their capabilities. If the system is not knowledgeable about learning and behavior problems and does not recognize that the offenders have educational handicaps, the youths may not receive appropriate treatment. They also may be unjustly prosecuted and convicted of a crime for which they are not guilty.

Wolfensberger (1969) describes several roles generally ascribed to the handicapped. They are (1) subhuman, (2) objects of pity, (3) sick, (4) menaces. Even though these roles may be inappropriate, they still are very prevalent in the general public perception of the handicapped. If the police officers, lawyers, or the courts also see LBP adolescents this way, such attitudes will have an adverse effect on the treatment of these youths. It is important that those involved with such youths have a thorough understanding of learning and behavior problems so they can make the appropriate decisions and allowances for these adolescents to ensure fair treatment.

Incidence

If criminal justice is "the study of the phenomena of crime by those agencies which society has developed to respond to that phenomena" (Morgan, 1977), how does the justice system respond to the "phenomenon" of the LBP adolescent offender?

The percentage of such offenders will vary according to the authors who write about them and the definition of standards assigned to their population. Keilitz, Zaremba, and Broder (1979) point out this discrepancy when they indicate the following source and prevalence of offenders: Duling, Eddy, and Risko (1970)—32 percent; Podboy and Mallory (1977)—49 percent; and Poremba (1967)—50 percent. This range of the prevalence of offenders can be attributed to the operational definition used of an offender, the geographical location, the racial composition, and the socioeconomic status of the offenders studied.

Comparing these figures to the usual level used to identify the size of the total learning and behavior problem population, namely, 10 to 15 percent, it can readily be seen that based upon incidence, there is a disproportionate representation. According to Ogg (1973), the actual number of handicapped offenders in correctional facilities varies according to the geographic region of the country, with the Midwest having as few as 2 percent of the prisoner population so handicapped and the South with as many as 27 percent of its prisoners thus identified.

Why does this occur? Why are there so many LBP individuals in the correctional system? Perhaps the answer lies in that system and what occurs when these adolescents enter it. According to Mattina (1977), the legal system functions in the following manner: Two competent attorneys argue the two sides in a case, a competent judge presides, a competent jury listens to the arguments, a competent forensic psychologist provides input if needed, and through all of these proceedings justice occurs. However, when LBP adolescent offenders are involved, the persons in this system may inadvertently treat them inappropriately because they lack knowledge and expertise about such individuals. These adolescents' legal rights, as established for all citizens, may be abridged.

The criminal justice system is complex. Figure 3-1 presents the steps in the process. LBP adolescents who have committed a felony usually proceed through this process; they are not exempt from it and are treated the same as any other adolescent offenders charged with felonies.

These LBP adolescents are trapped in a "Catch-22" situation because persons who operate the system lack an understanding of the nature of their problems. This can be attributed to the lack of special education training provided to police officers, attorneys, and judges. When individuals are arrested, they are read their rights, charged with the crime, and placed in jail. If the arrested person is suspected of being "different," a forensic psychologist is called in to determine: (1) the defendant's competence and (2) whether the individual knew the nature and quality of the crime.

These determinations usually are made through the administration of the Wechsler Adult Intelligence Scale (1955) or the Stanford-Binet Intelligence Scale (1973) and the forensic psychologist's observations. The psychologist then gives

Figure 3-1 Steps in the Criminal Justice Process

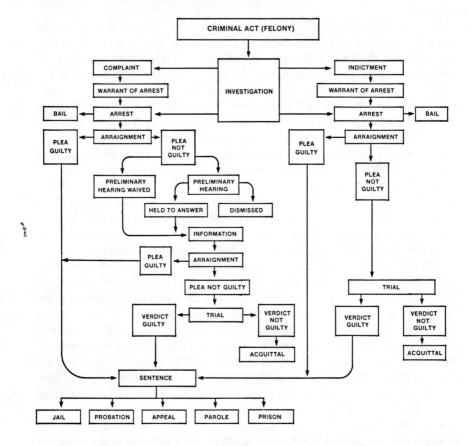

Source: Adapted from *An Introduction to the Criminal Justice System and Process* by Police Science Division, Campbell, Calif.: West Valley College, 1973, p. 12.

the attorneys and/or the judge an IQ score and a subjective evaluation. The inherent problems in this evaluative process are that, in all probability, the forensic psychologist may not be adequately acquainted with the concept of learning and behavior problems and does not understand the behavior and actions of the person involved. In addition, since lawyers and judges are not informed about the problems of these individuals and are not trained in interpreting intellectual evaluations, they tend to fix upon the IQ score.

This is where the "Catch-22" situation begins. The principals in the system usually do not know how to plead, defend, or decide a case when the offenders have a learning or behavior problem. Therefore, LBP offenders fall through the judicial slots and are not served properly by the system.

Legal Rights

What are the legal rights of LBP adolescents, and do the various parties in the system understand them? Not much is known about how informed police, attorneys, and the courts are on this subject. If they are uninformed, then these individuals may be sentenced to jail unjustly or may be placed in facilities that are not appropriate for either their condition or their crime. If the court is knowledgeable, the judge will, if the person is guilty, have several alternative correctional facilities in which to place the individual.

The question then arises, how informed are the police, attorneys, and judges about these conditions? According to Biklen (1977), Haggerty et al. (1972), and Schilit (1979b), these persons usually are uninformed about the handicapped and their conditions. They do not know what to look for, how to handle, or how to defend such individuals. This lack of knowledge may interfere with these persons' due process rights.

In a similar vein, do handicapped individuals comprehend the implications and rights assured them by the *Miranda v. Arizona* (1966) decision? It is crucial that LBP adolescents understand this. The language of the Miranda warning may be confusing, and the youths may not be capable of understanding it enough to protect themselves against self-incrimination or false incrimination. Like the rest of society, when LBP individuals come into contact with law enforcement agencies they have a certain amount of apprehension and fright. They usually behave in the same manner as more normal individuals. They will be nervous and may erroneously admit to something or anything they think will help get them out of the situation. The Miranda warning helps individuals exercise their due process rights. The Miranda warning, which must be read to a suspect at the time of arrest is:

You have the right to remain silent.

Anything you say can and will be used against you in a court of law.

You have the right to talk to a lawyer and have him present with you while you are being questioned.

If you cannot afford to hire a lawyer, one will be appointed to represent you before any questioning, if you wish one.

Do you understand each of the rights I have explained to you?

Having these rights in mind, do you wish to talk to us now?

(*Miranda v. Arizona,* 384 U.S. 436 (1966))

Based on these due process rights as stated in the Miranda warning, the most appropriate alternative would be for LBP adolescents to have a lawyer present before making a statement. This position was strengthened by the U.S. Supreme Court on May 18, 1981 in *Edwards v. Arizona,* 451 U.S. 477 (1981). The accused person, "having expressed his desire to deal with the police only through council, is not subject to further interrogation until counsel is made available to him, unless the accused himself initiated further communication exchanges or conversations" (p. 47) with the police.

It often is unclear what procedures should be followed by the police once an LBP adolescent has committed a crime and is apprehended. Should they take the person to the police station, to a legal aide office, home under parental guidance, to an institution until trial, or to a facility for youthful offenders?

Allen (1966) favors a youthful offender court that provides 24-hour service for such persons and affords them a place to go rather than the county or city jail. Under Allen's concept, from this placement the individuals would be sentenced if found guilty, or freed if acquitted. If found guilty, they would be sentenced and committed to a facility for habilitation rather than incarceration. The facility's staff would consider the offenders' level of functioning and type of handicapping condition and try to habilitate them to become useful members of society. These LBP offenders need assistance from judicial system personnel that may be beyond what normally is afforded to adolescents.

THE LBP AND THE PSYCHOLOGY OF CRIME

Adolescents with LBPs do not become criminals by happenstance. According to Coffey, Eldelfonso, and Hartinger (1974), criminal behaviors in adolescents and adults are products of circumstance, chance, culture, environment, and sociological and psychological conditioning and usually evolve from one or more of these factors. These are intertwined with the individuals' station in life, development, and personal associates. Frequently, persons who commit a criminal act under any of these circumstances are members of a group that engages in unlawful behavior only temporarily. Peer pressures influence these persons to take part in a crime they know is wrong and would not ordinarily commit.

The following sections analyze the psychological and sociological aspects of delinquency and criminality and their relationship to LBP adolescents. They cover (1) psychological and sociological explanations, (2) school failure rationale, (3) susceptibility rationale, and (4) the relationship between learning disabilities and delinquency.

Psychological and Sociological Explanations

Adolescents with LBPs tend to come into contact with the law because of a variety of reasons that have psychological or sociological underpinnings. These factors fall into four major categories:

1. the socioeconomic strata from which the individual comes
2. the person's level of suggestibility
3. the youth's ability to be manipulated and prodded into behavior by others who are more in control of themselves or are functioning at a higher intellectual plane
4. a decrease in the individual's functional intellectual ability because of the overlaid emotional disturbance or learning disability that may interfere with cognitive functioning.

The psychological and sociological explanations that follow usually are the reasons why LBP individuals come into contact with the law.

Many psychiatrically oriented criminologists consider criminality a product of a personality maladjustment. The socialization process is regarded as producing healthy or unhealthy personalities. Crime and delinquency are considered a correlate of the latter. Charles A. Murray, a noted writer on LBP adolescents and their interaction with the law, hypothesizes several causal sequences that could bring these individuals into contact with the criminal justice system. Murray (1976) feels it is not intuitively obvious that LBP individuals will become delinquent. He believes that a causal chain exists because handicaps produce effects that in turn contribute to other results that ultimately produce delinquency. Murray identifies two such causal chains: (1) a school failure rationale, and (2) a susceptibility rationale.

School Failure Rationale

The first of these familiar sequences links learning and behavioral disorders to school failure, to dropouts, and delinquency. Murray used "the school failure rationale" described by Berman (1975):

> The cycle begins with early problems at home. The child was showing perceptual and attention problems even prior to school but the behavior was written off as "ornery" or uncooperative personality. The child enters the early grades of school already accustomed to the fact that he won't be able to do things as well as expected of him, that he will fail, be humiliated continually. This prophecy is fulfilled in school as teachers, considering the child a behavioral problem, punish and ridicule him for failures or for behaviors that he cannot control. The child begins to think

of himself as a loser, as someone who can never hope to live up to what people expect of him. Rather than face the embarrassment of continual failure in front of friends and teachers, the behavioral signs become even more pronounced. Clowning around and general disruptiveness become ways which best insulate the youngster from having to face continual and repeated failure. He becomes much more successful as a clown or troublemaker than he ever could be as a student. He gets further and further behind, becomes more and more of a problem. Eventually he is suspended, drops out, or is thrown out of school to roam the streets, and inevitably the road leads to delinquency and is well under way. (pp. 45-46)

This rationale refers to three immediate problems that set the stage for LBP adolescents as potential criminal offenders: (1) adults perceive them as being disciplinary problems, (2) they are inherently handicapped in achieving academically, and (3) their peers perceive them as being socially awkward and generally unattractive and use them as a butt of many jokes. As a result, these individuals begin to live up to the label being placed upon them, i.e., a self-fulfilling prophecy begins to take shape. This leads to the school failure rationale (Exhibit 3-1) as described by Murray (1976). It is a complex process but all the circumstances are present in the school and, if activated, will lead LBP adolescents to delinquent behavior.

Susceptibility Rationale

Murray (1976) postulates a second line of arguments that links LBP individuals to delinquency and criminal behavior. It is a much briefer and a much more direct chain than the school failure rationale. In effect, this susceptibility rationale (Exhibit 3-2) argues that certain types of learning and behavior problems are accompanied by a variety of socially troublesome personality characteristics and that these traits contribute to individuals' perceiving themselves as less than complete persons and not capable of picking up on the social cues that are passed to them through their day-to-day interactions with other individuals.

In essence, by not being able to understand or misinterpreting the social cues directed to them, these individuals often create problems for themselves and especially with respect to law enforcement personnel. According to Murray, this susceptibility rationale for linking these individuals to delinquency is a causal chain suggesting that the adolescents begin with one strike against them if exposed to experiences that could lead to delinquent acts. That strike is that these individuals do not interpret the messages from the environment in the same way that more normal individuals would. Therefore, these persons are more susceptible to breaking the law than would those without such problems.

Exhibit 3-1 The School Failure Rationale

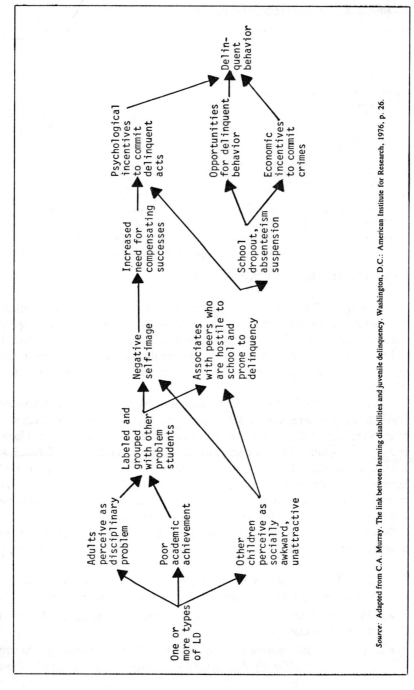

Source: Adapted from C.A. Murray. The link between learning disabilities and juvenile delinquency. Washington, D.C.: American Institute for Research, 1976, p. 26.

Exhibit 3-2 The Susceptibility Rationale

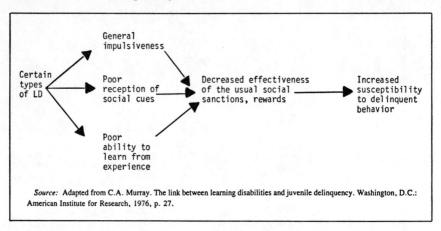

Source: Adapted from C.A. Murray. The link between learning disabilities and juvenile delinquency. Washington, D.C.: American Institute for Research, 1976, p. 27.

Learning Disabilities and Delinquency

According to Gregarus, Broder, and Zimmerman (1978), increased attention has been given in recent years to the possibility of a relationship between specific learning disabilities and juvenile delinquency. If there is such a causality relating to LBP adolescents, then special education should play an integral role in delinquency prevention. However, there was an apparent lack of empirical evidence on this issue.

As a result, in 1976 the National Institute for Juvenile Justice and Delinquency Prevention funded a research and development study, the purpose of which was to establish reliable data that would assist in a methodical development of informed policy and programs. The grant was awarded to the Association for Children with Learning Disabilities (ACLD) to design and conduct a remediation program for learning disabled juvenile delinquents to improve academic skills, change school attitudes, and reduce the delinquency of learning disabled teenagers who had been officially adjudicated as delinquents by a juvenile court.

Dorothy Crawford, Project Director of the ACLD research and development project, reported the results of this project in 1981. The research results were:

- The evidence for the existence of a relationship between learning disabilities and self-reported delinquency was statistically significant.
- Adolescents with learning disabilities reported a significantly higher frequency of violent acts.
- Learning disabilities were strongly related to official delinquency. The probability of being officially delinquent (on a national measure) was 9 of every

100 learning disabled adolescent males compared to 4 of every 100 non-learning disabled males. The probability of being an adjudicated delinquent was 220 percent greater for adolescents with learning disabilities than for their nonlearning disabled peers.

- The same probability applied for being taken into custody by the police.
- The incidence of learning disabled adolescents in the adjudicated delinquent group was 36 percent. This indicates that a substantial proportion of official delinquents are learning disabled. (p. 3)

These data indicate learning disabled adolescents as a high risk group in need of special services. They are at higher risk to be delinquents than their nonlearning disabled counterparts. The following comparative data give rise for concern among professional and parent groups:

- The large number of learning disabled delinquents could not be attributed to sociodemographic characteristics or a tendency to disclose socially disapproved behaviors.
- The data indicated that learning disabilities contributed to increases of delinquent behavior both directly and indirectly through school failure.
- For comparable offenses learning disabled adolescents had higher probabilities of arrest and adjudication than those without learning disabilities.
- Among adjudicated delinquents there was no difference between those with learning disabilities or not for being incarcerated.
- As officially nondelinquent boys advance through their teens, those with learning disabilities experience greater increases in delinquent activities.
- Learning disabled teenagers from families with higher parental education and occupational prestige and those that are white were most vulnerable to the effects of a learning disability. (pp. 3-4)

A relatively small proportion of the adolescent population is affected by learning disabilities, but it appears to be one of the important causes of delinquency. Because of this, a remediation program was implemented to attempt to reduce the incidence of delinquency among learning disabled adolescents. The methods and results of this program were:

- Instruction was directed to the adolescents' area of greatest deficiency.
- Fifty-eight percent of time was devoted to reading and language skill development and twenty-five percent spent on improving math skills.
- The learning disabled delinquents experienced greater educational improvement than their counterparts who were low achievers.

- There was significant improvement in intellectual growth with 55 to 65 hours of remedial instruction in one school year.
- There was a dramatic decrease in delinquency with at least 40 to 50 hours of instruction. The instruction was significantly effective in preventing or controlling future delinquency.
- A major factor in preventing delinquency was not academic skills improvement but seemed to be due to the nature of the relationship between the adolescents and the learning disabilities specialist.
- The model of instruction did significantly provide academic and intellectual growth and reduce delinquent activity; it did not significantly change school attitudes. (pp. 4-5)

Based on data provided by Crawford (1981), it appears that applied research, program development, training and technical assistance, and information dissemination are needed.

CRIMINAL BEHAVIOR IN LBP ADOLESCENTS

Individuals with LBPs are not exempt from criminal behavior. Morgan (1977) indicates that while practitioners are aware of adolescents who commit criminal offenses, they are unsure of the exact incidence for a variety of reasons: (1) categorical definitions are misinterpreted statistically, (2) methodology sometimes is not clear, and (3) diagnostic evaluations are not quantitative or qualitative. However, certain evidence indicates a high prevalence of learning and behavior problems in relation to individuals in correctional facilities.

Keilitz, Zaremba, and Broder (1979) and Morgan (1977) report the following prevalences of handicapping conditions in correctional facilities for disruptive youth: emotional disturbance, 16.23 percent; mental retardation, 7.69 percent; and learning disabilities, 10.59 percent. Morgan (1977) hypothesizes that up to 42.4 percent of incarcerated youths have some type of handicapping condition that facilitated or contributed to their coming into contact with the law. It should be noted that these figures do not include handicapped offenders not incarcerated; therefore, the actual incidence or prevalence of such LBP adolescents cannot be pinpointed accurately.

Further compounding the problem is the criminal justice system and its component parts (the police, lawyers, and judges) and their reactions to LBP adolescents. According to Schilit (1979b), persons in the criminal justice system are inadequately prepared to serve LBP adolescents because they are not trained in methods to handle, interpret, interrogate, try, prosecute, or habilitate them. Police officers usually are given a minimal amount of information about LBP adolescents in their basic training. Lawyers usually do not receive any training through a planned sequence of learning experiences about the handicapped and their relationship to the system. Attorneys who have become activists for adolescent offenders with handicapping conditions have done so on their own accord or through some circumstance that brought them into the situation.

Judges usually are as uninformed as attorneys. However, they are even less inclined to become trained to become aware of LBP individuals. They probably are the most unaware members of the system; yet they carry the greatest weight when it comes to sentencing individuals to a criminal justice facility, a community facility, or to probation. It should be noted that judges usually do not understand the IQ concept. They have indicated that if the IQ is low, the criminal offense involved is worse than that committed by an individual with a high IQ. Therefore, they hand down stiffer punishments for persons with a low IQ than for those with a high IQ.

Studies by Keilitz, Zaremba, and Broder (1979) and Schilit (1979a) report that criminal behavior exhibited by LBP individuals closely follows the Brown and Courtless (1971) findings. The studies describe seven types of criminal behavior. They rank the order of crimes committed by LBP adolescents as: (1) crimes against property, (2) misdemeanors, (3) crimes against persons, (4) sexual assaults, (5) physical assaults, (6) burglary, and (7) murder. In essence, what is being said is that LBP individuals do not commit certain types of crimes more frequently than others. Instead, they seem to parallel the crime ratios, criminal tendencies, and criminal behaviors of society as a whole.

MYTHS AND MISCONCEPTIONS

Many myths and misconceptions prevalent in society result in LBP offenders' being misunderstood and treated inappropriately. The myths and misconceptions can be categorized into three major areas (Biklen, 1977).

The first area is that these individuals cannot be educated adequately or helped to develop and change their behavior to keep them out of contact with the criminal justice system. Although this is untrue, the preservation of this myth has produced (and will continue to cause) much harm for these adolescent offenders. If the general public believes these persons cannot be educated, assisted, or helped, it follows that it also will not believe they can be rehabilitated. These adolescents usually can be habilitated if proper circumstances and training are made available.

A second myth is that LBP adolescent offenders have criminal tendencies. In reality, the individuals discussed here do find themselves in jail, and the incidence figures do indicate their number in correctional facilities is higher than might be expected. Why are so many of them in prisons? One reason usually given is that more of them engage in and get caught in criminal acts. This is difficult to prove. Rather, it may be because LBP adolescent offenders lack the sophistication of experienced criminals in avoiding discovery. They also are used as dupes and may quite unknowingly commit a crime because someone tells them to do so.

After they are arrested, they are much more likely to incriminate themselves by waiving their rights or by making a confession indiscriminately. Once these adolescents go to court they often have court appointed attorneys who may not serve them properly because they do not understand their problems. If these youths are convicted, the probabilities are that they will not appeal the case as average offenders might. All of these factors work against LBP offenders and produce a higher incidence of these youths in correctional facilities.

A third myth is that LBP adolescents cannot read or follow directions. Actually, most of them can do so very well. However, when they become involved with the police they have difficulty answering or following directions given to them. This usually is because they are frightened and confused and have never been trained, instructed, or schooled on how to handle themselves when confronted by the law. Therefore, it is important that those instructing adolescents provide learning experiences on the legal system and their rights under the Constitution. If this instruction is conducted throughout the students' school years, many future problems can be avoided.

If these adolescent offenders are to be helped, society must do away with many of these myths and misconceptions. It is important to get across the point that these individuals have the same rights under the law as those without such problems. Once this is made clear to the criminal justice system, the treatment of LBP adolescents should improve.

ADVOCACY: HELPING ADOLESCENT OFFENDERS

Advocacy has been developing since the late 1970s as an essential service needed for the handicapped. However, advocacy systems need to expand their services further so LBP youths can benefit from advocate intervention. In doing so it is imperative that advocates working with these adolescents be professionally trained and fully understand them, their own role, and their responsibilities to such youths. In addition, these individuals must know when, where, how, and why to intervene on behalf of these adolescents once they have encountered the legal system.

Advocates must know the duties, responsibilities, functions, and activities that are inherent with their role. They must be trained observers who have the capability of perceiving the programming activities or environment in an impartial and neutral manner and not on an emotional level. After reviewing a case, advocates must know what actions to pursue and which agencies would be most appropriate to contact to best assist the adolescents. Wolfensberger (1969) defines an advocate as "a mature, competent citizen representing, as if they were his own, the interests of another citizen who is impaired in his instrumental capacity or who has major expressive needs which are unmet and which are likely to remain unmet without special intervention'' (p. 20).

Without the special intervention of an advocate, many of these youths will be unable to take advantage of the wide range of services available to them. Advocacy is not just a duplication of services already offered by counselors, social workers, and other professionals. According to the National Association for Retarded Citizens (NARC) (1973), advocates are in a position to perform services over and above those that institutions and protective agencies can offer. They must be capable of determining the best possible way to assist their clients and then proceed to do so.

Advocates can get directly involved with programs that are within or outside the criminal justice system to make sure that the adolescents' every need is known and met. However, because they cannot be all things to all people, they must establish a set of criteria and a framework from which to operate. To be able to assist these adolescent offenders, they must be able to:

1. assist parental involvement in activities that directly impact on their son or daughter
2. develop a model and method of delivery of services to assist these LBP individuals
3. require agency accountability for delivery of social services
4. ensure that existing community services assist the individuals when they need it rather than referring them to a waiting list of a more appropriate agency
5. become ombudsmen for these individuals if they wind up in court
6. attempt to minimize their correctional facility placement whenever possible
7. create a parent/citizen council to assess policies and procedures of agencies for the purpose of introducing program modifications and accountabilities
8. ensure that adolescents' civil rights are not abridged
9. protect against the dehumanization and lack of human rights ensured to these individuals

According to Schilit (1977), advocates thus are catalytic agents. They place major emphasis on mobilizing resources already existing in the community that can assist these adolescents rather than creating new resources, programs, or agencies. Advocates also must protect these individuals against well-intended services that work for the interest of the system at the expense of the person. In certain instances, advocates may deem it necessary to confront the surrogate agency. However, such confrontation should occur only as a last resort after a series of efforts to obtain the resources offered by the agency.

In conclusion, advocates are not all things to all people. They must be selective in the tasks they undertake or assume; otherwise they will be inundated with responsibilities that will minimize their effectiveness and the number of LBP citizens they will be able to represent. Along these same lines, they must be careful not to alienate themselves through their interactions with the agencies from which they seek help and service. However, they must not be afraid to take a strong stand on issues that affect these adolescents or their role will become merely perfunctory and thus of no value to the individuals they represent.

PREVENTION THROUGH EDUCATION

One of the easiest and most effective ways to decrease the number of LBP adolescent offenders is to practice active primary prevention in the schools through instruction about the criminal justice system. Instruction should be provided to everyone in the legal system about learning and behavior problems and other relevant aspects of special education. This section discusses the schooling of LBP adolescents and the education of the police, attorneys, and judges with whom they may become involved.

Education of the Adolescent

LBP adolescents tend not to be knowledgeable about the law and the criminal justice system. Therefore, there is a definite need for them to be educated in these areas. Even when not coerced in the usual sense, they may be unable to understand police procedures and their consequences and therefore cannot make genuine decisions in relation to them. These individuals are more likely to be unaware of their constitutional right to refuse to answer incriminating police questions and to consult with an attorney; even when the interrogator advises them of these rights, they may be unable to appreciate their significance (Allen, 1966).

According to Allen (1969), LBP adolescents who may have committed a crime are particularly vulnerable to an atmosphere of threats and coercion, as well as to one of friendliness designed to induce confidence and cooperation. These youths may be hard put to distinguish between the fact and the appearance of friendliness. It is unlikely that they will see the implications or consequences of their statements as more normal persons would.

Historically, society has pursued three alternative courses with these adolescent offenders. It has (1) ignored their limitations and special needs, (2) changed traditional criminal law processes, and (3) grouped them with psychopaths, socio-paths, and sex deviants. This has been shown in several cases.

In *Commonwealth of Massachusetts v. Femino* (1967), a handicapped individual was arrested and interrogated after a murder. He was informed of his rights but unknowingly waived them. The arresting officers never asked for his educational records. The man confessed to the crime and his statement was used as evidence during his trial. He was convicted and appealed. His counsel contended that medical testimony of the defendant's low IQ and his being easily led should have been allowed into evidence. The contentions were denied and the individual was sent to jail.

In *United States v. Masthers* (1976), the defendant was accused of armed robbery and later tried to withdraw his original guilty plea on grounds of incompetence. Expert witnesses confirmed that the defendant had a learning disability. The defendant testified that, at the time of his guilty plea, he had not understood what the Constitution was, let alone knowingly waived his constitutional rights. On the basis of this testimony, the court vacated the earlier guilty plea and sentence, thus allowing the defendant to enter a new guilty plea based upon careful explanation, in simple language, of his rights. The court then sentenced him to the time he already had served.

A further example demonstrates how persons with learning and behavioral problems can be coerced into relinquishing their rights. In New York, a 20-year-old mentally handicapped laborer "confessed" to the murder of J.W. and her roommate, giving the police details of the crime that "only" the murderer could have known. Later, he was shown to have been innocent. The details of the crime, which were suggested to him, were supplied by the police after a prolonged questioning period. As his attorney carefully put it, "He would have confessed to the murder of Julius Caesar if they kept after him long enough" (Allen, 1966; p. 5).

Core Knowledge

There is a specific body of knowledge that should be transmitted to LBP students during their school years. It involves (1) the criminal justice system, (2) the types of violations of the law that exist, (3) the ways in which criminals are arrested, (4) the procedures that are followed when a person is arrested, (5) the ways in which criminals are punished, and (6) the ways a person leaves the criminal justice system after confinement in it.

Criminal Justice System. The students should have knowledge of the role of the police officer, the attorney (whether prosecuting or defending), and the judge, as well as the steps in the process as presented in Figure 3-1 supra.

Kinds of Violations. The students should be informed of the two kinds of laws (civil and criminal) and the two types of crime that can be committed when a law is broken (felonies and misdemeanors).

Ways Criminals Are Arrested. There are three ways criminals (or suspects) can be apprehended: (1) by the police, who may do so by ticket or an arrest warrant;

(2) by the judiciary or the courts, which can issue bench warrants for a person's arrest; and (3) by corrections' apprehension, usually when a person has violated parole or probation.

Procedures Followed after an Arrest. The procedures, once a person is arrested on either a suspected or an actual charge, are as follows:

1. The person is apprehended and charged with the crime.
2. The Miranda warning is read.
3. The individual contacts an attorney or one is appointed by the court to conduct the defense.
4. The suspect is "booked," i.e., personal information is recorded, finger-prints are taken, and the individual is placed in a holding facility.
5. The suspect is arraigned in an initial appearance before a judge. A formal notice of the charge is given, the person is advised of constitutional rights, and bail is set. If the crime is serious enough, bail will not be set.
6. A pretrial hearing takes place at which the defense and prosecuting attor-neys discuss the charge and decide whether the suspect is competent to stand trial if competence is to be an issue.
7. A jury is selected. If the case goes to trial, the jury decides the individual's guilt or innocence. If innocent, the suspect is released and the case is closed. However, if found guilty, the person is sentenced with a fine or imprisonment, or both.
8. Adolescents with learning or behavior problems should be informed that if they are found guilty, they have the right to appeal to a higher court. At that time, suspects may be released with or without bail to await action on the appeal.
9. If no appeal is requested, the person is sent to jail or to the penal reform facility.
10. Parole may be permitted if the suspect is to be released from imprisonment early. The person then must follow the parole board's instructions and report to the parole officer on the specified dates mandated by the court. Adolescents with learning or behavior problems should be warned that a violation of parole can result in revocation of that freedom and require imprisonment.

Ways Criminals Are Punished. Criminality and criminal behavior of adoles-cents who become offenders can be punished in three major ways: (1) They may be told to pay a fine. If they do not, they may be imprisoned. (2) They may be put on probation under the supervision of a probation officer. Failure to meet the condi-tions of probation can result in imprisonment. (3) They may be imprisoned. The amount of time spent in jail is decided initially by the judge at their trial but may be shortened by parole.

Leaving the Criminal Justice System. Individuals who have been charged with a crime never really leave the system. They may, in the future, be considered a suspect in a crime similar to the one in which they were involved originally. However, technically, they are out of the system if they are acquitted of the charge, pay a fine, or, after serving their sentence, are released from the correctional facility.

Educational Programs and Support Services

Riekes, Speigel, and Keilitz (1977) have developed the most comprehensive training program for special education students in existence. It is called *Law and Education Project*. This program was implemented in 1973 for educable mentally retarded and emotionally disturbed special education students and is used throughout the St. Louis public school system. It was the first such program in special education in the United States. A teacher/coordinator model is used in the program. The coordinator, trained in law-related education, contacts participating teachers at least one hour per week, varying from 7 to 20 weeks. The coordinator's role encompasses team teaching, provision of materials and trained resource people, and assistance with community involvement projects. Workshops and graduate courses have also been frequently offered to special education teachers. The trained resource people who volunteer their services are lawyers, law students, police officers, juvenile court workers, and consumer experts. The coordinator provides orientation for resource people about the program and students, in order to increase their effectiveness. The coordinator also works with individual teachers to develop effective law-related field trips to police facilities, courts, local legislative bodies, and consumer agencies. The program has proven to be successful.

Other agencies in the country that serve as clearinghouses to assist special education personnel in working with handicapped individuals, in terms of informing them of their rights and position in relation to the criminal justice system, include:

The American Bar Association
1800 M Street, N.W.
Washington, D.C. 20036
Attention: Commission on the Mentally Disabled

The American Civil Liberties Union
Juvenile Rights Project
22 East 40th Street
New York, N.Y. 10016

The Civil Rights Division
  U.S. Department of Justice
  1121 Vermont Avenue, N.W.
  Washington, D.C. 20005

The National Center for Law and the Handicapped
  1238 North Eddy Street
  South Bend, Indiana 46617

The President's Committee on Mental Retardation
  Regional Office Building #3
  7th and D Streets, S.W.
  Room 2614
  Washington, D.C. 20201

Education of Police Officers

The need for the police to be informed about adolescent offenders with learning and behavior problems is serious, especially since so many LBP adolescents have passed through the hands of these officers and now are part of the criminal justice system. Education of the police officers may prevent continuation of the mistreatment and misunderstanding that now exists. The police need more detailed information about these adolescents than they are receiving at their training academies. In general, police officers in training are required to take four to six hours in the various areas of special education. Unfortunately, these hours usually cover only how to transport a mentally ill or an aggressive person to a facility for evaluation. The police are not instructed in how to identify LBP adolescents or any other type of handicap, in procedures to deal with these individuals, or in how to modify their procedures in apprehension, transportation, and booking. This must be accomplished before LBP adolescents will be fairly served and protected by the legal system.

Police officers must be aware at the time of the initial contact that any adolescents they apprehend may have a learning or behavior problem. If so, they must understand that, when reading the Miranda warning, the suspects may not be able to understand police procedures and their consequences and therefore may be unable to make a decision that would be in their own best interest.

It also is likely that these LBP adolescents will be unaware of their constitutional rights to legal counsel, or their right to refuse to answer incriminating questions. This problem and the legal approach to retarded offenders are described by Bazelton, Boggs, Hilleboe, and Tudor (1963) in their report of the Task Force on Law: The President's Panel on Mental Retardation. The following succinctly summarizes the panel's position:

The retarded are particularly vulnerable to an atmosphere of threats and coercion, as well as to one of friendliness designed to induce confidence and cooperation. The retarded person may be hard put to distinguish between the fact and the appearance of friendliness. . . . Some of the retarded are characterized by a desire to please authority: if a confession will please, it may be gladly given. . . . It is unlikely that a retarded person will see the implication or consequences of his statements in the way a person of normal intelligence will. (p. 155)

Accordingly, LBP adolescents are as prone and capable of norm-violating acts as their normal counterparts. It is their behavior when being arrested and the type of incarceration forthcoming that should be of concern to professionals in educational and judicial systems.

Education of Attorneys

A three-year study conducted by Allen (1968), a professor of law and Director of the Institute for Law, Psychiatry, and Criminology at George Washington University, identified four principal factors attributing to why an adolescent's learning or behavior disability is not disclosed at or before trial by the defense attorneys: (1) the attorneys' failure to recognize the disability, (2) their insensitivity or indifference to the disability, (3) the uncertainty of how the legal system may apply to that disability, for example, determining the capability of their client to understand their actions, (4) the inappropriateness of the legal result if the fact of the disability is established.

Although the fourth factor is the result of an inadequate criminal justice system, the first three are primary concerns related to the education of lawyers. As noted earlier, there is a dire need for attorneys to be educated and experienced in the field of special education so they can identify and properly defend or prosecute LBP adolescent offenders.

Brown and Courtless (1971) provide an example of what has happened to mentally retarded offenders because of the lack of education on the part of both defense and prosecuting attorneys. They report five major findings that have direct impact on lawyers and their dealings with LBP adolescent offenders:

1. In 59 percent of the cases the handicapped offender entered a plea of not guilty. However, in 80 percent of the cases the original arrest charge was the same as the one on which the person was tried and convicted.
2. A confession or incriminating statement was obtained from the handicapped individual in two-thirds of the cases surveyed.
3. No pretrial, psychological, or psychiatric examination of the accused was made or a social history taken in 78 percent of the cases. When examinations

did occur, 11 percent were as a result of commitment for observation in a mental hospital. Most upsetting is the fact that in no case was there an examination requested or ordered during the course of the trial.

4. In 92 percent of the cases competency to stand trial and criminal responsibility were not raised.
5. In 88 percent of the cases no appeal was made, while in 84 percent postconviction relief was not requested.

These data portray a gloomy picture about conditions in the nation's courtrooms. It is the responsibility of the attorney or judge to request testing so as to be able to identify LBP adolescent offenders. As can be seen, the plight of these youths is rather desperate. Failure to identify a problem in an accused person means that a number of important legal issues that the defendant should raise go unconsidered. An attorney must be aware of LBP individuals' limitations in helping counsel investigate the case yet must construct a defense strategy and be an advocate. The ability of attorneys to protect these individuals from exploitation, abuse, or degrading treatment is questionable. An example of this is when a public defender, several of whose clients were in prisons and were identified as mentally retarded, asserted, "I don't recall that any of my clients were retarded" (President's Committee on Mental Retardation, 1976).

The *Gideon v. Wainwright* decision (1963) expanded the right of indigent accused persons to obtain court-appointed counsel. Public defenders now represent 69 percent of poor people with mental illness or learning or behavior problems who cannot afford private attorneys. For this reason, public defenders are in a key position in the criminal justice system for ensuring the proper training and treatment of these adolescent offenders. Haggerty et al. (1972) show that attorneys involved in criminal processes rarely know whether the accused person is handicapped. This lack of knowledge or awareness goes back to the law school curriculum, which does not educate or train law students in this area at all.

An unaware attorney is unqualified to provide the proper environment—psychologically, physically, and emotionally—for these adolescents. To rectify this, lawyers should be trained in the following six major areas:

1. identification of LBP individuals
2. how to handle or deal with LBP persons
3. whom to contact for special advice in presenting the case
4. awareness of the special circumstances affecting these youths in the event they are drawn into the legal system
5. awareness of what services are available in the community that can forestall or limit the adolescents' placement in a criminal justice facility
6. experience with LBP offenders so the attorney can distinguish fact from fiction and appeasement from accountability

It is through this type of training that LBP adolescent offenders will find justice in the legal system.

Education of Judges

A well-informed judge can expedite the movement of these adolescents through the criminal justice system with a minimal detrimental effect on their future. This can be accomplished if judges are systematically educated through a series of required continuing education workshops or courses at the state and national level. A closer working relationship with special education professionals can help keep judges current and provide a valuable resource for consultation. A system of this type would avoid all of the shortcomings mentioned in the section on education of attorneys. However, according to Schilit (1979b), judges have previously shown little inclination to be educated about handicapped offenders.

Schilit (1979b), in a study on the awareness of 100 police officers, 75 attorneys, and 35 judges in Buffalo and Erie County, N.Y., shows that these persons, once approached and counseled in the importance of their understanding LBP adolescents or other handicapped individuals they encounter, did indicate a willingness to learn about this subject and were actively seeking information. The study finds that:

1. 84 percent of the population surveyed indicated an interest in attending a one-day seminar on mental retardation and mentally retarded offenders
2. 65 percent of this population felt there should be mandatory training for all criminal justice personnel on mental retardation
3. only 14 percent of the respondents indicated they knew of any training programs or of colleagues trained in mental retardation.

Persons involved with the criminal justice system can be expected to take advantage of training in special education in the foreseeable future because of the emphasis on the handicapped throughout contemporary society.

SUMMARY

LBP adolescent offenders are in a "Catch-22" situation because of the lack of understanding about them that pervades the criminal justice system. Judges, attorneys, and police officers receive little if any training in this area. Therefore it is often difficult for professionals in the criminal justice system to treat the LBP adolescent differently from other adolescent offenders. Information and strategy provided in this chapter about the LBP adolescent offender within the criminal justice system will, perhaps, generate interest and improve existing conditions.

Improvement, possible with the collaboration and education of professionals from both special education and criminal justice, should prevent the LBP adolescent from falling into a Jean Paul Sartre *No Exit* situation.

NOTE

1. Although the training of police officers, attorneys, and judges in special education has been minimal, there is evidence of increased training activity. One such training program is conducted by Dr. John Nelson of the Department of Special Education at Arizona State University at the Phoenix, Arizona Police Academy. On a national basis, the National Association for Retarded Citizens of Arlington, Tex. has developed the *Police Training in the Recognition and Handling of Retarded Citizens* program.

Chapter 4

Communicating with Parents of LBP Adolescents

L. Kay Hartwell, Roger L. Kroth, and Douglas E. Wiseman

INTRODUCTION

Parents and professional educators must work together, utilizing a wide variety of strategies, to ensure that the total society understands its responsibility to the handicapped. This attitude, as expressed by Abeson (1978), is but one example of the positive trend and increased acceptance of parental involvement in the educational process of LBP adolescents.

The movement toward such positive involvement in the schools has led toward the development of exploratory and model programs for involving parents of adolescents in all areas of exceptionality. A number of contributing factors have been identified by Kroth (1979):

1. the enactment of legislation (in particular P.L. 94-142 and Section 504 of the Rehabilitation Act of 1973—P.L. 93-112) that clearly mandates parents' consent for testing and placement decisions, as well as their participation in the development of their children's educational plans
2. the influence of parent participation in early childhood programs, which has continued as these pupils progress through the system; these programs helped establish a pattern that encourages parents to continue active involvement once their children reach school age—and throughout their careers to high school
3. the changing nature of the focus of parent organizations from advocacy and procurement of services for young children to direct involvement in educational programming and, more recently, advocacy for secondary programs
4. the decreasing size of families, which perhaps has increased the opportunity for parents to attend to the needs of adolescents; also, by the time children are of secondary school age, there are not as many younger ones at home to keep parents from attending meetings

Still another factor has been the recognition of the advantages of structured parent involvement. The assumptions that parents of secondary level students do not care, are not interested, will not go to school—or that adolescents do not want their parents to visit the school—are being questioned.

In contrast to this positive trend, educators in the past emphasized parent involvement at the elementary age level only. Such activities revolved around monthly topical meetings for parents of the entire school, regardless of their interest or need, as well as traditional reports of progress (conferences) required by many schools. Many educators have not recognized the positive trend and the concomitant need for teacher or school support, information, or skill development for parents of LBP adolescents. In reality, parents of low-achieving or troubled adolescents are both apprehensive and fearful. The schools' ability to provide programs that will work to overcome low achievement in basic skills, academic coursework, and career and vocational education, is limited because these adolescents are nearing completion of formal schooling.

Alexander, Kroth, Simpson, and Poppelreiter (1982) identify several reasons that preclude parent involvement at the secondary level:

1. Parents, especially those of students classified emotionally disturbed, have a long history of conflict with the schools.
2. Parents are confused by the complex physical and administrative school structure.
3. The family structure often is complex, e.g., divorces, extended family arrangements, foster home placement.
4. Parent education programs lack continuity.
5. Parents suffer overkill in their exposure to behavior modification programs that do not identify other, more relevant parental/adolescent needs.
6. Parents suffer burnout because of the intensity and duration of their child's problems. Parents inadvertently are losing support services when they most need them because of the rush to mainstreaming.

Practitioners have been aware through research and program evaluations that parental involvement can aid the educational development of children and adolescents (Gordon, 1974; Hayden & Haring, 1976; Kroth, 1979; Kroth & Simpson, 1977; Lillie & Place, 1982; Shearer, 1976). However, the literature also includes descriptions of parental actions' interfering with positive child behavior and learning (Buscaglia, 1971; Cansler, Martin, & Valana, 1975). Parents also have been criticized, ridiculed, and blamed for the behavior of their children (Kroth, 1972).

This often has led to misconceptions and misunderstandings between parents and teachers. Recently however, Alexander et al. (1982) identified several variables that have contributed toward the development of a strong, positive, cooperative parent-school relationship. These authors believe the relationship has improved because parents are more knowledgeable about handicapping conditions and because schools are providing more direct services to parents. Other favorable trends are the development of standards for parent involvement and the availability of commercial training kits and books for teachers.

With this relatively new and positive partnership between school and home, teachers are challenged to plan, prepare, and initiate effective communication to establish helping relationships. A real problem surfaces at this point because many educators feel inadequate in working with parents since the teachers lack formal training in adolescent behavior management, remediation of learning problems, and counseling of parents. It is not enough for teachers to have good intentions, be caring, and have empathy; they also must have skills to relate effectively to parents on both an individual and a group basis.

Having presented a rationale and basis for the positive trend toward parent involvement of adolescents, the rest of this chapter covers (1) parent rights, responsibilities, and advocacy; (2) conferencing strategies; (3) increasing parent involvement in the schools; (4) a brief overview of three secondary level parent involvement programs; and (5) practical suggestions for dealing with current issues in parent involvement.

PARENT RIGHTS, RESPONSIBILITIES, AND ADVOCACY

The purpose of structuring parents' involvement is to include them in the continuing activities of their LBP teenagers' educational program. Educators and others believe that involving parents in such activities and roles as teachers' aides, assisting other parents, teaching academics to the adolescents, and planning the intervention program with teachers will enhance their feelings of self-worth. Their general understanding of youngsters will increase, and they will have a larger repertoire of experience and activity from which to draw when interacting with their own child (Becker, 1971; Kroth, Whelan, & Stables, 1970; Lillie, 1976). Therefore, teachers should assist parents in structuring and focusing their involvement. Practitioners should:

1. Assist parents in understanding the importance of being "informed parents." For instance, the more knowledgeable a parent is about standardized tests, the more informed questions s/he can ask about the child's program. Or, understanding a scope and sequence will assist in planning programs that are realistic.
2. Explain the screening, identification, placement, and annual review process to parents as it is carried out in your district school. Include who is involved, each person's role, and particularly the parents' role.

3. Role play or encourage the parent to ask questions about the educational program.
4. Encourage parents to speak up and ask for an explanation of terms they do not understand.
5. Involve interested parents in learning how to administer educationally related tests that teachers normally administer, such as the Peabody Individual Achievement Test (PIAT). They should be taught test observation skills as well.
6. Parents can serve as aides or tutors to other classes. This will increase their experience and knowledge related to problems of educating children.
7. Part of the parents' role is to be available for conferencing.
8. Parents should be encouraged to express what they specifically would like their child to learn.
9. Explore with the parent alternatives for involvement according to their needs and interests. (Kroth, 1979)

Parents often have legitimate reasons for not being involved in these educational programs to the degree educators feel necessary. Teachers and other professionals must be careful not to judge that nonparticipation is a lack of interest.

Parents of LBP adolescents require clear and accurate information for use in planning and monitoring the students' educational program. Faas (1980) indicates that parents have the right to know:

1. how to obtain services for their youngsters
2. when they can expect certain services to be available
3. what types and locations of services are available
4. that their written permission is required for both assessment and placement of their teenagers in special education programs
5. what procedures are used by local schools
6. that they have the right to see the school's records and files related to their son or daughter
7. what constitutes their adolescents' rights
8. that the law requires an individualized education program (IEP) be developed and written if their offspring is identified as having exceptional needs.
9. that they must be invited to participate in the meeting(s) at which the IEP is developed
10. what progress their teenager is making and how the school measures growth
11. that the educational progress of students with special needs must be reviewed at least once each year
12. that they have a right to request a review when they disagree with the school's findings or recommendations

Generally, it is the school's responsibility to inform parents of their legal rights and those of their adolescents. This information can be given through pamphlets prepared by parent groups, state departments of education, or the Office of Special Education (OSE), U.S. Department of Education. Information also can be provided through large and small group meetings, filmstrips, handouts, or newsletters.

The authors suggest a moderate approach to advocacy such as working within the system, maintaining open lines of communication, using group processes, negotiating in good faith, and many other positive approaches available to parents, teachers, administrators, and school boards. Stronger, less positive measures may be needed to ensure the rights of their adolescents. Biklen (1974) presents several methods of advocacy available to parents and teachers:

1. Demonstrations: publicize issues, serve as an easy approach for successful short-term action
   a. marches
   b. sit-ins
   c. phone-ins
   d. overloading administrative systems
   e. leafleting
2. Demands: can promote the winning of concessions and serve as effective community education tools
   a. list of grievances
   b. contracts
   c. list of consumer needs
   d. bill of rights
3. Letter writing:
   a. carbon copies to attorneys
   b. public letters
   c. letters to the editor
   d. newsletters
   e. bulletins
   f. letters of complaint/support
4. Fact-finding forums:
   a. town meetings
   b. community polls
   c. testimony before legislative panels, town councils, school boards
   d. seminars by expert panels
5. Communications: help educate the community, serve as a symbol that advocacy is alive and will influence the future

a. booklets
b. pamphlets
c. workshops
d. slide shows
e. resource guides

f. television debates
g. posters
h. phoning campaigns
i. advertisements
j. TV, radio public service announcements

6. Symbolic acts: call attention to a policy, practice, or need that deserves exposure—often sarcastically
   a. mock event
   b. theatrical rendition
7. Education:
   a. workshops
   b. teach-ins
   c. consciousness-raising groups
   d. consumer meetings
   e. newspapers
   f. television and radio appearances
8. Boycotts: difficult without injuring the party being advocated for but may be effective when brief (one week)
   a. economic boycotts
   b. stalling
   c. refusal to pay for services
9. Lobbying: can effect changes in laws and policies
   a. telephone calls
   b. petitions
   c. telegram campaigns
   d. public statements
10. Model programs: can create alternative social institutions to force changes
    a. group homes
    b. integrated day care
    c. special education
11. Legal advocacy:
    a. lawsuits
    b. legal memoranda
    c. legal rights booklets
    d. civil rights statements
    e. legal representation
12. Demystifying:
    a. translate research findings, diagnostic terms, testing procedures, and results into everyday language
    b. explain program structure, curricula methods, materials and special equipment or therapeutic intervention used

These advocacy methods are ways in which parents and teachers can structure their joint involvement. This includes (1) defining the parents' role in the educational process, (2) presenting information on parent-student rights, and (3) finding acceptable ways for teachers to serve as advocates for better programs, legislation, and increased funding. Teachers should advocate within the guidelines of their employing school or agency. They also should serve as resource persons to parent advocacy groups and their activities.

CONFERENCING STRATEGIES

Every professional having contact with LBP students has the responsibility to plan and work cooperatively with the parents to enhance the total educational program. A significant factor in this working relationship is the professionals' ability to communicate effectively. Parents usually know their progeny best and should be recognized as the true experts on them. Teachers thus have to learn to be consultants to parents. Too often, professionals have categorized parents as hostile, too demanding, not demanding enough, frustrated, uncooperative, or too involved, or have used other labels that may act as barriers to effective communication.

Teachers also must recognize that educational programs can be affected positively by parents' involvement and that the latter can be a resource to professionals. Therefore, care must be taken when structuring these communications and contacts to avoid negative interactions.

One specific area of parent-teacher communication involves school conferences. These are the most common means for sharing information. Kroth (1972) discusses two types of such conferences—information-sharing and problem-solving. These are similar in content, type of structure, and preparation.

Skills important to teachers in communicating and planning these conferences include techniques of communication, such as active listening; values clarification; knowledge of body language; family dynamics; and methods of involving the parents. This section discusses ways to structure a parent-teacher information-sharing conference to facilitate effective communication. Such conferences are effective when carefully preplanned by the teacher. The University of New Mexico/Albuquerque Public Schools Center for Parent Involvement has developed a *Conference Checklist* (Exhibit 4-1) to assist teachers in such structuring.

The form in Exhibit 4-2 is used for writing a detailed report on the parent-teacher conference and is signed by both parties. It then is made a part of the record on the development and operation of the IEP.

One way to assist parents in preparing for the meeting is to send them information on *Tips for Progress Conferences* (Exhibit 4-3).

Exhibit 4-1 Structuring the Parent-Teacher Meeting

Conference Checklist

Preconference

_____ 1.   Notify

   • Purpose, place, time, length of time allotted

_____ 2.   Prepare

   • Review student's folder
   • Gather examples of work
   • Prepare materials

_____ 3.   Plan Agenda
_____ 4.   Arrange Environment

   • Comfortable seating
   • Eliminate distractions

Conference

_____ 1.   Welcome

   • Establish rapport

_____ 2.   State

   • Purpose
   • Time limitations
   • Note taking
   • Options for follow-up

_____ 3.   Encourage

   • Information sharing
   • Comments
   • Questions

_____ 4.   Listen

   • Pause once in a while!
   • Look for verbal and nonverbal cues
   • Questions

_____ 5.   Summarize
_____ 6.   End on a Positive Note

Exhibit 4-1 continued

Postconference

_____ 1.   Review Conference with Student, If Appropriate
_____ 2.   Share Information with Other School Personnel, If Needed
_____ 3.   Mark Calendar for Planned Follow-Up

Source: Reprinted by permission of the University of New Mexico/Albuquerque Public Schools Center for Parent Involvement, Albuquerque, 1979.

Exhibit 4-2 Form for Official Record of Parent-Teacher Meeting

Parent Conference Report

_____   _____
        Name of Student   Date of Conference

_____
        Name of Parent(s)

CONFERENCE OBJECTIVES: (1)

                       (2)

                       (3)

INFORMATION RECEIVED:

OBSERVATIONS:

CONFERENCE SUMMARY:

                       _____
                       Teacher Signature

                       _____
                       Parent(s) Signature

Source: The University of New Mexico/Albuquerque Public Schools Center for Parent Involvement, Albuquerque, 1979.

Exhibit 4-3 Guidelines for Preparing Parents for Meeting Teachers

Tips for Progress Conferences

What Good Is a Conference?

A teacher-parent conference is a two-way exchange of information about your child. A scheduled conference is a good time to exchange ideas and inquire about your child's school progress. If there is anything worrying you about your child's work, or if anything is bothering you about school procedures, you will have the opportunity to discuss it at the conference time.

For good conferences to happen, there are several basic assumptions which you and the teacher must make.

It is realistic to assume both of you want your child to succeed, that neither wants to push the child too fast, that both agree learning goes on at home as well as at school, and most importantly, that the goal of both is the best possible education for your child.

How To Get Ready for the Conference

1. If you have small children, please get a babysitter or someone to watch after them.
2. Please be on time. The teacher may have another scheduled conference.
3. Ask your child if he has any questions he would like you to ask his teacher.
4. Jot down what you want to learn about your child from the teacher.

Questions You Might Want To Ask the Teacher

1. Is my child progressing up to his ability?
2. How is my child achieving in specific subjects?
3. What books is he using?
4. Does he participate in group activities?
5. Does he get along with other children?
6. Does he obey the teacher?
7. How can I help at home?
8. How has he done on any tests taken this year?

Questions the Teacher May Want To Ask You

1. What is your child's general reaction to school?
2. How does he spend his time after school? What are his hobbies, interests, abilities?
3. How is his health? Does he seem to have any problems?
4. What is his response to rules and responsibilities at home? What type of discipline works best at home?
5. Does he have time set aside daily for reading, study, or homework?
6. Does he have a quiet place to work?

Exhibit 4-3 continued

At the Conference

1. Arrive on time. Stay only as long as you are scheduled—if necessary, reschedule for a later date.
2. Keep the attention focused on your child and how you can assist both student/teacher.
3. Inquire about concerns that you have regarding your child's school progress.
4. Volunteer information that might help the teacher understand your child, health, etc.

After the Conference

1. If you have later or further questions, feel free to contact your child's teacher or the office.

Source: Reprinted by permission of the University of New Mexico/Albuquerque Public Schools Center for Parent Involvement, Albuquerque, 1979.

MODEL FOR INCREASING PARENT INVOLVEMENT

As noted earlier, since the late 1970s there has been increased interest in developing structured parent involvement programs in the schools. At the secondary level, however, few models have been available. As with remediation programs, it seems that the elementary school models do not transfer adequately to the secondary level. This section discusses a conceptual model, defines various levels of parent involvement, looks at alternative efforts, and briefly reviews four model programs at the secondary level.

A comprehensive involvement program for a project or a public school system consists of more than informing parents of their rights or teaching them how to modify behavior. It also includes recognizing their strengths as well as their needs. The *Mirror Model for Parental Involvement* (Figure 4-1) proposed by the University of New Mexico/Albuquerque Public Schools Center for Parent Involvement, Albuquerque, New Mexico, provides for a variety of levels of involvement based on those strengths and needs. It is based on assumptions that parents of exceptional young people, regardless of the handicap, are not a homogeneous group and that the role of professionals is to be consultants to them.

Sensitive special educators need to look carefully at the characteristics and family structure of the parents in the target population. Even well-meaning, carefully designed parent education programs may put too much stress on that family structure. Excessive attention to one family member may mean that others are neglected. Some families may be made to feel guilty because they do not participate when their major objective is to provide food and clothing for their offspring.

The top half of the mirror model looks at the services that professionals can provide to parents.

Figure 4-1 Mirror Model for Parental Involvement in Public Schools

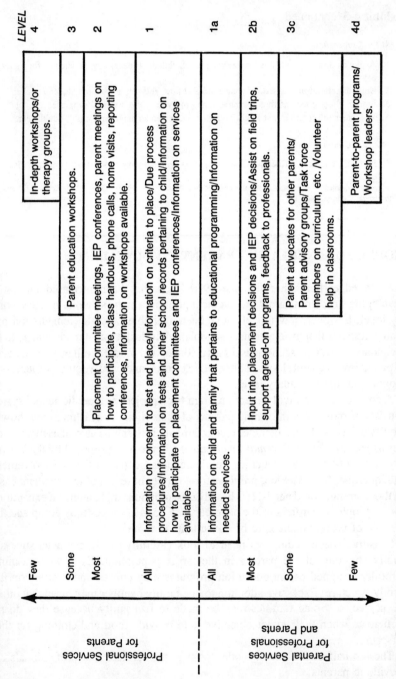

LEVEL		
4	Few	In-depth workshops/or therapy groups.
3	Some	Parent education workshops.
2	Most	Placement Committee meetings, IEP conferences, parent meetings on how to participate, class handouts, phone calls, home visits, reporting conferences, information on workshops available.
1	All	Information on consent to test and place/Information on criteria to place/Due process procedures/Information on tests and other school records pertaining to child/Information on how to participate on placement committees and IEP conferences/Information on services available.
1a	All	Information on child and family that pertains to educational programming/Information on needed services.
2b	Most	Input into placement decisions and IEP decisions/Assist on field trips, support agreed-on programs, feedback to professionals.
3c	Some	Parent advocates for other parents/ Parent advisory groups/Task force members on curriculum, etc. /Volunteer help in classrooms.
4d	Few	Parent-to-parent programs/ Workshop leaders.

Professional Services for Parents

Parental Services for Professionals and Parents

Source: Reprinted by permission of the University of New Mexico/Albuquerque Public Schools Center for Parent Involvement, Albuquerque, 1979.

Level 1

It is the responsibility of professionals to be sure that all parents know what they are consenting to when their teenagers are being considered for or are placed in special environments. All parents should know that they can dissent from placement and what avenues (due process) are open to them if they disagree with the professionals. Parents should know that they can review records and that they have the responsibility as well as the right to participate in IEP planning. In some instances, educators may assume incorrectly that parents are aware of this information because their adolescents have been in the program over a period of time; such an attitude must be avoided.

There are a variety of ways to communicate information to parents. Face-to-face contact is the desired mode. Professionals may need to make home visits, schedule meetings or group sessions at times convenient for parents, and send them letters, newsletters, and handbooks. Attention must be paid to the parents' native language. Filmstrips and handouts available from organizations such as the Council for Exceptional Children also are helpful.

From a psychological as well as ethical point of view, it is better for the parents to get information from the professionals who work with their progeny than to hear it from other sources. This establishes a level of trust and a stance of openness between the parties. The major responsibility for seeing that parents are informed usually lies with project directors or directors of special education. However, coordinators, teachers, counselors, and psychologists often are the deliverers of these services.

Level 2

Most parents need and appreciate being involved in these educational plans and progress. Some may not be able to attend conferences because of work schedules, distance, or demands at home. Others may not respond to written communications, but this does not necessarily mean they are not interested.

Again, there are a number of means of communicating with them. Teachers may use daily or weekly report card systems and telephone calls to provide progress information. Many parents learn to fear telephone calls, notes, and requests for conferences from school personnel because they typically have been negative. When the reports tell of good events as well as bad ones, they indicate that educators are able to recognize and reinforce the positive as well as the negative. Systematic, frequent reporting systems range in design from simple to complex, some requiring parental feedback and some no feedback. The important thing is to keep parents informed and, thus, involved.

Some teachers develop classroom-oriented handbooks that explain procedures and identify personnel; others provide a periodic newsletter. Teachers working at live-in institutions have put together scrapbooks with pictures and student work that are sent to the parents once or twice a year.

Teachers originate many of the activities in Level 2 to keep parents involved through sharing information, even if they cannot visit the school or are too far away for home visits.

Level 3

Some parents will be able to become involved in education workshops that lead to skill building. Not all, or even most will need such training; even if many do require the skills, a number will not be able to take advantage of the sessions because of other demands on their time and energy. An important question for educators to ask themselves is, "Would we be able to take the time from our busy schedules to participate in the parent education programs that we have designed?"

Usually, parent education workshops are short and rather intense, with specific objectives and assignments. Monthly parent group meetings are more appropriately regarded as a Level 2 activity since they primarily are informational presentations and a large attendance is expected.

These workshops usually are limited to less than ten participants. A great deal of involvement and interactions with skills are demonstrated. These workshops may involve specific topics such as management techniques, communication skills, parent/youth participation games, student study, and learning to test or evaluate their own teenagers. The workshops may include four or five sessions over several weeks. The groups should be formed according to interests or identified needs expressed by parents or staff, and not simply required of all parents.

It is most desirable that the teacher be involved in the design and presentation of the workshop, with assistance from a support person. The teacher usually knows the parents because of activities in Levels 1 and 2 and has established a feeling of trust.

Level 4

A few parents may need therapy of some sort in addition to the activities in the first three levels. Although such parents often draw the attention of professionals because of the intensity of their reactions to the situation, they probably constitute only a rather small percentage of the total population if the activities in the first three levels are carried out. Their anxieties often are reduced when they obtain information and skills and learn to arrange their lives in manageable terms.

Most school districts and projects do not have qualified personnel available to provide the in-depth psychological services. Personal counseling often is not seen as the responsibility of the school system. It then becomes necessary for school personnel to be able to refer parents to the appropriate services.

It is difficult to estimate the percentages of involvement at each of these four levels. However, past experience indicates that educators should expect very close to 100 percent involvement for Level 1, 80 to 85 percent for Level 2, 40 percent for Level 3, and 10 percent for Level 4. These percentages are likely to vary according to the population and the various projects. They also may vary if involvement over a long period of time is necessary. For instance, a high percentage of parents of deaf children may be involved in skill training (Level 3) for preschoolers but may feel little need for education groups in the middle school years. By carefully analyzing the characteristics of the families and their histories of involvement, meaningful activities can be planned.

The mirror side on the bottom half of the Mirror Model presents the strengths that parents can bring to the process. The program should not be built solely on a deficit (parental needs) model.

Level 1a

Merely by living with their youngsters, all parents know more about them than professionals do. It may take skillful questioning by the professionals to find out this information, and it may take the development of a level of trust between both sides before parents are ready to share information.

When a case history is taken from the parents in preparation for placement, great emphasis often is placed on demographic data and medical and physical information. While this is important, it may be more important to find out how the teenager learns. What did the parents do to teach such abilities as how to walk, talk, throw balls, work on cars, etc.? Does the adolescent learn best by being shown or by being told? What turns the student on or off and what are the major interests?

If parents can be regarded as individuals who have taught their progeny a number of things, then parents and professionals can solve problems together in the future. Parents know things that professionals need to know.

Level 2b

Most parents can become actively involved in planning and implementing these educational programs. It is possible to write the parents into the IEP as deliverers of specific services, just like any other adult in the program. Parents can provide such services as listening to their teenagers read, regulating TV watching time, reinforcing daily or weekly report card systems, and playing games with them to develop language or math skills.

Most parents can be expected to help at some time or other with classroom activities. This might include aid on a field trip, talking to a class, making cookies, or making phone calls to or providing transportation for other parents. These often are one-time activities but can be a very important part of a total involvement program.

Level 3c

Because of their interest, time available, special knowledge, or skills, some parents can become much more involved than others in the total program. Some might volunteer to work in the classroom for specified periods; others might collect information or write and produce a newsletter for other parents; some might work in the resource center, showing films and filmstrips, cataloguing materials, and checking out materials. Some parents may serve on curriculum task forces, working with professionals to determine what skills should be taught and when.

It must be reiterated that parents are not a homogeneous group. Some have advanced degrees or special skills in developing materials and designing equipment. They may be doctors, lawyers, engineers, electricians, mechanics, or typists. If their skills can be recognized and brought to bear in the education of LBP adolescents, they can benefit many besides their own. While some may have trouble accepting their own teenager's condition, they could prove to be valuable resources.

By carefully analyzing the characteristics and strengths of parents, programs can capitalize on talent that often goes untapped. Because practitioners tend to become concerned about parents' deficits or needs, they want to teach them something rather than learn from them. It is up to educators to look for creative, meaningful ways to involve parents; those who are needed and feel needed can be productive in many ways.

Level 4d

A few parents may want to become involved as educators for other parents. A number of professionals are apprehensive about this, fearing that parents, because of their own emotional involvement, will not be able to be good teachers. Although this may happen, it is not usually the case.

A number of communities have had parent-to-parent programs that are quite successful. These usually serve as support for parents to whom a handicapped child has just been born or who are faced with enrolling their child in special education. A parent or parents who "have been there" meet with those facing the new situation. A variation of this is to have parents of secondary level children meet with those of elementary pupils who are in transition to the new level. Similarly, parents of those who have left an institutional setting may meet with those who are considering the move. Most of these programs are successful. Professionals can be helpful in meeting with parents who are interested in this activity, discussing their motivation, sharing techniques for helping, and creating situations where these meetings can happen.

There are a number of steps that should be considered when placing parents in this role. They should go through the program as participants, then should assist the leader with a group; the leader then should help the parents with a group, and finally the parents are ready to take over. This procedure seems long and may not be necessary for all parents, but it does expand the number of cases with which they come in contact before they begin running a group. It also builds their confidence as leaders.

There are at least a few parents in any target population who have the time, interest, knowledge, and skill to be extremely helpful to others. In some cases, they prove more helpful than professionals. Practitioners can expand their base of parental involvement by becoming trainers of trainers and thus using parents effectively in the education of others.

WAYS TO INVOLVE PARENTS

Since there are a number of levels at which parents can be involved (Exhibit 4-4), it is necessary to determine the quality and quantity of participation desirable or required. Since parents' participation generally is considered a voluntary activity, they usually need clearly communicated objectives for their involvement.

Parents of LBP adolescents are concerned about the welfare and future of their teenagers. Throughout their classroom career, parents have felt the problem would go away or be dealt with effectively by the school. As the child has grown closer to the end of adolescence, parents appear to have increased need for additional support from the school. This is evidenced by the number of contacts they initiate with the schools and by their attendance in structured programs for involvement at the secondary level.

Primary to developing structured programs for increasing parents' participation is the assessment of their strength and need for school involvement and support. One example of collecting information on needs for school support is a question-naire such as Exhibit 4-5.

Parent involvement will increase as needs are identified and alternatives for participation are developed and implemented. A few parents (Figure 4-1, supra) can provide assistance as volunteers, as teaching parents, or on advisory commit-tees.

Benefits of increasing parent involvement are numerous. Among those men-tioned by Kroth (1975) are:

- Parents can realize that they are not the only ones with a particular problem.
- Parents can share their strong emotions with others who understand. Feelings of quiet or anger regarding a handicapped youth often are alleviated when they are expressed in a group meeting. The realization that other members of the group have similar feelings seems to have a positive effect.
- Parents can share solutions. They will often listen to solutions to problems from other members of the group more readily than they will from an outside authority.

Exhibit 4-4 Steps toward Parent Participation in Programs

Ways To Involve Parents

	Objectives	Advantages	Disadvantages	Consideration
Written Reports	- Keep parent continually informed of child's progress	- Easy to do - Personal - Maintain contact - Proud parent can show them to others	- May not show growth in low-functioning child - May not provide teachers with feedback - Cannot understand how parent interprets the information	- Must be written at parents' reading & informational level - Teacher must be willing to do regularly
Informal Notes	- Highlight special events	- Personalized - Do not have to be maintained - Proud parent can show them to others	- Easy to put off or forget	- Are you doing it for all children? - Budget for materials
Newsletters	- Keep parents informed of program news, special events, etc.	- Can include information applicable to all parents in a single communication	- Difficult to write because of varying level of parents' intelligence	- Should have universal appeal - Use short, high-interest items - Try to include most of the children's names

Scrapbook	- Shows child's growth with examples, i.e., pictures, child's work, written notes	- Personalized - Highly motivating - Pictures often more meaningful than words	- Time comsuming - Can be expensive	- Might be organized around skills - How to share it with parents without losing it/or how to keep it up to date if possible, keep it
Telephone	- Information sharing or problem solving	- Easy - Personalized - Can cover greater territory than with written word or video - Quick feedback	- Cannot read body language as well as in person - Cannot show or demonstrate	- Prepare parents for phone call, i.e., arrange time and purpose of call - Review in your own mind the purpose of the call - Prepare notes to work from during the call
Video and Movies	- Show parents child's accomplishments	- Personalized - Pictures can be more meaningful than words	- Expensive - Require viewing equipment - May take a long time to get samples needed	- Is the material self-explanatory or does it need a good interpretor? - Might include key personnel as well as child

Source: The University of New Mexico/Albuquerque Public Schools Center for Parent Involvement, Albuquerque, 1979.

Exhibit 4-5 Questionnaire on Parent Needs for School Support

Child Information

1. Birthdate: _____
2. Sex: (   ) Female   (   ) Male
3. Age when learning problem discovered: _____
4. Who discovered the learning problem? _____
5. Is your child taking medication that effects learning and/or behavior?
   (   ) Yes   (   ) No   If yes, what is the name of the medicine? _____
6. Class Placement: (   ) Sophomore   (   ) Junior   (   ) Senior
7. Teacher: _____
8. Language spoken at home: _____
9. Number of years student has been in special education: _____

Parent/Guardian Information

1. Your relationship to the child: ____ Mother
   ____ Father
   ____ Guardian _____
   ____ Stepparent   (specify relationship)
2. Mother's age: _____
   Mother's educational level: _____
   Mother's occupation: _____
3. Father's age: _____
   Father's educational level: _____
   Father's occupation: _____
4. Guardian's/stepparent's age: _____
   Guardian's/stepparent's occupation: _____
5. Have you ever been in a parent training group specifically designed for parents of handicapped children?   (   ) Yes   (   ) No

What type of training did you receive?

	How helpful was the training?			
	Very Helpful	Helpful	Not Very Helpful	No Help
( ) workshop for handling behavior problems	1	2	3	4
( ) workshop on education of handicapped	1	2	3	4
( ) workshop on drugs and alcohol	1	2	3	4
( ) general information on school programs	1	2	3	4
( ) specific information on school programs	1	2	3	4
( ) other _____	1	2	3	4

1. Are you interested in a series of meetings with a group of parents to discuss common problems of parents in rearing children today and in planning for their future?
   (   ) Yes   (   ) No

Exhibit 4-5 continued

2. The best time to meet is: ( ) Mornings ( ) Afternoons ( ) Evenings
3. The best days for me are: ( ) Monday ( ) Tuesday ( ) Wednesday
                            ( ) Thursday ( ) Friday ( ) Saturday
4. I would like the meetings to last: ( ) 45 min. ( ) 1 hour ( ) 1½ hour
                                      ( ) _____
5. I would like to meet: ( ) once a week
                  ( ) once a month ( ) twice a month
                  ( ) once during each semester ( ) _____
6. The best place to meet would be: ( ) at school ( ) in a home
                            ( ) at a church ( ) _____

7. I would like to receive information by attending:
PLEASE CHECK AS MANY WAYS AS YOU WOULD LIKE
- ( ) large group sessions
- ( ) small group sessions
- ( ) independent study
- ( ) field trips
- ( ) discussion and sharing
- ( ) presentation by leaders
- ( ) role playing (acting out)
- ( ) discussion of ready materials
- ( ) parent/student sharing
- ( ) films, tape recordings, slides
- ( ) _____

8. What would encourage you to attend parent programs?
PLEASE CHECK AS MANY WAYS AS YOU WOULD LIKE
- ( ) interest in topic
- ( ) free materials
- ( ) baby-sitting provided
- ( ) transportation arranged
- ( ) college credit
- ( ) honorarium ($)
- ( ) trading stamps
- ( ) helping my child in school
- ( ) _____
- ( ) _____

9. The following are some ideas for parent programs.
PLEASE CHECK AS MANY TOPICS AS YOU WOULD LIKE
- ( ) community resources
- ( ) laws relating to education and work
- ( ) chemical dependency (drugs/alcohol)
- ( ) human sexuality
- ( ) learning/social characteristics
- ( ) behavior management
- ( ) listening and communication skills
- ( ) talking with professionals
- ( ) planning educational programs
- ( ) adjustment from elementary school to junior high

Exhibit 4-5 continued

```
                                            ( ) adjustment from junior high
                                                school to senior high school
                                            ( ) adjustment from senior
                                                high school to the work world
                                            ( ) _____
                                            ( ) _____
10. Other topics I would like discussed.
    _____  _____  _____
11. People I know who would be good resource persons.
    Name: _____ Topic: _____
    Name: _____ Topic: _____

I WILL BE ATTENDING PARENT MEETING ( ) YES    ( ) NO ON DECEMBER 6
at 7:30 p.m.

                                            _____
                                                   Parent or Guardian
```

THREE MODEL PARENT INVOLVEMENT PROGRAMS

Parent involvement programs have been significant components of elementary school special education programs for several decades. However, in those years, efforts in involving parents of LBP adolescents were infrequent and little publicized. In the latter part of the 1970s, with the impetus of the Child Service Demonstration Centers (CSDC) and Handicapped Children Model Programs (HCMP), secondary program models—including those for parents—have been developed, implemented, and evaluated. Three such models—the Mesa (Arizona) Demonstration Resource Center, the Billings (Montana) Demonstration Program for Specific Learning Disabilities, and the Houston (Texas) Model Demonstration Center for Secondary Learning Disabled Students—are still in operation and serve a range of students with learning and/or behavior problems. Descriptions of the three models follow.

The Mesa Demonstration Resource Center

Mountain View High School in Mesa was the site of a joint project involving Arizona State University and the Mesa public schools. The CSDC developed a comprehensive, six-component program for LBP adolescents and other low-achieving students. The major thrust of the project was providing alternative services within the school program to avoid or prevent failures in class. One of the components focused on parent involvement in the special education program.

The Mesa public schools have been strongly committed to parent involvement, so that element seemed appropriate for providing a supportive setting for the project goals. The first year of the three-year effort was a false start that provided both the project and school staffs with valuable insights in developing the program. The project hired a full-time professionally educated parent trainer who had the responsibilities of developing a program, coordinating activities, and running workshops. Although the third-party evaluation of the program was positive, reduced participation by parents suggested that their needs were not being met.

Two major corrective modifications were introduced:

1. The management of the program was given to the special education staff at Mountain View High School. The teachers and project staff jointly agreed on activities that would constitute a comprehensive program and teachers were reimbursed for their out-of-school efforts. Rather than having all teachers performing all activities, they were assigned according to their strengths and interests.
2. Three general levels of involvement were established to individualize parent participation: awareness of available information, knowledge acquisition, and skill acquisition.

Awareness was basically regarded as a first level of support for the parents. The information presented was general and appropriate for large groups. Awareness activities included a newsletter and information/communication meetings such as a parent-teacher dinner and were designed to keep parents informed of the project and optional opportunities for participation.

Information or knowledge acquisition was the second level of support. This level accented the active parent involvement of gathering information relevant to the decision making necessary for educating their youngster. The special education teachers gathered a comprehensive collection of resources and materials that included career education opportunities, recreation and training programs, community and agency resources, and annotated bibliographies on family-related topics. These resources served as a library or parent center and included workshop audiotapes, videotapes, written training modules, and books and journals.

Miniworkshops for small groups of parents were developed to increase their role in the educational process, with teachers as leaders. Follow-up activities were assigned to ensure that parents used the information from the workshops.

Skill development, the third level of support, consisted of monthly meetings for four to six parents so they could learn to use specific abilities they had requested, such as communication, behavior management techniques, and procedures for development of IEPs. The parents role-played and practiced the new skills on each other. The teachers followed up with questionnaires and telephone calls on how the skills were being utilized.

The project emphasis shifted from general to individualized participation over the three years. Individual "Parent Support Plans" were prepared for each couple. It was felt by both sides that the emphasis on individualization and the teacher-parent management of the program were the major reasons for its success.

The Billings Demonstration Program

The Billings Public School CSDC resulted from joint parent-administration efforts to improve the program for specific learning disabilities. The emphasis was on regular and special education teacher training at the inservice level. The project site was located at Arrowhead School.

A strong component of the project was parental involvement and training. The first step was a parent needs assessment, undertaken jointly by the Association for Children with Learning Disabilities (ACLD) and the faculty of the schools. It was decided to focus the parent involvement component on affective concerns such as awareness of the feelings, frustrations, and anxieties of learning disabled students, particularly at home, at school, and with peers.

At each of the junior and senior high schools, three two-hour meetings were held during a three-week period. Invitations to participate were sent by each building principal and were followed up with telephone calls from the special education teachers. The first workshop had the theme of the adolescent at school, the second of the adolescent at home, and finally, the adolescent among peers. The content of the workshops was directed toward teaching skills to facilitate parenting, such as communicating, organizing family meetings, and setting family goals.

The effective communication established between parents and teachers in the workshops was applied to individualized interaction and training throughout the year. This resulted in positive parent attitudes toward school personnel and their child's participation in classes.

The Houston Model Demonstration Center

The University of Houston and the Houston Independent School District worked cooperatively to establish a CSDC model program for secondary learning disabled students in the Spring Forest Junior High School. The program was titled the "Synergistic Classroom." Synergism implies that many forces are necessary to assist the learning disabled students and that the end product is greater than the sum of its individual parts. The program taught the students intellectual and affective strategies for dealing with the academic and social demands on them.

The school and parent programs were coordinated to run concurrently in The High Intensity Learning Center. This was a specialized strategy-building program designed for student-parent-teacher involvement covering a 12-week period. Following completion of structured activities at the Learning Center, the students were cycled into other follow-up options that would respond to their individual needs.

The program was centered on the Learning Center, with one parents' meeting each week. The theme was that parents, student, and teacher made up a team that must succeed for the betterment of all the participants. The team directed its energies to three major concerns: (1) coping with alienation and frustration, (2) providing a sound knowledge base, and (3) teaching affective skills.

The weekly meetings had three segments: (1) a home/school exchange of ideas and information, (2) the creation of plans to facilitate the development of a strong support group, and (3) lessons to encourage a sound and comprehensive knowledge base and to develop skills needed for parenting. During this 12-week period, the special education counselor made home visits to talk with the family. These visits were both communication icebreakers and training sessions, depending on the family's needs or desires. The parents were asked to sign a contract for active involvement in the program, particularly for areas that related to the home.

Follow-up telephone calls by teachers encouraged parent attendance and opened new lines of communication. The project focus was on individual needs, including the student, the parents, and the teacher. The parents and the teachers were encouraged to complete forms once each week so all participants could keep apprised of progress. The project was rated highly by the parents and had a high degree of participation.

These three model parent involvement programs had a number of factors in common:

1. a focus on individualization
2. parent advisory committees that planned jointly with school personnel
3. content relevant to and selected by parents
4. a strong support system for parents
5. the goal of teaching both information and skills
6. structured and unstructured meetings
7. a high expectancy for more parent-school interaction and communication
8. a goal of increased parent participation

STRATEGIES FOR PARENT INVOLVEMENT

There are a number of issues that pertain to parent involvement. How teachers and other school personnel deal with them depends on personal philosophies and previous experiences. The following section addresses each of the identified issues and provides suggestions for strategies that might be used to resolve each one. The strategies are not intended to be all-inclusive; rather, they are intended to stimulate practitioners to generate additional means of working effectively with parents for the welfare of LBP adolescents.

There are several key areas of parent-teacher-student involvement. The teacher must be prepared to respond to and have knowledge about these areas, which are discussed next.

Parents As Resources for Other Parents

There are several advantages in utilizing parents as resources for other parents. They seem to be more willing to accept the support and counsel of others with similar problems than of those who "don't know what it is like to have an LBP youngster." There is a need, too, to identify those who have been effective in working with other parents through advocacy groups. Another method is to train parents in leadership activities. The following strategies are suggested for teachers:

1. Selecting as resources those who have participated in parent training activities or workshops to develop skills such as communication or teaching academics to LBP students.
2. Training parents as resources in a structured manner such as (a) using those who have participated in training, (b) having them assist as group leaders, and (c) having them lead a group with support assistance or no assistance.
3. Suggesting to parents they can be resources to others during the identification, staffing, and placement process.
4. Using parents to provide referral information to others seeking professional services related to their teen-ager's problems.
5. Using parents as listeners for others who have family problems related to the presence of an LBP youngster.

Therapy for Parents in the Public Schools

The provision of therapy for parents in the schools is a controversial issue. While it is recognized that a few parents of LBP youths will need therapy or counseling, most educators do not feel that it falls within the domain of school-related services. Unless specifically written into a project, most school systems do not employ qualified family therapists. It also could be argued that this is a duplication of community services. However, there are several strategies that can be used to assist parents:

1. compiling a directory of services (they already exist in some large communities); special education personnel can help parents by identifying serv-

ices that are germane to their needs; the directory also should list qualified private psychologists, counselors, or therapists

2. conducting an informal meeting at which a number of agencies that provide counseling or therapy present their programs to a group of parents
3. developing a slide-tape program with pictures of the various agencies, a short narrative, and brochures that could be viewed by parents at their convenience

Parents' Follow-Through at Home

After analyzing such family characteristics as knowledge base, time constraints, energy level, and inclination to be involved, teachers must determine whether it is desirable and feasible to involve the parents. If they are to be involved in home instruction, teacher strategies can include:

1. writing the parents into the IEP; they can be designated as providers of services just like any other persons
2. reinforcing the parents on a systematic basis such as with notes, letters, telephone calls, certificates, copresentations at conferences, articles in newspapers, pay (in some instances), or an honor roll board
3. removing the adolescents from the program; most public schools will not do so if the parents refuse to follow through at home, but some special programs may require parent participation

Training Teachers To Work with Parents

Almost everyone agrees that teachers, parents, and students benefit from the teacher's involvement with parents. Until the recent increase in parent involvement training programs in universities, workshops, and staff development programs, few teachers had the training, experience, or expertise to structure and plan for such involvement. To follow the suggested strategies listed below, teachers could:

1. Conduct a self-assessment related to activities they generally perform with parents, rating themselves by using an (A) for a general awareness level; a (K) for a more in-depth knowledge or skill level, or an (S) for having the skill needed to perform the function. The suggested functions are those needed to plan, communicate, and work effectively with parents:
   A. Act as the advocate for student and parents in all IEP-related and other pertinent matters.
   B. Schedule parent conferences that provide progress reports, information, goals, and objectives;

(1) Progress reports
   a. Collect academic, social data
   b. Set up conference format agenda, plan logistics
   c. Select modes of presenting data
   d. Suggest listening skills (choice of modes)
   e. Recommend study skills
   f. Report differences between formal and informal assessment strategies
(2) Transmit information/program goals, etc.
C. Make home visits and hold telephone conferences.
D. Work as part of the multidisciplinary team (especially in facilitating parent involvement and comfort).
E. Assist the parent to mainstream the student into school, family, and community life.
F. Consult with individual parents regarding implementation of school program.
G. Supervise parent volunteers.
H. Develop and implement a responsive program to meet parent needs.
I. Act as an advocate for the program, selling it to parents.
J. Act as a resource, referral, and information person.
K. Listen, communicate, provide emotional support to families.
L. Provide parent education (teach behavior management, etc.).
M. Work with parent and other educationally related advisory groups.
N. Identify and understand family dynamics, cultural differences, values, etc.

2. Use a variety of resources to increase skill levels in each of the areas indicated in the self-assessment:
A. Request inservice training from the school district related to developing skills in working with parents.
B. Attend presentations at national and state conferences providing examples of effective parent programs.
C. Take a university course in counseling, communication skills development, active listening, or family systems.
D. Review textbooks on the subject of teacher-parent communication or relationships and read books written by parents of the handicapped.
E. Review commercial programs such as the following:

- *Even Love Is Not Enough: Children with Handicaps*, by Parent Magazine Films, Inc., 52 Vanderbilt Avenue, New York, NY 10017, 1975.
- *Keeping in Touch with Parents: A Teacher's Best Friend*, by Leatha M. Bennett and Ferris O. Henson, Learning Concepts, 2501 N. Lamar, Austin, TX 78705, 1977.

- *Managing Behavior: A Parent Involvement Program*, by Richard L. McDowell, B.L. Winch and Assoc., P.O. Box 1185, Torrance, CA 90505, 1976.
- *Systematic Training for Effective Parenting*, by Don Dinkmeyer and Gary D. McDay. American Guidance Service, Inc., Circle Pines, MN 55014, 1976.
- *The Art of Parenting*, by Bill R. Wagonseller, Mary Burnett, Bernard Salzberg, and Joe Burnett, Research Press, Champaign, IL 61820, 1977.

F. Meet or telephone parents early in the school year to open lines of communication that do not involve problems or crisis situations.
G. Gain experience by teaming up with the counselor, school psychologist, or school social worker in working with parents; this gets more of the school staff involved and helps spread the emotional and scheduling strain for both teachers and parents.
H. Volunteer professional skills to local parent advocacy groups for work on special projects.

Physical Child Abuse, Death, Family Problems

Because of the growing emphasis on providing services to all handicapped students, particularly in rural areas, special teachers face many more complex problems that traditionally have not been the responsibility of the schools.

Some complex problems are common to all adolescents. No attempt is made here to develop a comprehensive list of these problems or their solutions. While the problems may not be common or frequent, most teachers will have contact with similar situations during their professional lives. Problems and suggested strategies are discussed in the following material.

Child Abuse

1. Determine the procedure in the school district and in the state for reporting suspected child abuse.
2. Note observations, dates, and comments by the student.
3. Report suspected abuse, then follow up with the agency to determine what action it has taken.

Death of a Student

1. Locate local resources for inservice training or information related to the topic of death and dying for teachers, parents, and students in the school.

2. Identify resources in active parent advocacy groups or community churches that have dealt with this problem.
3. Read and/or identify books, articles, and films for use with parents, other teachers, and students.

Family Problems

1. Do not try to accept ownership of interpersonal family problems but listen sympathetically while seeking resources to assist in resolving situations.
2. Identify family counseling resources in the community or a person in whom the family has confidence, such as a member of the clergy, family friend, or relative to assist the parents.
3. Assure confidentiality in all cases; this is extremely important for professional reasons and for the faith and confidence of the parents with whom teachers work.

Other issues could be considered here, but those discussed generally are concerns that teachers have expressed and/or are reviewed in the literature.

SUMMARY

The approach to parent involvement presented in this chapter is based on assumptions of mutual trust and respect between the two sides. Professionals must recognize the effect that positive parent involvement can have on an LBP student's educational program. They also must respect the parents' rights and needs and provide support through structured programs based on individual needs.

Several factors have led to the increased need for structured parent involvement programs: (1) recent legislation, (2) results of research indicating the positive effects of such programs, (3) teacher recognition of the importance and advantages of these efforts, (4) parent advocacy groups' pushing for support for low-achieving adolescents, and (5) the emerging role of the teacher in student advocacy.

Parent rights and responsibilities and parent-teacher advocacy activities were discussed and resources were presented for both sides. Effective communication between parent and teacher is critical to both advocacy and educational programming for LBP adolescents.

Educators are optimistic about the future of the involvement of parents of LBP secondary students. The strength of this trend will benefit students' educational programs. The idea that parents do not want to be involved with the schools and that teachers do not see the benefit of parent participation is false. It is to be hoped that this trend toward structured parent-teacher involvement will encompass all adolescents—those in general education as well as those in programs for LBP students.

Part III

Curricula, Classroom, Strategies, and Validation

The therapeutic and self-restructuring medium in the public schools remains the curriculum. Serious students of the special educational instructional process are faced with two haunting questions: First, what do they have to work with in their classrooms? Second, how valid and helpful are the masses of scientific materials that pour in on teachers?

The answer to the first question lies in part in the classroom environment. Chapter 5 addresses the teaching environment, the curricula, and the content and process of delivering instruction.

The special education curriculum process is based on the individualized education program required by P.L. 94-142. Chapter 6 dissects that process into several components. Chapter 7 introduces two major special education teaching approaches—remediation and tutoring. Chapter 8 looks at the content-related aspect of secondary special education methodology. It examines entry into the curricular process by setting the initial instructional objective through criterion-referenced assessment. It then uses mathematics as an instructional subject, developing an example of sequenced objectives based on informal assessment.

Chapters 9 and 10 bring up the question of scientific inquiry, which involves teachers' second major question every time they prepare a lesson. Commercial publishers have flooded special educators with materials, and teachers generate large quantities of them. The question is: which, if any, of these are the most effective and most efficient with LBP students? The answer is that educators' need to service LBP adolescents has far outstripped the available scientific data to support the effectiveness of these commercially produced materials. These chapters examine the curricula, student-task interaction, and the learning process. They force secondary special educators to examine the data collection issues relating to the science of instruction. Unless teacher education programs become more sophisticated—training the teachers to be capable of evaluating the effectiveness of materials through scientific methods of inquiry—the effectiveness of such materials will continue to be questioned.

Chapter 5

Classroom Organization and Synthesization

Michael J. Fimian, Mark S. Zoback, and Bruno J. D'Alonzo

INTRODUCTION

At the high school level, there are a number of different types of service delivery options available for students with learning and/or behavior problems. Several were discussed in Chapter 1. The availability of these options makes it possible to select a course of action for each student that will be the least restrictive and most productive. The single category resource room and variations thereof is the most common option in secondary schools, but recent trends indicate that the cross-categorical room is becoming popular.

For LBP students, the resource room is a viable alternative. Of course, this administrative arrangement, as with any other educational environment, must be appropriately staffed, operated, and supervised if the students' needs for a specialized education are to be achieved. Numerous writers, including D'Alonzo, D'Alonzo, and Mauser (1979), Deno (1970), Lerner (1976), Reger (1973), Sabatino (1972), Sindelar and Deno (1978), Wiederholt (1974), and Wiederholt, Hammill, and Brown (1978) have cited the importance of the resource room concept and environment as the most promising alternative to placement in segregated special classes or in regular classes without support services.

This chapter provides information on basic classroom organization and synthesization, assuming that teachers will have their own rooms for LBP students.

This is primarily a "nuts and bolts" approach to establishing an optional learning environment for secondary aged LBP students. It is not a rigid plan that teachers must accept in place of strategies they have developed over years of working in a specific room or school. Rather, it is designed as a guide to environmental changes and organizational innovations that can make a difference between a smoothly running classroom in which learning can take place and one characterized by teacher and student stress and missed educational opportunities.

123

The chapter discusses such basic, yet crucial, considerations as: (1) the physical environment of the classroom, (2) appropriate equipment and materials, (3) use of space, (4) storage requirements, (5) the organization of the learning environment, (6) recordkeeping, (7) curriculum selection, and (8) communication with other school personnel.

ORGANIZING AND SYNTHESIZING

"Where do I start?" is a question teachers often ask at the beginning of each school year. When newly certified teachers first enter their own classrooms, they must make major decisions and address numerous activities in a relatively short time. For some fortunate teachers that may mean two weeks or more; for many, however, it amounts to 72 hours or less.

During that time, educators must equip and furnish the classroom, organize the available space, and sometimes anticipate expanding or modifying the area to meet classroom, student, and teacher needs. In short, they must organize the physical environment.

In addition, they must organize the learning environment, including surveying and analyzing each student's needs; establishing instructional objectives; organizing assessment and datakeeping systems; selecting curricula; choosing, ordering, and/or making instructional materials; organizing and storing all materials; and organizing teacher, support staff, and student time in relation to morning and afternoon activities.

Once class is in session, they must synthesize the instructional and physical environments, including scheduling, developing curricula, assessment and consultant activities, and establishing recordkeeping systems capable of professional communication.

The term classroom organization refers to any planning or preparation activity before the entrance of either students or support staff. Synthesizing and implementing means putting into action what was organized earlier. Just as in a research study in which a series of activities must be planned ahead of time, so, too, must teachers design the physical and learning environments they will put to use later in the classroom. In this chapter, both organization and synthesization are subsumed under the term "classroom management." These include welding together human resource environments, curricula, and the administrative procedures.

ORGANIZING THE PHYSICAL ENVIRONMENT

When organizing a classroom's physical environment, a number of activities must be addressed in a brief time. These include equipping and furnishing the classroom and organizing its space. Equipping and furnishing the classroom is a topic rarely, if ever, found in a special education textbook. The success of this activity will depend a great deal on the teacher's ingenuity, creativity, and access to resources.

Basic Classroom Equipment

It is never too soon to begin thinking of the numerous pieces of equipment needed to create an environment that will conform both to educators' institutional style and to the intellectual and emotional needs of students. Creativeness and ingenuity are most valuable.

In addition to individual desks and chairs for each student, the teacher, and any aide(s), some other basic equipment is needed:

- a large rectangular table or other large flat surface suitable for games and activities involving large groups of students
- tables of various sizes and shapes (kidney, oblong, square, rectangular) for a variety of needs (group lessons, learning centers, activity centers)
- chairs for each of the learning centers as well as a few extra for placement near the teacher's desk or the bookshelves
- bookcases of varying sizes to store games, books, and other student-accessible materials and as partitions to separate instructional/activity areas
- cabinets (file and storage), which also can be used for partitions as well as for storing student files, test materials, and small valuable pieces of equipment; a lock on the file cabinet would be extremely useful
- bulletin boards, chalkboards, mirrors, and wastebaskets

Once conventional channels of obtaining equipment such as purchasing or borrowing have been exhausted, teachers should determine what additional equipment would enhance their classrooms and how they might be able to acquire it. Three effective nonconventional means of acquisition are: (1) asking for donations, (2) finding recycled articles and equipment, and (3) creatively using common and easily acquired materials, such as discarded containers, crates, and boxes. People often are willing to donate an old couch or armchair. Old rugs or carpets can improve acoustics and enhance the looks of the classroom while defining floor sections.

Basic Expendable Materials

Most of the materials needed should be available in the school. Teachers should compile a list by determining what already is in their rooms, what they still need, and what they would like to have. Then, when preparing the budget for the coming year, or if money becomes available, the teacher will be prepared to submit a requisition.

Organizing Classroom Space

The physical arrangement of the classroom is crucial to the education of LBP students. Therefore, it should be given much thought and consideration. In addition to representing the teacher's personality, the floor plan should reflect individual instructional needs and the types of tasks that will be taught. Since different tasks often require varying environments, it is not unusual to have a number of different environments in one classroom. Each partitioned area may reflect a certain programming function—reading in a highly structured cubicle, for instance. Flexibility in layout will permit immediate or rapid reorganization of an area for any type of activity. The arrangement of furniture and other classroom objects is discussed in detail later in this chapter.

Room Location

High school special education teachers usually have little to say in the location of their classrooms. If possible, however, they should try to acquire a room that is close to classes of similarly aged nonhandicapped peers. This will facilitate mainstreaming efforts while establishing peer tutorial arrangements using non-handicapped students and improving access to regular school activities.

The classroom also should be accessible to the central office or guidance offices. Resource teachers tend to receive more messages than most classroom teachers, so proximity to a telephone or intercom is important. Also important is the proximity of the classroom to student restrooms. The general rule is that the closer the restroom, the fewer problems encountered with special education students.

When possible, the rooms should receive a good amount of sunlight. Nothing brightens the visual, emotional, and psychological aspects of a classroom more than a good dose of sunlight for several hours a day.

Use of Horizontal and Vertical Space

One of teachers' most important jobs is to create an atmosphere that will foster both emotional and intellectual growth. The horizontal (or floor and ceiling) and vertical (or walls) arrangement of space should demonstrate function while creating an environment that facilitates pupil learning and growth.

Although teachers spend much of their time throughout the classroom, the location of their desks is important. Thomas (1975) suggests having a "teacher station" in the center of the classroom while Hewett (1968) proposes that the desk be at the front of the room and adjacent to a chalkboard. Another suitable location is a rear corner, from where teachers can observe the classroom dynamics without calling attention to themselves.

Similarly, the aide's location should not attract students' attention. However, it should be situated with functionality in mind. When adjacent to the teacher's desk, the aide can perform similar functions. Students also will perceive this location as a centralized unit. When located across the room from the teacher's desk (Figure 5-1), the aide can perform the same duties while maintaining control over additional activities and student behaviors in that part of the classroom.

Learning and activity centers have been shown to be an extremely useful and logical means of organizing a classroom (Hewett, 1968; Thomas, 1975; Volkmor, Langstaff, & Higgins, 1974). Learning centers are areas in which academic and intellectual skills are taught directly; activity centers are areas where intellectual skills are taught through student initiated and directed learning experience. The organization of space should demonstrate a distinct separation between each of these centers yet maintain the image of one classroom. This is a challenge that requires much planning and a willingness to make changes on the spur of the moment.

Career Resource Center

Especially at the senior high school level, one activity core will be the career resource center, an integral component of a total development program. Such a center is designed to provide career information to students and must have current, accurate, and readily understandable information and materials.

Meerbach (1978) suggests the following as useful functions of an effective career resource center: (1) collection, analysis, and storage of career information and materials; (2) retrieval and dissemination of such information and materials; (3) counseling and personal assessment; (4) placement service; (5) work-study coordination; (6) curriculum development; (7) teacher resource; (8) community resources coordination; and (9) a community resource.

The materials and equipment needed to ensure a successful center include:

- career reference books
- occupational files
- college catalogs and directories
- technical school information
- student interest inventories
- microfilm
- reader-printer
- filmstrips

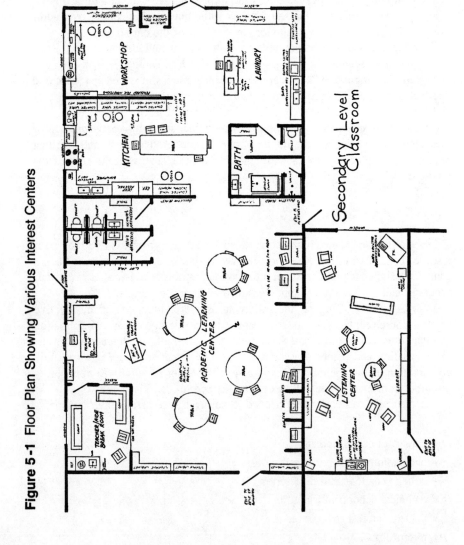

Figure 5-1 Floor Plan Showing Various Interest Centers

Career personnel such as counselors, vocational and trade school personnel, community business, and industrial and professional people also must be available to serve as resource persons to students and teachers. Additional career information systems should be available to students within the school district.

Computerized career guidance systems can be helpful when available. These include the Guidance Information System (GIS), the Oregon Information Access System (OIAS), the Computerized Vocational Information System (CVIS), the System for Interactive Guidance and Information (SIGI), and Project Discover. These programs have the capacity to store, instantaneously retrieve, and update masses of data related to public and proprietary schools as well as 21,741 occupations identified in the *Dictionary of Occupational Titles* (1977). They provide feedback, review, and personalized assistance to counselors or handicapped individuals.

When considering the problems of making efficient use of horizontal and vertical space in the classroom, teachers should:

1. Stand in each corner of the room and take a good, long look.
2. Evaluate the strengths and weaknesses of the existing plan for floor space, or location of furniture, chalkboards, bulletin boards, walls, windows, and ceiling.
3. Involve the students, if possible, by soliciting their suggestions (after all, it's their room, too).
4. Let their own objectivity, the students' ideas, and everyone's imagination run its course.

Later, once an ideal, logical, and functional classroom arrangement has been established, teachers should not hesitate to change it when a new idea or need presents itself.

Flexibility in Furniture Arrangement

Since teachers must be ready to alter the shape and function of the classroom as the behaviors and needs of students change, the planning of the use of the space should be both fluid and flexible. Change often is required on a moment's notice for the scheduled exercise time, play rehearsal, or group dance activity. Teachers will appreciate such flexibility foresight when, within three minutes, they can have 200 square feet of empty space in the middle of the room. Through careful placement of movable partitions and easily shifted furniture, needed space can be created rapidly on a temporary or long-term basis.

Pupil Space Requirements

Just as teachers need a space that is theirs alone, so too do the students. This space should include the desk at which work is done, the drawer in which work materials and personal possessions are kept, and a locker in which coats and sweaters are hung. In addition to recommending a minimum of 100 square feet per student, Hewett (1968) suggests acquiring 2' × 4' tables for each student. A table this size allows the student to spread out work materials. The greatest advantages are that the teacher can combine the tables, vary the distance between them, and reposition them quickly to reorient pupil attention to different parts of the room. Again, teachers should choose the equipment that best fits their needs and those of the students.

The need for pupil space extends beyond the table and chair to the entire classroom. Eventually, every student demonstrates a preference for certain parts of the room. Teacher awareness of personal "territorial preferences" is most important just before some students display aberrant behavior. This often can be circumvented by allowing the students to go where they are most at ease.

Storage Requirements

Thus far the discussion has focused on classroom organization in terms of individual student and teacher needs. In addition to accommodating each person's need for space, teachers also must organize and store their own materials. Their location will be important for their rapid and efficient retrieval and, later, their return to storage.

At least one file cabinet is needed for filing IEPs, tests, data, programs, instructional sequences, treatment sheets, unit plans, and articles. These files also may contain past and present evaluation reports, correspondence, IEP forms, school stationery, and other related materials.

Light, Ventilation, and Acoustic Considerations

When planning classroom design, teachers should pay some attention to three often-neglected elements: lighting, ventilation, and acoustics. These can have profound effects on students' emotional stability and learning ability.

The major purpose of proper classroom lighting is to produce an environment in which the students, barring visual defects, are able to see anything and everything with minimal discomfort and distraction. Teachers should become aware of the environmental determinants of lighting such as the color of walls, ceiling, and floor; the location and size of windows; the placement of lighting fixtures; and the effect of each of these on specific learners working on various tasks.

The sides of the classroom should be noted. It has been determined that, with typical ceiling fixtures, the light level at the sides of a room is less than 50 percent of that in the center (Sampson, 1970). If teachers are planning paper-and-pencil, reading, or other activities demanding moderate to high levels of illumination, these should be conducted four or more feet from the walls. Additional lighting such as a wall lamp or spotlight will increase the amount of highly illuminated space that can be used for instruction. Hellman (1982) presents a synthesis of the research on the effects of lighting and light on humans that should be of interest to special educators.

Even though carpets look nice, act as acoustic deterrents, and serve as environmental markers, it also has been found that dark ones can reduce ceiling illumination by as much as 50 percent (Sampson, 1970). Light-colored rugs, although harder to care for, are suggested for some areas of the room. Windows add to the beauty of a classroom but also present difficulties in maintaining a comfortable light balance. It is important that the room have adequate shades or blinds that will vary the amount of light being admitted (Scagers, 1963).

As for acoustics, the classroom ideally should have acoustically tiled ceilings and walls, with the floor covered with a carpet or large rug. The less noise students have to deal with, the less potential there is for distraction. When organizing a room, teachers should identify areas that: (1) will produce the most noise (e.g., the creativity center), and (2) will require the greatest amount of quiet (e.g., the library). These should be at opposite ends of the room and separated by as many partitions as possible (Figure 5-1, supra). At least one tall partition should be used near each of the noisiest areas.

ORGANIZING THE LEARNING ENVIRONMENT

Once the physical environment has been organized, it is time to start considering the learning environment. In many cases, organizing both occurs concurrently, particularly if time is short. For instance, while teachers may be arranging bulletin boards and awaiting the arrival of extra desks (e.g., physical environment organization), they may have to review curricular materials, organize the instructional materials, and review, survey, and analyze the needs of each student in the classroom (e.g., learning environment organization).

In organizing the learning environment (Figure 5-2), teachers should: (1) survey and analyze each student's needs; (2) establish instructional objectives; (3) organize assessment and datakeeping information; (4) select appropriate curricula; (5) select, make, or order instructional materials; (6) arrange and store instructional materials; (7) schedule teacher, pupil, and support staff time; and (8) set up miscellaneous activities.

Survey and Analysis of Student Needs

Before learning is to begin, educators must know where to start teaching. This entails surveying and analyzing each student's needs. To do this, teachers should locate and examine each student's central file. If difficulty is encountered, the school district should have a copy of each. The file will contain the previous year's

Figure 5-2 Decision Points in Organizing Learning Environment

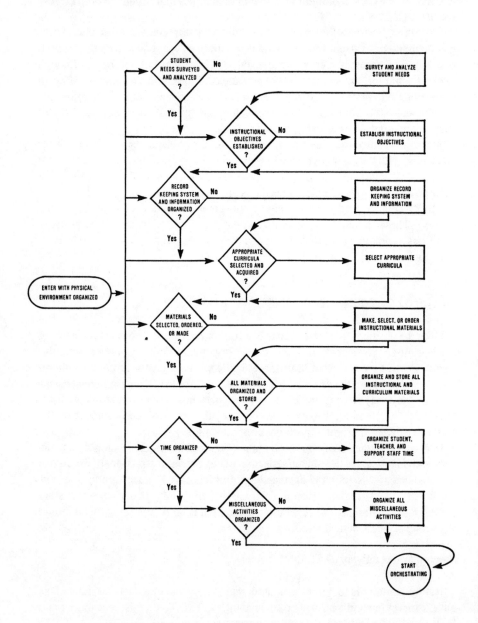

IEP for each student. Which skills were learned and how fast they were acquired should be noted and recorded. Two questions should be investigated: What curricular materials were used to teach each? What were last year's recommendations for this year's instruction? Familiarity with these recommendations will help when the time comes to teach and to write this year's IEP.

Each LBP adolescent's test results last year should be reviewed. These usually are reported in terms of norm-referenced test (NRT) and criterion-referenced test (CRT) results. The NRT results provide a general perspective on each student's intellectual functioning, achievement gains, and strong and weak performance areas; CRT results yield specific information on unknown and already known skills. Student-by-student lists of skills to be reviewed and those to be taught should be compiled. Teachers should determine whether any of these NRTs and CRTs should be used again to test the student at the beginning of the school year. Some district or school policies may require that this be done.

Before testing students, some preparations must be made. Teachers should choose which measurement instruments to use, obtain the appropriate protocols (directions scoring sheets), and familiarize themselves with the manner in which each is to be administered and scored. It is helpful to organize the blank protocols in one folder per student, with the folder labeled in the following manner and placed in a central file in the classroom:

Assessment Info—Month, 198___

Student's last name, first name

Acquiring written parental consent prior to testing is essential. Testing, assessment, and student evaluation are complex procedures that require much forethought and planning. Further information regarding these topics appears in Alper, Newlin, Lemoine, Perrine, and Bettencourt (1973); Buros (1972); Gronlund (1973); Hammill and Bartel (1982); Howell, Kaplan, and O'Connell (1979); Howell and Kaplan (1980); Smith (1974); Snell (1978); Valett (1969); and Chapters 8 and 9 of this book. The data from the use of both CRTs and NRTs with handicapped students should provide more than enough information to start preparing for instruction.

If last year's teacher used some form of instructional data collection or other recordkeeping system, it should be analyzed to determine which programs and which of their parts were successful in teaching the student. Overall, evaluation information summarized in the IEPs will help decide: (1) which directions should be taken in future class activities; (2) what assistance and specialized materials and procedures must be provided for individual students; and (3) what educational progress has been and, therefore, can be made.

Just as important as knowing what should be taught is knowing the students themselves. While reviewing each student's file, teachers should record personal information on an information sheet such as Exhibit 5-1, but teachers may want to develop their own or the school or district may have one that they prefer be used. If so, an information sheet may already have been filled out and included in the student files. These should need only review and updating. If possible, teachers should either contact the parents to solicit their suggestions or visit the students and their families at home before school begins and note any student physical limitation(s) that may require modifications in instructional approach—e.g., partial or total loss of sight or hearing, cerebral palsy. Either the file or the parents can provide information on items and activities that were reinforcing for the adolescents and that can be prepared, purchased, or initiated during the first week of school.

Establishment of Instructional Objectives

Once each student's IEP and folder have been reviewed, teachers should have enough information to start specifying and organizing the individual's instructional objectives for the upcoming year. (This assumes, of course, that the data and information from last year's IEP and recommendations for this year's instructions are both reliable and valid.) Later, current student tests will yield additional instructional information. For the present, however, there should be enough information available to establish instructional objectives for each adolescent. Since the IEP is the accepted vehicle for organizing and communicating such information, it is suggested that the state, district, or school IEP format be used from the first day for data recording, flow, and communication. If a format has not been authorized, then one should be chosen immediately or a form developed containing all of the needed subsections. Sample format and other IEP preparation information may be found in Arena (1978); Hudson and Graham (1978); National Association of State Directors of Special Education (1978); Turnbull, Strickland, and Hammer (1978); and Chapter 6 of this book.

In some cases, the school district may have adopted a packaged system that will provide continuing or formative evaluation data. This should prove valuable when writing the IEP. Annual or summative evaluations also may be available for each student. The school secretary, principal, director of special education, or director of pupil personnel in the district can say whether such a system exists. It is important that all teachers make certain they are aware of the deadline for IEP development for the state and/or district. In any case, they:

1. should not reinvent the wheel but should use last year's instructional suggestions as a foundation and springboard for this year's program
2. should describe specific student performance levels, stating both instructional goals and objectives, and establish priorities for teaching across the three domains: cognitive, psychomotor, and affective (Bateman, 1971)

Exhibit 5-1 Model Information Sheet Based on Student Files

Name _____ Date _____
Age _____ Birth Date _____
Hair Color _____
Eye Color _____
Height _____
Weight _____
Parent or Guardian's Name(s)

_____

Parent or Guardian's Address

_____
_____
_____ (Zip) _____

Parent or Guardian's Telephone Number

_____

Physical Limitations (If Any):
  Sight _____
  Hearing _____
  Epileptic Seizures _____ Frequency _____
  Physical _____

Medication:

_____ _____ _____
_____ _____ _____
_____ _____ _____

Behavior Problems:

_____ _____ _____
_____ _____ _____
_____ _____ _____

OTHER

Signed By: _____ Program Director
            _____ Program Coordinator

Miscellaneous:
  Independent Play Skills _____
_____
  Leisure Time Activities _____
_____
  Interacts with Peers/Adults _____
_____
  Prevocational Skills _____
_____

Exhibit 5-1 continued

Communication:
  Verbal (Speech) _____

  Nonverbal _____ (Sign Language) _____

  Receptive Language Skills _____

  Expressive Language Skills _____

Behavior Problems
  (Procedures, If Any) _____
  _____
  _____

Medical Concerns _____
  _____

Sleeping Habits _____
  _____

Type of Clothing Most Beneficial for Student _____
  _____

Foods (Likes, Dislikes) _____
  _____

Likes, Dislikes (In General) _____
  _____

OTHER

3. should draft objectives in observable and recordable terms, including an agent (or student), the behavior (or action or verb statement), the conditions (or givens) under which the behavior is to occur, and some criterion(a) for acceptable performance (Howell et al., 1979; Kibler, Barker, & Miles, 1974; Mager, 1962; Mager & Pipe, n.d.; McAshan, 1974; Popham & Baker, 1970)
4. should include this information on the appropriate IEP form

A copy of this should be left in the classroom and should be examined periodically and modified if necessary throughout the academic year. The advantages of using objectives are evident as they: (1) allow the teacher to select, substitute, and rearrange course topics into instructional sequences; (2) facilitate individualization efforts; (3) improve evaluation of instruction; and (4) help in the formulation of skill-based instructional groups (Bateman, 1971; Hawkes, 1971; Richey, 1979).

Organizational Recordkeeping Information

During the first week of school teachers are responsible for obtaining certain information, such as: (1) pretest and other recorded data; (2) material from each student's file and IEP; and (3) miscellaneous legal, medical, and permission forms.

Pretest and Other Data

The establishment and organization of instructional objectives go hand in hand. Similarly, the continuing collection of evaluation and other types of information require some means of organization if the data are to be analyzed easily. How efficiently teachers collect and organize the data is determined in part by the types of questions asked and information acquired and in part by the means by which these details are assembled. The types of questions asked and related methods of recording data are outlined in Exhibit 5-2. These are discussed at length by Howell et al. (1979), and Snell (1978), and by Fimian and Goldstein in Chapter 9 of this text.

Exhibit 5-2 Questions Asked and Data Collection Method

Question Asked	*Data Collection Method Used*
(a) How long does the behavior occur?	(a) duration recording system
(b) How often does the behavior occur?	(b) frequency or event recording system
(c) Does the behavior continue to occur for a long period of time?	(c) continuous or anecdotal recording system
(d) At what rate, or how fast, does the behavior occur?	(d) rate recording system
(e) How much teacher assistance, across time, must be provided to allow the student to perform a given task?	(e) points-scored recording system
(f) What percentage of correct/incorrect or appropriate/inappropriate responses occur in a given sitting?	(f) percent correct/incorrect or appropriate/inappropriate recording system
(g) How many behaviors occur, each of which results in a lasting product (e.g., the *number* of pages read, puzzles completed), given a preestablished time period?	(g) recording of direct measurement of achieved tasks

Data recording methods vary from classroom to classroom. However, Smith and Snell (1978) suggest as minimum procedures that teachers should: (1) describe the target behavior in observable terms, (2) identify the characteristics of that behavior and select the appropriate measurement procedure (Exhibit 5-2), (3) select an evaluation design to test the effect of intervention on the behavior, (4) specify any condition for observation that will yield an accurate measurement (e.g., when, where, and for how long the behavior will be observed), (5) construct a data recording form or specify the method of data collection, (6) collect the data through observation, and (7) display the data graphically.

These and subsequent data analysis and communication techniques are discussed elsewhere (for example, see Howell et al., 1979; Howell & Kaplan, 1980; McCormack, Chalmers, & Gregorian, 1978 ; and Chapter 8, infra). It should be kept in mind that the modification of a student's behavior is the primary goal of this process.

Confidential File and IEP Information

The acquisition and organization of information from these sources have been discussed. Every attempt should be made to safeguard the confidentiality of this material.

Miscellaneous Information

It is the teachers' responsibility to obtain, as early as possible, various legal, medical, and permission forms from each student's parent(s) or legal guardian(s). First it must be determined what forms must be completed after checking with school administrators, nurse, and other related professionals. When possible, these forms should be hand-delivered to the parents (possibly during the home visit) with a request that they be returned promptly.

It is important to be aware of policies that might affect the student's attendance since many states require certain medical and dental interventions such as vaccinations within one month of the start of school. This information should be related to the parents and, if necessary, they should be reminded with a letter and/or telephone call. Once these forms are returned, this should be indicated by a checkmark next to the student's name on a list prepared for this purpose, and a check on the forms themselves. The forms are placed in the student's file immediately and ancillary service personnel (e.g., nurse, psychologist) are informed that the completed documents have been obtained.

Selection of Curricula

Before reviewing and selecting various curricula, teachers should look at the materials that either have been used with their students in the past (these may be noted on last year's IEPs) or that are available and readily attainable within the school or system or a local special education resource center (a call to the district or state office of education can determine whether and where there is one).

In either option, teachers may borrow and use curricular materials for some period of time; however, loaners are provided for only a month or two, so it is essential to plan appropriately. Borrowing materials on a short-term basis may not be particularly valuable from the standpoint of long-term instruction but will prove important if these are needed to tide classes over until previously ordered items arrive. This option also allows teachers to review materials at no cost and can help them decide whether or not to purchase them. Unless teachers are familiar with specific materials, they should not purchase them based only on their catalog advertisements; instead, they should be obtained on a review-before-deciding-to-purchase basis. This will save time and money in the long run.

Charles (1976) developed the following list of materials usually supplied by the school district:

construction materials	flat pictures
drawing materials	motion pictures
painting materials	filmstrips
models and displays	recordings
collections and specimens	duplicated materials
maps and globes	magazines and newspapers
charts, diagrams, and graphs	professional books
posters	encyclopedias and other references
drawings and paintings	textbooks
photographs and transparencies	supplementary books
curriculum guides	reading programs
language kits	math kits
motion picture projectors	science kits
filmstrip projectors	chalkboards
slide projectors	bulletin boards
opaque projectors	flannelboards
overhead projectors	paper cutter
projection screens	lettering sets
phonographs and tape players	microprojectors
tape recorders	microscopes
duplicators	Language Masters (pp. 178-179)

Subject Choice

The choice of subjects will vary from classroom to classroom, student to student, and teacher to teacher. Tool skill areas such as reading, mathematics, spelling, writing, and language are universals for most handicapped students (Hammill & Bartel, 1982; Howell et al., 1979; Perry, 1974). Self-care, music, art, language arts, sensorimotor functions, cognitive development, prevocational and vocational training, motor skills, and social skills represent less frequently taught but perhaps equally important curricular areas (Perry, 1974).

Some students will not be capable of mastering the tool skill areas such as reading and mathematics; instead, training in social skills, prevocational skills, gross and fine motor skills, and language may prove more important in meeting their needs. Again, what will be taught or not taught will depend primarily upon the needs of the individual students. Many will take specific subjects such as English, history, or biology in a variety of settings as listed in Exhibit 6-1 (infra).

Availability of Materials

According to Charles (1976), there are several ways in which materials can be used by teachers: (1) to catch and hold the students' attention, (2) to allow for tangible operations and manipulations, (3) for motivational purposes to encourage activity, (4) to allow for student observation, (5) to extend the students' experiences, (6) to provide new experiences, and (7) to depict and summarize concepts.

Most teachers have a wide selection of instructional materials available from several sources. Availability is no small matter; if teachers do not already have what they need, and cannot acquire it through conventional means, they might have to resort to alternate choices. Once sources such as the classroom, school, district, and local and state materials centers are exhausted, it is time to consider two other options. The first is to make the materials. However, because of extensive use of teacher time and the expense involved, this generally is not a good idea. Much time already will be spent writing programs based on specific objectives and modifying existing curricula. As often as possible, the development of total curriculum programs should be left to the specialists.

The second and more frequently chosen option is that of purchasing the materials. Teachers should check with their principal or director of special education to determine the school year planning budget and the possibilities for acquiring additional money, if needed. It must be remembered that this amount has to be distributed across eight or nine months. It is wise to get the opinions of professionals who have had experience with these materials, then consult a number of catalogs. The prices of items should be noted and the overall cost of the desired materials then compared to the yearly budget. The total cost may be distressingly high. To return to financial reality, teachers should review their original list and differentiate between necessities and frills. This will demonstrate that a surprising number of apparent "needs" actually are not all that essential.

Before ordering the materials, it is important to remember: (1) sales taxes and shipping add to the overall cost; (2) the order must be cleared with immediate supervisors, who may have insight into the availability of materials as well as special school system procedures regarding their acquisition; (3) any order—even a "rush"—may take months to be delivered, so materials ordered in September should not be expected to arrive before Thanksgiving; and (4) one reason the budget is so small may be that last year's "thoughtful" teachers used this year's money to order materials in the late spring for their successors' use in the fall. If the materials have not been placed in the teacher's room, they may be stored in central receiving somewhere.

When reviewing curriculum materials for purchase, a number of points should be kept in mind. Numerous variables related to the curriculum to be used, the students to be taught, and the teacher who will instruct will determine the appropriateness of given courses for a specific situation (Exhibit 5-3). Once these variables have been considered from the general case standpoint, a specific review of the materials should follow. Wilson (1978) groups these as follows: (1) bibliographic information and price; (2) instructional area and skills, scope/sequence; (3) component parts of the material; (4) reading level of material; (5) quality; (6) format; (7) support materials; (8) time requirements; (9) field test and research data; and (10) method, approach, or theoretical bases. Additional concerns and criteria are outlined in the National Education Association's booklet *Selecting Instructional Materials for Purchase: Procedural Guidelines* (NEA, 1972).

Commercial Materials

A number of authors have compiled extensive lists of curricular and instructional materials—a task beyond the scope of this chapter. To determine which materials would be appropriate for review, and which publishers produce them, any of the following sources can be helpful:

- Wilson (1982) reviews some 500 curricular programs on areas such as reading, vocabulary, spoken and written language, mathematics, and perceptual-motor skills. Each material is rated in terms of its function (primary, elementary, intermediate, junior and senior high, and in some cases, normed grade level) and the publisher's name. She also lists names and addresses for approximately 125 publishers, curriculum groups, and vendors.
- Blake (1974) provides extensive lists of materials and programs in each of the following areas: oral language, reading, written language, arithmetic, and personal-social skills.
- Perry (1974) and Valett (1969) offer additional lists of curricular sources.
- The staff at the curriculum laboratory at the local state university or special education resources center should be able to provide numerous references for, and samples of, curriculum materials.

Exhibit 5-3 Curricular, Student, and Teacher Variables To Be Considered in the Purchase of Curricular Materials

Curricular Variables
  1. Content area targeted
  2. Specific skills to be taught
  3. Theories and techniques associated with the concepts
  4. Methodology employed
  5. Modifiability of materials

Student Variables
  1. Needs of the student
  2. Current functioning level of the student
  3. Group potential across students
  4. Preference of programming or presentation style
  5. Preference of presentation methods
  6. Physical, social, and psychological characteristics of the student

Teacher Variables
  1. Teacher preferred philosophy and methods of instruction
  2. Teacher preferred instructional approach
  3. Time constraints that preclude curriculum use
  4. Training that may be needed
  5. Previous training history of the teacher

Source: Adapted from Judy Wilson. Selecting educational materials and resources. In D.D. Hammill & N.R. Bartel (Eds.), *Teaching children with learning and behavior problems* (3d ed.). Boston: Allyn & Bacon, 1982, 411-413.

Instructional and Other Materials

The previous section discussed the review, selection, and acquisition and/or purchase of curricular materials. Some materials used in the classroom every day have little or nothing to do with established or marketed curricula. These include teacher-developed or adopted instructional matter, play or leisure articles, audio-visual items, housekeeping equipment and supplies, and health and first aid supplies.

Instructional Materials

Instructional materials are acquired in a number of ways. The simplest, least time-consuming, but costliest method is that of ordering manipulatives and instructional materials from educational catalogs. These usually are available already from other teachers, in the main office, or the district special education office. The considerations discussed earlier in reference to buying curricular items hold true in this case, too.

The most time-consuming, yet least costly, acquisition method is for teachers to make as many of the materials as their time and resources allow. If a ready supply of waste items discarded by businesses, factories, and others is immediately available, they constitute a valuable source of raw materials. For example, one of the authors of this chapter, in the early 1970s, once entirely supplied a classroom—including all the furniture, partitions, and most of the instructional materials—for a total cost of a little more than $100. Those were early 1970s dollars, but even with inflation, the total a decade or so later still would be less than $200.

A median compromise between these two options involves browsing through a major materials outlet (there usually is at least one in every large city). Teachers can requisition through their school district all materials they cannot make, and can study and draft plans in a small notebook for those they can make. Aside from a reasonable outlay of materials and time, all else that is required of innovative teachers is a bit of creativity, elbow grease, and sometimes even sweat.

Instructional materials include an extensive number of purchased or teacher-developed items that can be used in conjunction with curricular matter. In the high school resource room, materials used in the regular class setting in which the students normally would be enrolled should be available to the special education personnel assigned to the youths. If the students are assigned to a self-contained special education program, the teacher may borrow materials from the learning center, purchase them through normal requisitioning procedures, make them, or obtain them on loan from the community library, business, industry, agencies, or professional enterprises. Charles (1976) lists community sources of free and inexpensive materials:

> airlines and travel bureaus for posters, itineraries, leaflets
> telephone company for leaflets, dry cells, wire
> lumber yards for sawdust, wood samples and scraps, plastic
> hardware stores for metal, scraps of various kinds
> food stores for cartons, boxes, cardboard, packing material
> department, food, and drug stores for old window displays and
>   advertising materials
> Salvation Army for inexpensive children's books and games, old cloth-
>   ing for costumes
> National Dairy Council for pictures and posters of dairy products
> local newspapers for old newspapers, samples of print and type
> carpet stores for carpet and drape samples and remnants
> pharmacies for plastic bottles, tongue depressors
> television repair shops for discarded resistors, transistors (p. 184)

Audiovisual Materials

Audiovisual materials usually are costly to purchase, moderately difficult to maintain, and used with a frequency that suggests they are better copurchased and coemployed with one or more other teachers. Teachers can ask around the school to find out what is available and what the staff feels is needed. Suggested and often-used materials are: manuscript and cursive alphabets, art items, cassette recorders, cassettes, charts, films, filmstrips, filmstrip viewers, globes, listening station equipment, maps, overheads, overhead projectors, pictures, movie and slide projectors, radio, record players, records, screens, slides, tapes, television, View Masters with reels, microcomputers, telelecture units, computerized educational programs, electronic video games, etc. The selection, acquisition, utilization, and care of audiovisual materials are discussed at some length by the NEA (1972).

Housekeeping Equipment

Housekeeping materials may be kept either in the classroom or in a janitor's closet. These may include push and corn brooms, buckets, cleansers, dishpan, dustpan, mop, sink strainer, sponges, towels, and wastebaskets. Extreme caution should be taken when storing cleansers and soaps in the classroom. Alkalies, lyes, poisons, or other fatal chemicals or dangerous equipment never should be stored anywhere other than in a locked janitor's closet.

Health and First Aid Materials

Health and first aid materials may or may not be stored in the classroom. School, district, or insurance regulations will determine this. Band-Aids, gauze, handkerchiefs, Merthiolate, medicated soap, tweezers, blankets, and a cot are commonly needed items. If they cannot be stored, teachers must know the location of and how to attain quick access to the first aid cabinet.

Organizing and Storing Materials

The way materials are stored in the classroom will contribute to how, and how often, they are used. Placing materials in the back of deep shelves, in the bottom of standing lockers, or on the top of tall cabinets will limit their accessibility. In some cases, however, as with general classroom materials or first aid supplies, this may be desired. In general, all materials, including curricular items, should be categorized and shelved by subject area as soon as they arrive. Categorization schemes could include assigning one shelf for speech matter, one or more for academic or programming materials, one for gross- and fine-motor items, one for special materials, and one for special curricular materials such as reading or mathematics programs. Each shelf should be labeled so the staff and students know where to return the materials. Small items are best kept in labeled shoeboxes. Larger space-consuming materials such as television sets are best stored in a locked closet to prevent theft.

Instructional materials specific for one type of task or related to an activity center are best kept at the activity center. For instance, on a table or carrel allocated for a language training center, any or all of the following materials may be found: typewriter, Language Master, tape recorder, individual filmstrip projector and selected filmstrips, and a library of assorted reading materials (Valett, 1969). Teacher-developed instructional programs, articles, IEPs, lesson plans, and other flat materials are best kept in a filing cabinet or box or crate.

SYNTHESIZING THE INSTRUCTIONAL ENVIRONMENT

Establishing Communication

In many special education settings, a team approach has been adopted. Therefore, the specialist professionals who participate are important insofar as they may act as role models and provide advice concerning the teachers' professional behavior. They are important to the students insofar as they will be directly involved in providing or delivering some kind of services to them. (The administrative staff usually provide the resources and personnel to teach; teachers, therapists, and aides actually deliver those services on a direct pupil-contact basis.) Without all this support, aid, and understanding, the teachers' job may not develop as rapidly or extensively as it could otherwise. Conversely, without teachers' support, assistance, and understanding, the effectiveness of the specialist professionals' roles will be equally limited.

It cannot be stressed enough that lines of communication be established during the first week and fostered every week thereafter. It must be kept in mind, for instance, that support staff members don't really work for the teachers; like the teachers, they work for a common employer and the students to whom they are assigned. In short, functioning as a team requires certain professional characteristics on the part of all. These include (1) the willingness to give and receive constructive criticism, (2) the ability to work closely and cooperatively with others, (3) the commitment to provide and improve upon the education services delivered to each student, and (4) a willingness to share responsibility for the decisions of the team (Richey, 1979).

If teachers cannot adopt or exhibit these characteristics, they are not prepared to function as team members and therefore should not. If a job requires team membership, therefore, it is best that teachers examine their own feelings and attitudes on this relationship before accepting such a position.

To facilitate communication, teachers should meet with team members early and often. During the first week, it is helpful to invite them into the classroom, show them what has been going on, and solicit their advice and suggestions. They should be asked about what they do and how they do it. They will want to find out what the students are like and to discuss any peculiarities of working in the particular school. The dimensions, qualities, and professional characteristics that make a team approach successful should be discussed. These include cooperation and accommodation, professional strength and knowledgeability, and the diversity of perspectives that a number of professionals can contribute to any school staff.

Implementing the Daily Schedule

Implementing the daily schedule takes a certain degree of skill and expenditure of energy on the teachers' part. Many a teacher will relate stories about the annual struggle to reduce classroom inertia by building momentum. Just as a car starts from a stationary position and starts to pick up speed, so do classrooms. Unless the driver steps on the accelerator, the car won't reach a desired speed. Similarly, unless teachers make efforts to adhere to the classroom routine, model behaviors to maintain and strengthen the existing schedule, praise staff members and students who are always prompt, keep the transition periods short, and spend much of the time in actual instruction, their classroom may never reach desired speed.

If the school does not have a bell system, teachers should adopt some method of keeping informed of when the periods begin and end (e.g., an alarm clock, timer, wristwatch alarm). It also is important to make sure that all staff members involved in the classroom are aware of the teacher's schedule and how they fit into it. If it is impossible for them to meet that schedule, it should be changed for their convenience. Allowing them first priority when the daily class schedule is set up should facilitate this.

Implementing Assessment Activities

After the students have arrived, it is time to consider their evaluations. In many cases, teachers will know a great deal about what to teach from studying the youths' IEP files and last year's final test results. Based on this information, teaching for at least part of the school day should begin right away. The balance of the noninstructional time may be used for evaluation, using information in each student's folder and/or other appropriate measurement tools. When testing, teachers should remember the following:

1. Some tests—norm-referenced tests, for instance—have established and formal procedures for their use; other tests—typically criterion-referenced tests—may be given on a much more informal basis.
2. Schedule all assessment activities for the morning. Many students will not yet be acclimated to the school year schedule, and will fatigue quickly. Testing tired students may result in biased results.
3. Spend some time with your students before assessing them. If using a "Hi-I'm-your-new-teacher-glad-to-meet-you-sit-down-and-take-this-test-for-me" approach does not bias the test data, it may color your students' perceptions of you as a teacher.
4. Explain to the students why you are giving them each test. Also, be sure they know that it is not meant to put them "on the spot" and that it is acceptable to admit those things they do not know. In all cases, monitor observable manifestations of fatigue, test anxiety, and possible confusion regarding their expected test performance. (Howell et al., 1979)

Implementing Curricular, Teaching Activities

Many teachers and their classrooms have an inertia problem at the beginning of the school year when it comes to implementing curricular and educational activities.

During the first week of school, teachers should develop each student's IEP. This time-consuming process is alleviated by many of the preparatory activities that already have been conducted. What remains is to put each student's instructional goals and objectives in writing in a fashion that says "This is what we are (I am) going to teach this student this year." The best time to start this is after the pupils have arrived and while pretesting procedures are being conducted or completed. For suggestions on developing, monitoring, and evaluating IEPs, note Arena (1978), Hudson and Graham (1978), National Association of State Directors of Special Education (1978), Turnbull, Strickland, and Hammer (1978), and Chapter 6 infra.

If the curricula that are to be used in the classroom have not been thoroughly reviewed, now is the time to do so. Teachers should ask themselves the following questions: What special provisions in terms of materials, time, and faculty behaviors are required to implement the curricular learning experiences? Are there enough materials so they can be used concurrently by a number of students? If not, can the schedule be rearranged so that the curriculum can be used in subsequent periods? Are all necessary materials available that will allow teaching to start immediately?

Teaching means many things to many people. In this chapter, the term is limited to the actual instructional interaction that occurs between teacher and students.

Although this sounds like a simple process, it actually is very complex. In light of this, Bateman (1971) suggests addressing certain core attributes of instruction before getting "fancier" in classroom presentations. "Teaching" from this perspective is: (1) obtaining and maintaining pupil attention; (2) presenting concepts through clear and nonconfusing terms and presentations; (3) eliciting clear and unambiguous responses from each adolescent, whether in group or individual instruction situations; and (4) reinforcing and/or correcting student responses immediately and diplomatically. Nonstructured and impromptu situations should be anticipated and met as they arise to allow for spontaneous learning in the classroom.

Implementing Behavioral Programs

Too often the behavioral program is represented in the same negative light as are management programs. That is, given a problem child, what do teachers do with the adolescent? The authors and others (McCormack, 1978; Walker, 1979) suggest that, in light of both appropriate and inappropriate behavior on the part of each student, teachers anticipate establishing proactive (or positive management and reinforcing) as well as reactive (or problem management and intervention) behavioral programs, as needed, with all students. Should teachers anticipate problems? Yes, there may be some. Should they anticipate only problems? By all means, no. Being prepared for anything, negative or positive, reinforcing or intervening, is the mark of a good teacher.

The purpose of any behavior management program is twofold: (1) increasing the duration, frequency, or strength of appropriate classroom behaviors while at the same time (2) decreasing the duration, frequency, or strength of inappropriate behavior. Techniques commonly used to increase the frequency, duration, or strength of any behavior are: (1) employing positive support in the form of activity reinforcers, consumables, manipulables, visual and auditory stimuli, social stimuli, and/or tokens; (2) employing avoidance or escape situations; and (3) demonstrating appropriate behavior via shaping, modeling, or imitation techniques. Techniques commonly used to decrease these factors are: (1) extinction; (2) punishment; and (3) time out.

Any reinforcing event can be described in terms of a number of parameters: (1) schedules of reinforcement that describe how often and at what time the step is used in any given situation; (2) an amount of reinforcement that varies from situation to situation—too much, too early will satiate the student, whereas too little, too late may not have an effect on modifying the behavior; (3) the timing of the reinforcing event that will have an effect on how much the behavior is modified—the sooner the reinforcement follows the behavior, the greater its effect upon that behavior (Fimian, 1978). Any of the following source materials can be helpful: Ayllon and Azrin (1968), Bandura (1969), Harris (1972), Neisworth and Smith (1973), Skinner (1974), Sulzer and Mayer (1972), Walker (1979), Walker and Buckley (1974), and Watson (1973).

PULLING IT ALL TOGETHER

A variety of additional activities should be implemented, starting during the first week and continuing throughout the school year. These are outlined in the checklist in Exhibit 5-4. Key questions to be answered follow.

Is the physical layout of the classroom appropriate for what is needed? Has the classroom been equipped and furnished with everything that is needed? If not, have the needed items been ordered, assuming this can be done with the budget? Is the horizontal and vertical space used efficiently, yet presented appealingly? Is any expansion or other modification of the present space anticipated during the upcoming year for which arrangements should be made now, or equipment and furnishings purchased? If any of these remain outstanding questions by the end of the first week, a review of the section of this chapter "Organizing the Physical Environment" is in order.

Have all concerns related to the organization of the classroom as a learning environment been addressed by the end of the first week? Has the teacher started to survey and analyze each student's needs, to establish instructional objectives for each one, and to organize a recordkeeping system? Has the teacher selected appropriate curricula, obtained/made/ordered selected courses and other instructional materials, organized and stored these in easily accessible places, and set up short-term classroom activities via a daily schedule and long-term teaching and professional activities via a monthly reminder?

Some of these activities must be started and completed during the first week, while others must be started during the first week but realistically may not be completed for weeks or even months. Which are most important for the classroom? And when should they be initiated and completed? As the answers to these questions vary from classroom to classroom and teacher to teacher, only each individual educator can tell for sure.

The checklist in Exhibit 5-4, however, should help in addressing and meeting these considerations, activities, and deadlines. The checklist offers a number of first-week organization and synthesization activities as outlined in previous sections of this chapter. These activities, listed on the left, are rated in terms of (1) each one's order of priority, and (2) the goal date to complete each activity. Once each activity has been prioritized as being either very, moderately, or of little importance, a realistic goal date should be set for the completion of that activity.

Exhibit 5-4 Checklist for Organizing First Week's Activities

Activity	Status		Priority			Goal Date for Completion
	y	n	1	2	3	
Classroom Organized?						
Classroom equipped & furnished?						
Space organized?						
Learning Environment Organized?						
Student needs surveyed & analyzed?						
Instructional objectives established?						
Recordkeeping system organized?						
Curricula selected & acquired?						
Materials selected, ordered, made?						
All materials organized & stored?						
Time organized?						
Miscellaneous activities organized?						
Instructional Environment Synthesized?						
Professional communications established?						
Daily schedule implemented?						
Assessment activities implemented?						
Curricular and teaching activities implemented?						
Behavioral programs implemented?						
Is it all pulled together?						

Status Key

y = yes, this activity has been completed

n = no, this activity has not yet been completed

Priority Key

1—very important

2—important

3—it can wait

SUMMARY

Special education teachers at the high school level never should assume that their newly assigned classroom will meet their preconceived expectations. Many of the components described in this chapter represent the ideal, or what is perceived to be the ideal, for effective education to take place. It is quite possible that the teacher may have access to various materials or be assigned to an acoustically sound, well-ventilated, and properly lighted classroom. This type of assignment generally is the exception rather than the rule. In light of this, it is the teacher's responsibility to make the best of an often less-than-perfect situation. For that reason, a number of make-do suggestions have been offered.

Suggestions have been provided on organization of the physical, learning, and instructional environments. Implementation of these points depends mostly on the teacher's ability to be creative and adaptable. An additional quality that would help is the ability to be persuasive, particularly in communicating needs to the proper authorities so they may obtain the needed hardware, software, physical, instructional, and learning environments that teachers have identified and feel are necessary to be effective in their work.

Chapter 6

IEPs for LBP Adolescents

Bruno J. D'Alonzo and Michael J. Fimian

INTRODUCTION

On November 29, 1975, President Gerald Ford signed into law a $7.8 billion measure to assist the states in the education of their handicapped children. This law—Public Law 94-142—called for a greatly strengthened federal commitment to ensure the provision of free and adequate educational services to all children in this country, regardless of their handicaps. Nearly two years later the final rules and regulations for implementing the law were published (Federal Register, August 23, 1977). This milestone represented half of a decade's efforts by sponsors, parent groups, lobbyists, and other supporters to help meet the educational needs of handicapped children and adolescents.

This chapter presents not only a variety of concepts related to a key part of that act—the individualized education program (IEP)—but also a procedural analysis to help practitioners develop, monitor, and evaluate IEPs for their students. In so doing, this chapter consists of seven major sections: (1) the IEP defined, (2) an IEP rationale, (3) related concepts, (4) Stage I: developing the IEP process components, (5) Stage II: developing the IEP product, (6) Stage III: from the Individualized Implementation Plan (IIP) to the daily lesson plan, and (7) Stage IV: monitoring and evaluating the components of the IEP.

The ideas and strategies that follow are adaptable to a variety of secondary school systems. Their successful implementation involves integrating the instructional aspects of quality, comprehensiveness, practicality, and realism for these young people.

THE IEP DEFINED

What is an IEP? It is many things to many people. For some, it is an intriguing programmatic and monitoring concept; for others, it is unnecessary and excessive paperwork. The authors of this chapter represent the midground. Having written many IEPs, we may not appreciate the paperwork; on the other hand, we do appreciate both the concept of and need for such advanced planning in written form. The intent here is that by keeping the paperwork to an effective minimum, the concept of the IEP still may be maintained in both the spirit and letter of the law.

The basic principle of providing an appropriate education based on the unique needs of each adolescent with learning and behavior problems is the crux not only of the issue but of the law. This individualized education is achieved principally through the IEP.

A written IEP contains several key concepts: individualized, education, and program. Individualized means that the written program describes the educational needs and services for one person, not a class or group of students; education specifically refers to special education and related services that require specially designed instruction to meet the unique needs of handicapped young people; program means a written statement of what actually will be provided to the individual, as distinct from a plan that provides guidelines from which a program must be developed subsequently.

What, specifically, is an IEP? It is defined in the law, and regulations, as follows:

(a) A written statement of the student's present levels of educational performance;

(b) A statement of annual goals, including short-term instructional objectives;

(c) A statement of the specific special education and related services to be provided to the child, and the extent to which the child will be able to participate in regular educational programs;

(d) The projected dates for initiation of services and anticipated duration of the services; and

(e) Appropriate objective criteria and evaluation procedures and schedules for determining, on at least an annual basis, whether the short-term instructional objectives are being achieved. (Federal Register, 1977; § 121a.346, p. 42491)

The spirit and intent of the act provide flexibility to permit the IEP developers to include more than the legally required data. However, to meet compliance standards, the IEP must include at least these five components, which represent the minimum standards.

Development of a program consists essentially of two components: the IEP meeting and the IEP document. Their purposes and functions as stated in the policy clarification document are as follows:

1. The IEP meeting serves as a communication vehicle between parents and school personnel, and enables them, as equal participants, to jointly decide what the child's needs are, what services will be provided to meet those needs, and what the anticipated outcomes may be.
2. The IEP process provides an opportunity for resolving any differences between the parents and the agency concerning a handicapped child's special education needs; first, through the IEP meeting, and second, if necessary, through the procedural protections that are available to the parents.
3. The IEP sets forth in writing a commitment of resources necessary to enable a handicapped child to receive needed special education and related services.
4. The IEP is a management tool that is used to ensure that each handicapped child is provided special education and related services appropriate to the child's special learning needs.
5. The IEP is a compliance/monitoring document which may be used by authorized monitoring personnel from each governmental level to determine whether a handicapped child is actually receiving the free appropriate public education agreed to by the parents and the school.
6. The IEP serves as an evaluation device for use in determining the extent of the child's progress toward meeting the projected outcomes. (Federal Register, § 1981, p. 5462)

ASSUMPTIONS UNDERLYING THE IEP

An attitude exists, if one agrees to comply with P.L. 94-142, that professionals must adopt the IEP. The question might be raised as to why, because they are professionals, they should do so. This requires outlining at least some of the basic premises underlying the use of the IEP (Morgan, 1977):

- *Premise One: The IEP concept provides a unique opportunity to restructure educational evaluation as a more useful process.* No longer can testing and assessment procedures be used solely because practitioners are required to test and assess students; rather, they are used to provide professionals with relevant and appropriate instructional information.
- *Premise Two: The IEP concept provides a unique opportunity to restructure educational evaluation as a fair and equitable process.* By supporting the concepts that all learners are normal to at least a certain degree, that all differ from one another in varying degrees, and that these differences are normal, professionals can emphasize Premise Three more effectively.

- *Premise Three: No two learners are alike.* Because of this, the IEP should emphasize that handicapped students differ from one another in terms of their needs, capabilities, and receptivity to alternative instructional methods. In so doing, teachers move from the realm of theory to that of practice.

- *Premise Four: School should not be a contest.* Ultimately, competition in the classroom should have only one purpose—improving the individuals' coping with a given task in comparison to their previous performance. However, that improvement need not emerge only through competitive situations. Based on this premise, evaluation becomes more important in that it compares individuals' present and past performances, and less importantly with other students. Evaluating how well Pupil A can do today in comparison with yesterday, last week, last month, and last year, will provide much more instructionally relevant information than by determining how much poorer or better Pupil A did today than Pupil B.

- *Premise Five: The IEP concept will make educators more effective, and therefore, better professionals.* One of the major results—and criticisms—of the IEP is that special education teachers and support staff must spend more time planning for instruction than actually teaching. Some professionals feel they must spend an inordinate amount of time on planning—time that can be put to better use actually teaching the students. Morgan (1977) notes that such a criticism "fails to recognize that exceptional learners require carefully planned and sequenced instructional programs. By specifying instructional goals and objectives and by regularly monitoring learner performance, the probability of successful intervention with handicapped children is substantially increased" (p. 3). In the long run, therefore, the time spent developing IEPs should prove beneficial for each handicapped learner as it will make the task of teaching that much more effective and efficient.

- *Premise Six: The IEP concept will make professionals more accountable.* Given the availability of more effective professionals—because of advanced knowledge, training, and fiscal and legislative support—compliance with the IEP will make them more accountable than previously. In the pre-IEP era special education was responsible for a number of shortcomings (Morgan, 1977), among them:

  1. Many special education programs have been terminal rather than transitional for the handicapped.
  2. Re-evaluation of the student for least restrictive placement has not generally been the primary procedure and this has denied them access to equal educational opportunity.
  3. Services have been promised but not delivered.
  4. The professional role for intervention by teachers has not been defined or carried out.

5. Parents traditionally were excluded from instructional decision making. (p. 5)

Morgan (1977) comments, "It has been said that the trouble with special education is that it isn't special and it isn't education. Careful adherance to the IEP development and implementation process will go a long way toward making the previous statement the exception instead of the rule wherever special education programs are discussed" (p. 3). These six premises are by no means the only reasons educators should be utilizing the IEP concept. There are others, but these are the most important.

PRINCIPAL CONCEPTS OF P.L. 94-142

Thus far, the IEP has been discussed as a concept and as a document, the first representing the spirit of the law, the second the letter. Where does the IEP fit in the entire picture of providing legally mandated services to exceptional children and youths? IEP concepts and terms discussed in this section, including related concepts in the Federal Register (1977), are the following:

Assurance of Students' Rights

1. All students have the right to a free and appropriate education.
2. All students have the right to a nondiscriminatory evaluation.
3. All students have the right to due process of law.

Procedural Safeguards

1. An IEP must be in effect at the beginning of the school year or, for newly identified handicapped students, an IEP meeting must be held within 30 calendar days after placement in special education.
2. Each student should be and will be served in the least restrictive environment.
3. A periodic review of the IEP must be conducted at least once a year and during a formal meeting of the multidisciplinary team.

Parental Right of Involvement

1. Parents have the right to participate in the development of their child's IEP.
2. Parents have the right to sue if dissatisfied with the IEP development team's recommendations.

3. Parents have the right to due process if they feel their child is not being served appropriately.
4. Parents have the right to access to information on their child.
5. Parents have the right of privacy for information on their child.

Nondiscriminatory Testing

1. Testing must be done in the student's native language or other mode of communication, unless it is not feasible to do so, and be administered by trained personnel in conformance with the instructions provided by their producer.

Least Restrictive Environment

1. This assures handicapped students the right to be educated with their normal peers unless valid evidence is available that partial or full removal is necessary.

One of the most important developments involving the concept of the least restrictive environment is the provision of a continuum of educational services (Turnbull, Strickland, & Brantley, 1982). A continuum of services most often is translated into a range of delivery of service environments needed to ensure the appropriate placement of the handicapped secondary school students. The 11 most common of such placement options available are presented in Exhibit 6-1.

Due Process

1. Due process is defined as a formal, impartial proceeding that is convened at the request of either a parent or guardian of a handicapped student or of a school district.
2. An impartial due process hearing usually is held whenever differences involving the education of the handicapped student cannot be resolved by less formal procedures.

The process generally followed in placing adolescents with learning and behavior problems in special education is presented in Figure 6-1.

During this process the parents must be fully informed about their child's status and the proposed action to be taken by the educational agency. This information must be transmitted in written, spoken, or other mode of communication and must be in the native language of the parents. If the student is 18 or older, this information must be transmitted in an identical manner.

Exhibit 6-1 Continuum of Service and Placement Options

Service Option	Descriptor(s)	Summary
Self-contained special education class placement	Segregated; most restrictive	The student is placed in this segregated environment as an individual or as part of a group of individuals with a similar handicapping condition, or as in recent years a new option has emerged, that of placement in a cross-categorical program containing adolescents with mild learning and behavior problems. Instruction, treatment, or therapy is provided by a special educator or therapist.
Part-time, self-contained special education placement and Part-time, self-contained general education placement	Segregated Segregated	Same as above, but also includes part-time placement in a general education classroom setting with a subject specialist providing instruction to an individual or group of individuals with a similar handicapping condition.
Departmentalized special education placement	Segregated	Same as self-contained special education class; however, subjects are taught by special educators with subject area specialization (e.g., English, history, vocational education).
Part-time, self-contained special education placement, and Part-time, general education placement	Segregated Integrated	Same as self-contained special education class, but also includes part-time placement in general education with nonhandicapped students (integrated).
Part-time departmentalized special education placement and Part-time general education placement	Segregated Integrated	Subjects are taught by special educators with subject area specialization (e.g., mathematics, English, history), and additional part-time placement in general education with nonhandicapped students (integrated).

Exhibit 6-1 continued

Service Option	Descriptor(s)	Summary
General education placement with part-time remedial academic, skill development, and tutorial resource placement	Integrated	The student is placed in a general education classroom and spends time periods during the week in a resource room. Instruction is provided by a special educator. Remedial academic instruction, basic skill development (e.g., reading, writing, language, computational skills) and tutorial instruction in specific subject areas are provided.
General education placement with consultative or itinerant resource teacher assistance	Integrated	The student is placed in a general education subject area. General education subject specialists are assisted by special educators and instructional aides in ways to provide appropriate methods, materials, special adaptations, management, and learning experiences for the handicapped student.
General education placement on a full-time basis	Integrated; least restrictive	The student is placed in the general education program and needs minimal or no special instruction or support. The teacher needs minimal or no special assistance.
Special alternative program or school placement	Segregated	The student is placed in a specially designed program or school outside the usual special or general education classroom. These environments are designed to meet the unique needs or problems manifested by such students. All the other previously described environments may not be appropriate. Special educators, therapists, counselors, and general educators work as a team to

Exhibit 6-1 continued

		provide appropriate educational services. This may include the following types of programs: homebound, hospital, residential, instruction in a mobile van, parent involvement, sheltered workshops, or crisis intervention.
Special summer school placement	Segregated and/or Integrated	The student is placed in a special summer school program for diagnostic and assessment purposes, special skill instruction, vocational and career development, therapy, recreation, physical education, or subject area enrichment. A team of specialists works with these students on an individual or group basis, segregated from or integrated with nonhandicapped students.
Community college and/or university placement	Integrated and/or Segregated	Special provisions are made for placement of the student in courses or program during high school years for specialized instruction, therapy, or treatment. Special educators, therapists, and/or general educators provide instruction for the handicapped in a segregated and/or integrated environment.

Source: Reprinted with permission from B.J. D'Alonzo, "Developing Secondary School Individualized Education Programs," in B. Weiner (Ed.), *Periscope: Views of the individualized education program.* The Council for Exceptional Children, © 1978.

Figure 6-1 Network Procedure for Placement of Exceptional Students

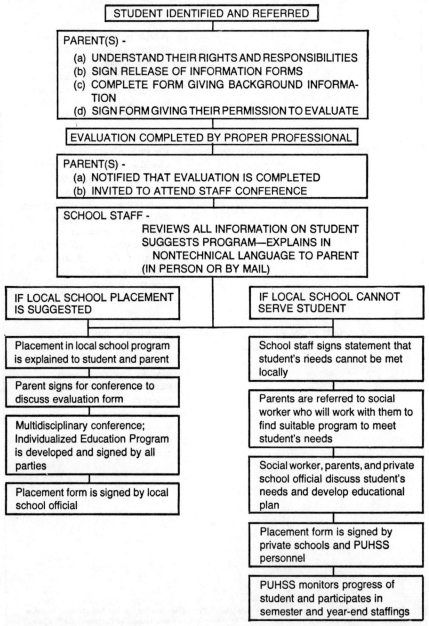

STUDENT IDENTIFIED AND REFERRED

PARENT(S) -
  (a) UNDERSTAND THEIR RIGHTS AND RESPONSIBILITIES
  (b) SIGN RELEASE OF INFORMATION FORMS
  (c) COMPLETE FORM GIVING BACKGROUND INFORMA-
      TION
  (d) SIGN FORM GIVING THEIR PERMISSION TO EVALUATE

EVALUATION COMPLETED BY PROPER PROFESSIONAL

PARENT(S) -
  (a) NOTIFIED THAT EVALUATION IS COMPLETED
  (b) INVITED TO ATTEND STAFF CONFERENCE

SCHOOL STAFF -
          REVIEWS ALL INFORMATION ON STUDENT
          SUGGESTS PROGRAM—EXPLAINS IN
              NONTECHNICAL LANGUAGE TO PARENT
          (IN PERSON OR BY MAIL)

IF LOCAL SCHOOL PLACEMENT IS SUGGESTED

IF LOCAL SCHOOL CANNOT SERVE STUDENT

Placement in local school program is explained to student and parent

School staff signs statement that student's needs cannot be met locally

Parent signs for conference to discuss evaluation form

Parents are referred to social worker who will work with them to find suitable program to meet student's needs

Multidisciplinary conference; Individualized Education Program is developed and signed by all parties

Social worker, parents, and private school official discuss student's needs and develop educational plan

Placement form is signed by local school official

Placement form is signed by private schools and PUHSS personnel

PUHSS monitors progress of student and participates in semester and year-end staffings

Source: Reprinted with permission from *Parent-Teacher Guide to Exceptional Student Programs.* Phoenix Union High School System (PUHSS), Phoenix, Arizona (1980).

Multidisciplinary Approach

As stated in § 121a.344 (Federal Register, 1977) the IEP should be developed in a meeting attended by at least the following participants:

1. A representative of the public agency, other than the student's teacher, who is qualified to provide, or supervise the provision of, special education services to the student.
2. The student's teacher.
3. One or both of the student's parents, subject to § 121a.345 (or legal guardian).
4. The student when appropriate.
5. Other individuals, at the discretion of the parent or agency.

DEVELOPING THE IEP PROCESS AND PRODUCT

This section analyzes the nuts-and-bolts concerns and activities essential to the development of the IEP. First, developing the IEP process involves the seven essential steps outlined in Figure 6-2. This model contains the elements necessary to assist teachers through the orientation, planning, referral, IEP preparation, monitoring, and review activities. Second, developing the IEP as a product or written document is discussed in light of the development activities outlined in the diagram.

Stage I: Developing the IEP Process Components

The seven-step procedural model in Figure 6-2 is applicable to the development, implementation, and evaluation of IEPs in most secondary education situations. Specific procedures vary from state to state, district to district, and school to school. This model represents the minimum procedural activities mandated by P.L. 94-142. Because of this, it is generally appropriate for all IEP situations.

The process starts before the teacher meets future students and continues throughout the remainder of that school year or until the adolescent leaves or is placed in another classroom. This means that the process does not stop after the documents are signed by all concerned, and it most certainly should not stop by filing the document away and out of sight. The seven activities in the IEP process are: (1) orientation and planning, (2) referral of the student, (3) preliminary assessment, (4) IEP preparation, (5) individual program planning, (6) instruction of the student, and (7) monitoring and review of the IEP.

Figure 6-2 Procedural Model for IEP Use

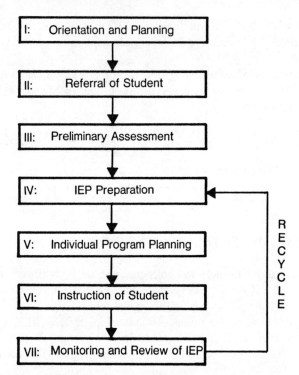

Source: Reprinted with permission from D. Morgan and M.J. Fimian. *The IEP Primer: May the Forms Be With You,* unpublished manuscript, Arizona State University, 1979.

Activity 1: Orientation and Planning

If teachers feel uncomfortable with their level of knowledge on federal legislation, participation in a general orientation on P.L. 94-142 is advised. There usually are persons in district or state offices whose job it is to communicate this information to the persons involved with the IEP.

The teacher then either should plan the overall details of the IEP system that is going to be used or, if a system already is in place in the school or district, should become acquainted with such procedures as early as possible. When reviewing the system that will be used, obtaining answers to the questions in Exhibit 6-2 can be helpful.

The teacher next should orient the parents to P.L. 94-142, the use of IEPs, and such elements as targeting instructional behaviors and prioritizing student objectives (Allen, Budd, Fowler, Peterson, Rowbury, & Thompson, 1978).

Exhibit 6-2 Questions To Ask about the IEP

1. What specific form(s) will be used for recording the IEP?
2. What specific persons will be responsible for developing IEPs?
3. How will parent participation be solicited and encouraged? (e.g., personal contact, telephone, letter)
4. What support or guidance will parents need so they may participate effectively in the decision-making process?
5. Under what conditions will it be appropriate to include the student in the development of the IEP?
6. How will agreement be reached among those responsible for the development of the IEP content?
7. Will other persons be included in the implementation of the IEP?
8. When will educational planning occur for new admissions?
9. When will initial educational planning occur for students currently in the program?
10. What specific persons will be responsible for evaluating whether instructional objectives are being met?
11. What criteria and schedule will be used in evaluating educational plans?
12. How will evaluation data be utilized?
13. How soon after development of the IEP will an educational program be initiated?
14. When will annual case review and updating of the IEP occur?

Activity 2: Referral of Student

This process begins when the student is referred to either the school or district office as one with potential exceptional needs. Referrals may be made by:

Parents of the student   Concerned community members
Private professionals   The student
School personnel   Community agency personnel
District personnel

Referrals may be received by:

Teachers   School psychologists
Counselors   District personnel
Principals

To determine how a referral is made in the local school, the teachers should contact their school or district office.

Next, either the administrator, receiving agent, or referral committee should collect and review existing information on the student and, if necessary, conduct an initial screening to determine whether the referral is both appropriate and warranted. In some cases, the student may not meet the state or federal definition of an individual with exceptional needs. The referral then may be returned, with reasons for the refusal and suggestions for possible educational and instructional alternatives.

Activity 3: Preliminary Assessment

If the referral is accepted and there is a need for more information about the student, the person's behavior, and academic performance and abilities, a preliminary assessment is made. This is necessary as a basis for making informed placement and instructional decisions. Because of federal statutes, the following steps must be undertaken:

1. The school must send a written notice to the student's parents, stating the reason for the assessment, the types of assessment to be done, and requesting their consent to conduct assessment activities.
2. The consulting members of student's review team are chosen.
3. Assessment responsibilities are assigned to appropriate staff members.
4. Assessment is scheduled and completed through the administration of checklists, standardized tests, criterion-referenced tests, and interdisciplinary evaluations; conducting informal observations and evaluations; collecting anecdotal records; and obtaining pertinent information from the parent.
5. Assessment summaries are completed and compiled.
6. Assessment summaries are reviewed for appropriateness and completeness.
7. Further need for assessment is determined. (West, Gobert, & LaCount, 1978, p. 154)

Activity 4: IEP Preparation

Once the assessment information is collected, the next step is to develop the IEP. Federal law now requires that schools provide an IEP for each student who is, or will be, receiving part-time or full-time special education services. This requires that the student study team and the parents meet as a group to share the assessment information, develop and write the IEP, and decide on the youth's placement. These activities may or may not necessitate meeting more than once.

The parents must be informed of the meeting and invited to attend. At the meeting, all assessment information and evaluations are examined, with oral reports by all team members in their areas of expertise.

Based on the assessment information, the IEP is developed and written in at least rough form. During the meeting, the following activities take place: (1) the present level of student performance is summarized orally and in written form; (2) the annual goals are determined and prioritized; (3) short-term objectives are written for each annual goal; (4) support services, the individuals responsible, amount of time, expected duration, and review dates are specified for each short-term objective; and (5) criteria for evaluation are specified.

Once the assessment information has been summarized in at least a rough version on the student's IEP form, it is time to consider placement options. Placement recommendations should be based upon factors such as (1) the goals, objectives, and services indicated on the IEP; (2) state eligibility requirements; (3) the least restrictive environment; (4) the resources and placement options available; and (5) the entry level of the student. Both the placement recommendation and the percentage of time the student will spend in the regular classroom should be stipulated on the IEP. Also at this time, the parents should be informed of their rights and those of their child. Finally, parental consent should be obtained prior to placement. Later, if program continuation is indicated, the parents are to be informed of this. If a change of placement is recommended, parents must be informed and their consent obtained.

Most school systems have not differentiated their elementary and secondary IEPs. Exhibit 6-3 displays a comprehensive IEP that may be useful in secondary schools.

Activity 5: Individual Program Planning

Once the IEP has been developed, but before instruction begins, certain activities should be undertaken by the child study team. It should:

1. rewrite the IEP goals into sequential short-term objectives, if this has not been done already
2. identify methods of and obtain materials for instruction, based on the stipulated goals and objectives
3. develop appropriate data systems to monitor progress
4. plan a new (or modify an old) class schedule and structure activities on the basis of objectives
5. develop home programs with the student's parents, if needed
6. assign specific responsibilities to those who implement the IEP
7. assign administrative and support services
8. establish timelines and deadlines for periodic pupil performance and IEP review for the balance of the school year

Exhibit 6-3 Individualized Education Program—Form 1

Meeting Purpose

Date ____

____ Multidisciplinary Conference

____ IEP Meeting

____ Annual Review

____ New ____ Continuing ____ Change ____ Transfer ____ Termination

IEP Process Checklist

Date ____

____ Initial Referral Made
____ Parents Notified (Evaluation)
____ Parent Approval Obtained for Evaluation
____ Nonacademic and Academic Observations Completed
____ Student Evaluation (formal and informal) Completed
____ Parents Notified and Invited to Multidisciplinary Conf.
____ Multidisciplinary Conference Held
____ Parents Informed of Rights
____ IEP Placement and Program Recommendations Made
____ Parental Permission for Placement Obtained
____ Parents Informed of Appeals Procedure
____ Parents Notified of and Invited to IEP Meeting (if separate)
____ IEP Meeting Held (if separate)
____ Program Entry Date Selected
____ Annual Review Date Selected
____ Reevaluation Date Selected
____ IEP Completed
____ IEP Signed by Meeting Participants

Identification Information

Student's Name _____ I.D. Number ____

Sex ____ Birthdate ____ Age/C.A.[1] ____ Grade ____

Mother's Name ____ Home Phone ____ Business Phone ____

Address ____

Father's Name ____ Home Phone ____ Business Phone ____

Address ____

Child's Address Is: ____ Same as Mother's ____ Same as Father's

Ethnic Group ____ Language or Mode of Communication
In the Home ____ Of the Child ____

District of Residence ____

Exceptional Characteristics - Eligibility ____ Severity ____

Primary Special Education Placement: Regular or Vocational Placement

____ District Program	____ Nonpublic	____ Regular	____ Vocational
____ Joint Agreement	____ Residential	____ Full-Time	____ Vocational-
____ Program	____ Day	____ Regular	Technical
____ Regional Program		____ Part-Time	
		____ Alternative	

Transportation Handled By: Transportation Type:

____ District   ____ Other (specify)   ____ Regular

____ Joint Agreement   ____ Special

Health Information (Report of Medical History and Current Health Status) ____

Yearly Class Schedule

	Time	Subject	Teacher
First Semester			
Second Semester			

Immunization is: __ Complete   __ Not Complete

*Last Vision Screening:	Pass ___	Not Pass ___	Date:	
*Last Hearing Screening:	Pass ___	Not Pass ___	Date:	
Last Medical Evaluation:	Pass ___	Not Pass ___	Date:	

*Completed at time of evaluation or within previous six months.

Significant
Findings   Vision _____
And
Current   Hearing _____
Health   Physical _____
Status: Medication _____
               Side Effects (if any) _____

Doctor's Name _____   Phone _____

1. CA = chronological age

Exhibit 6-3 continued: IEP—Form 2

Case Study Evaluation

	Preassessment Information		
	Major Concerns	Person Noting Concern	Dates
Reason for Referral			
Significant Teacher Observations (Special and Regular Teachers)			
Assessment of Learning Environment			
Significant Parental Input or Concerns			
Social-Personal Developmental Study (Adaptive Behavior and Cultural Background)			
Review of Academic/Vocational History			
Significant Test Data from Previous Administrations			
Other Agency Involvement (Past or Present)			
Interview with Youth			

List All Positive and Negative Forces Affecting the Student in Home and School Environment

Supportive	Constraining	Motivating	Frustrating

Exhibit 6-3 continued: IEP—Form 3

EVALUATION PROCEDURES (Based on Areas of Major Concern)
(see Form 2)

*Types of Assessment Information
Standardized Tests. Normed/Criterion
Rating Scales
Observations: Formal/Informal
Interviews
Checklist
Informal Assessment

Area	Types of Assessment Information*	Standardized Test (Name Instrument)	Date Administered	Persons Responsible for Evaluation
Math: Computation				
Reasoning				
Reading: Recognition				
Comprehension				
Spelling				
Prevocational/Vocational				
Speech				
Listening Comprehension				
Written Expression				
Expressive Language				

Receptive Language			
Visual Perception			
Auditory Perception			
Social/Emotional Behavior			
Gross Motor			
Fine Motor			
Self-Help Skills			
Other (Specify)			

Exhibit 6-3 continued: IEP—Form 4

Present Levels of Educational Performance (Significant Findings and Interpretations)		
Summary Academic Strengths	Level of Performance (Attach addt'l. pgs. if nec.)	Describe Performance (observable behavior)
Summary Vocational Strengths	Level of Performance (Attach addt'l. pgs. if nec.)	Describe Performance (observable behavior)
Summary Social Development	Level of Performance (Attach addt'l. pgs. if nec.)	Describe Performance (observable behavior)
Summary Personal Development	Level of Performance (Attach addt'l. pgs. if nec.)	Describe Performance (observable behavior)

Student Interests:

Student Motivation To Achieve:

Exhibit 6-3 continued: IEP—Form 5

Student's Name _____

Goal 1: _____

	Persons Responsible	
Name		Position
_____		_____
_____		_____
_____		_____
_____		_____

Short-Term Instructional Objectives	Needed Resources	Criteria for Successful Performance	Evaluation Procedure	Evaluated by Whom?	Date Objective Evaluated

Exhibit 6-3 continued: IEP—Form 6

__ New
__ Continuing
__ Change

__ Transfer
__ Termination

__ Multidisciplinary Conference
__ Initial IEP Meeting
__ Annual Review

Student's Name

Participants	Print Name	Signature	Position
Parent(s)/Guardian			
Rep. of the Local District of Residence			
Teacher(s)			
Member of the Evaluation Team			
Child (where appropriate)			
Spec. Ed. Director (Designee) (__ Yes __ No Designee)			
Others Involved in Evaluation			
Rep. of Nonpublic School			
Interpreter			
Other			

The following were explained:

Yes   No

___   ___   Multidisciplinary Conference — Recommended Placement — IEP Meeting

___   ___   I/We have received a copy of my child's individualized education program.

___   ___   I/We agree with the conference recommendations including placement.

___   ___   I/We agree to waive the ten (10) school day preplacement period (initial or change).

___   ___   I/We agree with the proposed evaluation(s).

___   ___   Legal rights, including the right to object to placement, were explained and offered in writing.

Date   Signature of Parent(s) or Guardian

Date   Signature of Staff Member Preparing Conference Report

Exhibit 6-3 continued: IEP—Form 7

Annual Review Meeting

Evaluation of Present Year

	Name of Person Evaluating Child's Achievement	Position

Evaluation Data for Determining Whether the Child Achieved the Short-Term Objectives

1. Summary of Formative Data (daily recorded progress) (charts or forms used to record achievement of short-term objectives)

2. Last of Summative Data (summary at the end of the program period) (types of assessment information, e.g., achievement or posttests, informal assessment, scores, dates)

3. Perceptions of Program Effectiveness
   a. Parent Opinion

   b. Student's Opinion

   c. Opinions of Those Working with the Student

Revisions and Recommended Changes for the Next Year

1. Complete/Revised Information on Form 1. (For each of the following items, record the information on a blank duplicate of the noted form.)
2. Present Level of Educational Performance (Form 4)
3. Annual Goals (Form 5)
4. Special Education (Form 5)
5. Related Services (Form 5)
6. Extent of Participation in Regular Education Program (Form 5)
7. Short-Term Instructional Objectives (Form 5)
8. IEP Participants at Annual Review (Form 6)
9. Explanation of Parental Rights (Form 6)

Source: Reprinted by permission from Southern Illinois University, Department of Special Education, 1981.

Activity 6: Instruction of Student

Until this step, all activities have been of a planning nature. It is time now to actually start teaching and providing learning experiences related to the goals and objectives listed in the IEP. Instruction should reflect the list of short-term objectives usually included in the individual implementation plan (IIP). These usually are written to last for an instructional period of a couple of weeks to one month, are generated from the long-term or annual goals, include a list of instructional materials and resources that will be used to help the student obtain the desired level of performance, and stipulate criteria for acceptable performance.

Activity 7: Monitoring and Review of IEP

This step takes longer to implement than any of the others. Once instruction begins, the IEP is to be used throughout the entire year. Over time, it may be modified in minor ways—usually in terms of listing changes of materials or staff, the addition of instructional objectives, or the deletion or modification of short-term objectives that have proved to be unrealistic to teach the student.

This also is the time during which the teacher and therapists come to know the student on intimate instructional terms by becoming familiar with the skills and concepts that the youth may or may not know, the learning style, and acquisition rate. Given this knowledge, the team can predict more precisely what the youngster may or may not learn, as well as better estimate how long a student will take to learn a certain set of skills. The more the staff members come to know both the student and what the adolescent is capable of, the more proficient they become in writing and rewriting the IEP.

Of course, monitoring and reviewing entails certain staff activities throughout the year. Among these are to (1) review daily and/or weekly performance data frequently; (2) review long-term and short-term objectives every other week; (3) conduct a formal team staffing and parent conference at least once in the fall and spring; (4) conduct a formal posttesting during the last month of the school year; (5) write a year-end report and performance summary for each student; and (6) develop the outline for next year's IEP or develop the IEP itself. This chapter discusses procedures for writing and evaluating the IEP in more detail later.

Stage II: Developing the IEP Product

The results of student assessment should be compiled in one central document—the IEP. Since federal law requires certain specific information to be included in the document, IEP forms usually are developed or adopted by the state, district, or school in which the student has been placed (Exhibit 6-3, supra). The forms include summaries of the assessment and placement information presented at the team meetings.

What type of information is required by P.L. 94-142 and for good IEP program planning? The ten steps in Exhibit 6-4 constitute a helpful guideline. They are discussed in the following sections.

Step 1: Statement of Present Performance

When compiling and reviewing the student's assessment information, educators must keep the following principles in mind. First, assessment information determines eligibility. P.L. 94-142 states who is eligible, yet it is the state statutes that usually dictate how to decide whether or not students should receive services. Just because youths have passed through the referral and assessment stages does not necessarily mean that they automatically are classified as handicapped. If they do not meet some predetermined criteria for exceptionality, they are not "handicapped." Also, because students may have received special education services last year does not automatically ensure their continuance this year. Only further assessment and team meetings will determine this. Second, assessment should be individualized according to the students' present functioning levels. Third, assessment is a continuous process. Fourth, assessment information comes from multiple sources such as tests and formal and informal observation. Fifth, labels do not indicate performance levels. Sixth, assessment should be culturally and linguistically unbiased. Finally, assessment should be sensitive to the child's handicapping condition (Higgins, 1977).

Exhibit 6-4 Ten Steps in Developing the IEP Document

1. Formulate a statement of the student's present level of educational performance.
2. Formulate a statement of annual goals.
3. Formulate short-term instructional objectives.
4. Formulate a statement of the specific special educational services to be provided.
5. Determine the date when those services will begin and the length of time the services will be given.
6. Describe the extent to which the student will be able to participate in regular educational programs.
7. Provide a justification for the type of educational placement the student will receive.
8. Provide a list of the individuals responsible for implementation of the IEP.
9. Provide an outline of objective criteria, procedures, and timelines for evaluating whether the short-term objectives are being achieved.
10. Compile all information on the appropriate form(s).

Source: Adapted from *Federal Register*, "Rules and Regulations Implementing Part B of the Education of the Handicapped Act," § 121a.346, August 23, 1977, p. 42491.

Assessment information should be reported in a language that is understandable to all team members, including the parents of the students. For professionals, this may mean translating their jargon. For parents, this means making the effort to learn about and understand certain basic educational concepts.

Finally, the team should document the individual standardized diagnostic techniques used in the assessment and report the results of the evaluation procedures. After it has been determined that certain students should be evaluated, it must be decided which type of evaluation is appropriate to assess the stated problems. The evaluation is conducted in the students' primary language after obtaining the written consent of the parent/guardian.

If the student problems appear to be limited to articulation, voice, or fluency, the evaluation should include at least: (1) a current audiometric screening, (2) a review of the student's academic history and classroom functioning, (3) an assessment of the functional skills, and (4) an assessment of the speech problem by a certified speech and language pathologist.

For students who are homebound or hospitalized, the evaluation must include: (1) certification by a competent medical doctor that the youths will be unable to attend regular classes for at least three months, (2) an assessment of the current educational level, and (3) such specialized evaluations as are required to understand the specific problems involved.

For all other handicapped students, the evaluation must contain in writing, but be not limited to: (1) the reason for referral; (2) educationally relevant medical findings; (3) their educational history, including documentation of efforts to educate them in the regular classroom; (4) determination of whether their educational problems are related to or resulting from educational disadvantage; (5) development of their history, including information concerning their primary language, cultural background, school achievement, and physical, social, and emotional development; if the primary language of the home is other than English, a home visit must be made to help check these items; the home visit must be conducted only with parent/guardian permission; (6) the types of tests that were administered and their results; (7) recommendations for specific goals and instructional objectives based on current levels of performance needs; (8) the results of a current vision and hearing screening; and (9) an educational evaluation.

In the case of evaluation for work experience, each exceptional student enrolled in such a program should be at least 16 years old. At the time of work-experience program placement, the student should be given a vocational evaluation that assesses aptitudes, interests, and special needs in relation to job placement, leading to development of a vocational plan. The plan describes the goals of the work experience program, including the provision of an education curriculum adjusted to the abilities and needs of the individual student. Assessment data should be used to obtain instructionally relevant information such as: (1) functional levels of performance, or statements describing what the student can and cannot do; (2) rate or strength of performance—how well the student can perform certain tasks in terms of speed, accuracy, or rate; and (3) learning style, or how the student deals with problems and tasks and how the person learns best (Morgan, 1977).

When summarizing the assessment information on IEPs, the team should:

1. list specific skills the youths have acquired, or have yet to acquire
2. list the students' strengths in terms of what skills they can and cannot use
3. avoid vague generalities that may be interpreted differently by various individuals (example: "Appears to be emotionally disturbed")

The team often will find that once the assessment data have been organized, they are to be compiled on the IEP form in a space not much bigger than a large postage stamp. When dealing with such limited space, the team should not resort to giving only performance scores and related test names or abbreviate summary statements by making them too vague or general. If necessary, a summary sheet should be appended to that page of the IEP form, noting this in the space available under the "Summary of Present Levels of Performance" section (IEP Form 4 in Exhibit 6-3, supra). If this first step in the development process is characterized by a lack of precision and carelessness, the rest of the IEP will follow suit.

Step 2: Statement of Annual Goals

These should describe the educational performance to be achieved by the end of the school year, given the services outlined in the IEP.

To develop appropriate and realistic goals for the coming school year, the team must start where the student is at that time—that is, based on present level(s) of academic performance. Such factors as age, grade, amount of education to date, learning strengths and weaknesses, and the student's and family's short-term and long-term plans all must be considered during goal setting. How much will the student learn in one year? The multidisciplinary team will use its professional judgment based on the supporting data available on the adolescent's present level of educational performance to determine appropriate long-term goals and short-term objectives. This is the very best it can do, given the lack of more accurate predictive measures.

Further steps in the selection of long-term goals are establishing priorities, goals, and objectives. When establishing priorities, the team should note any critical instructional or behavioral areas that need more attention than others. As these will become high-priority items, they should be discussed at the meeting by both the professionals and the parents. Stating an appropriate number of goals comes more easily with practice and familiarity with the student. If too many goals are set, none of them may get taught; too few goals can mean that the IEP may need to be rewritten after one month of instruction. Morgan (1977) suggests an optimum of three to five goals per student. The number of objectives generated for each goal statement should represent a manageable number, too. Three to five objectives per goal, for three to five goals, means an IEP with 9 to 25 objectives. More objectives and goals always can be added later.

Step 3: Short-Term Instructional Objectives

Short-term instructional objectives, usually found (but not required) in the individual implementation plan (IIP) section of the IEP (Form 5 in Exhibit 6-3), are much more specific than the related set of annual goals. Based on each of the annual goals, several (usually three to five) short-term objectives are generated. Short-term objectives are milestone steps between the present level of functioning and where the team hopes the student will be by the end of the year, as specified by the annual goals (Hayes, 1977). Of what do short-term objectives consist? The following are instructional components:

1. *Who?* The team should state the range of the student.
2. *What?* The team should state the specific behavior or response that the student must perform to demonstrate skill acquisition. Each behavior must be stated in observable and measurable terms.
3. *Under what conditions?* The team should describe the environmental or instructional situation in which the youth will perform.
4. *How well?* The team should state the criteria for mastery or acquisition of the desired response. Defining successful performance sometimes is difficult, so it is essential to be specific.

These short-term objectives should represent the most critical and highly prioritized needs while including all the related skills or behaviors that the student might reasonably be expected to acquire by the end of the instructional period. This time period is specified on the IEP and usually is the remainder of the school year (West, Gobert, & LaCount, 1978). This often proves difficult the first year of writing IEPs, or the first year of working with a new student. Not surprisingly, many teams find their educational prognosis to be more reliable during their second year with a given student.

While writing instructional goals and objectives, teachers frequently refer to a predetermined list of curricular areas. The student's assessment results, given in light of some curricular framework, facilitate the generation of goals and related short-term objectives. Predetermined curricular areas are available either in program form such as the *Behavioral Characteristics Progression Strands* (1973) or *Instructional Based Appraisal System* (Meyen, 1976), in the form of specific district curriculum guides, or as commercial programs specific to one or a few major curriculum areas such as reading, mathematics, or spelling. A thorough guide to this process is *Teaching Children Basic Skills: A Curriculum Handbook* by Stephens, Hartman, and Lucas (1978).

Before the short-term objectives are entered on the IEP form, they should be arranged in such a way that their relationship to the annual goal is evident and that they are ordered in either a simplest-to-most-difficult or first-to-be-taught to last-to-be-taught order.

For instance, the following are annual and prioritized goals:

Goal 1: To assist the student in awareness of the sources for locating information.
Goal 2: To assist the student in the use of a table of contents (Meyen, 1976)

If Goal 1 is the prioritized area, the teacher should include in order the related short-term objectives on the IIP sheet for that specific annual target. It should be remembered that short-term objectives are just that—short-term. In this case, short-term refers to several periods of time during the school year.

Given Goal 2, to assist the student in the use of a table of contents, the teacher specifies a number of short-term objectives:

1. The student will be able to locate specific information listed within the table of contents, given a textbook, with 90 percent accuracy.
2. The student will be able to use the table of contents to tell what page a story begins on when given the title of a story, nine out of ten times.
3. The student will be able to locate a title in the table of contents and tell how many pages long it is, given the title of a story, with 90 percent accuracy.
4. The student will be able to tell how many chapters, units, stories, etc., are in the book when given a table of contents, with 100 percent accuracy and within ten seconds.
5. The student will be able to tell the title of the story found on a given page by looking in the table of contents, with 90 percent accuracy, at a rate of five story titles per minute. (Meyen, 1976)

Once the annual goals and short-term objectives have been completed, it is time to start arranging for the provision of needed special education and related services.

Step 4: Special Education and Related Services

One of the most important issues to resolve in the team meetings is to determine and list the types of services the student will need. Usually, this is done by reviewing and considering: (1) the IEP objective by objective, (2) all available evaluation information, (3) the student's present level(s) of performance, (4) least restrictive environment options, and (5) the eligibility criteria for exceptional youths.

There appears to be some confusion regarding individual interpretations of the original proposed rules regarding the IEP content area of "educational services to be provided" and the final rules. The original rules required "a statement of the specific education and related services to be provided to the child determined without regard to the availability of those services." The final regulations (§ 121a.346(c)) deleted the clause "determined without regard to the availability of those services."

In short, the developers of the IEP must keep in sharp focus the spirit and letter of the law in the interpretation of the terms free appropriate public education, special education, and related services.

Step 5: Services' Start and Duration

The dates should be listed on an objective-by-objective basis as they occasionally will vary from one to another. Program termination dates usually correspond to the annual IEP review date, which typically occurs toward the end of the school year. If nothing else, the program termination date will be the same as the student's last day of class.

Step 6: Student Participation in Regular Program(s)

The possibility for participation in regular curricular or extracurricular activities increases significantly when placement is made in a physical facility housing regular education programs. Activities in which the student with learning and/or behavior problems traditionally have been integrated are homeroom, assemblies, lunch programs, athletic events, intramural sports, music, art, drama, physical education, home economics, industrial arts, and driver education. Since the core academic courses, including vocational education, have not always been open to these students, it is not always possible to integrate them into these classes. If the placement seems warranted, however, every placement possibility should be explored.

Step 7: Justification for Educational Placement

This requires that the team pass judgment upon and provide a rationale for a placement recommendation. The written justification must be included in the IEP, determined at least annually, and account for a number of factors. The placement must be based on: (1) the IEP; (2) proximity to the student's home, in the school the person would attend if not handicapped, unless otherwise indicated in the IEP;

(3) state and local criteria for eligibility; (4) the services needed and the capabilities of those available, the most appropriate and productive placement when all other factors have been considered; and (5) consideration of any potential harmful effect on the student or the quality of services needed (§ 121a.552).

It is relatively easy to physically place most adolescents with learning and behavior problems in a general education classroom. The question the IEP developers must ask is, "Will the student gain the maximum educational benefit from such a placement, or would a more restrictive one be more appropriate?" If the student can benefit and is qualified for a specific educational placement, the team must always keep in mind that the adolescent has a right to such placement.

Step 8: Individuals Responsible for IEP Implementation

Effectively communicating implementation responsibilities within the team is an important step in ensuring the provision of quality services to the student. When all team members are aware of their specific responsibilities, little confusion occurs once the plan is implemented. For this reason, each team member should review the IEP objective by objective. Then the IEP coordinator should stipulate which staff member is responsible for implementing which objective. Finally, this should be documented in the IEP on an objective-by-objective basis.

Step 9: Judging Progress toward Objectives

P.L. 94-142 establishes legal requirements for the periodic review and evaluation of the IEP. This requires that the team thoroughly and periodically review both the student's progress and the IEP in order to answer the question, "How will we know if the goals and objectives have been met?" To state that "the team has decided" or "it is the expert opinion of the team" is not satisfactory.

To establish the criteria objectively, a statement of the conditions under which the student's performance will be assessed and the standards for mastery must be described. The statement must be in specific terms so that any evaluator can determine whether the objective has been achieved (Morgan, 1977). Furthermore, this should be done on at least an annual basis.

If the short-term objectives have been written correctly, each should contain criteria for acceptable performance. In this case, the teacher notes this in the IEP. If the objectives have been written without the criteria, these should be included in the appropriate place on the form.

Step 10: Information Collection on Forms

This activity represents the stage of pulling it all together. Usually, one team member is assigned the responsibility of gathering, compiling, and writing the information on the IEP format at least in rough form. This may be the special evaluation teacher, the IEP chair, or a delegated representative.

Once the teacher has established the IEP content, the next major step is the actual writing of the document. There are four general but often overlooked steps in producing this document.

First, the writer produces a rough copy of the student's IEP (possibly in pencil). This should include the IEP cover sheet, the short-term objective page, and any other forms the district or school may require. The plan should be put away for a couple of days, then reviewed with a somewhat fresher perspective.

Second, any modifications, deletions, or additions should be made during the second review and before the child study team meets to go over the plan.

Third, since the information on the cover sheet generally is personal data and therefore not subject to modification by the team, this sheet can be finalized and typed before the meeting. At that session, summary information is added and the parents choose to sign or not sign the cover sheet. The annual goals or short-term objective pages should not be finalized yet. They will be modified, added to, or deleted from these forms before the final typed copy is prepared.

Fourth, after the child study team has met to put it all together, annual goals and related short-term ones are reviewed for modifications, additions, and/or deletions. The IEP receives a final review for comprehension, cohesion, and internal consistency, and is then typed.

Stage III: From IIP to Individualized Instruction

Effective teachers follow a process in lesson development that is quite natural and routine. They tend to select activities based on previous experiences or because they "know it is right." But how do they know the activity is as appropriate as it appears? Many teachers unconsciously take their activities through a series of steps to determine their applicability. But they have difficulty delineating those procedures because the process is so natural an aspect of teaching.

The procedure for preparing daily lesson plans consistent with the IEP goals is really quite simple. Any procedure requires relatively strict adherence to the steps but also leaves a little room for that individual touch. This procedure consists of four components.

Component 1: Short-Term Goal and Task Analysis

Teachers should:

1. Select a short-term goal from the IEP. It must, of course, be one in which the adolescent already has mastered all requisite skills. If they have not been mastered, then they should be included as instructional objectives and prioritized.

2. Analyze the skills involved in that goal. The specific skills and objectives involved in goal mastery must be identified. Most short-term goals are not specific, measurable, or broken down into their smallest parts.
3. Sequence the skills. Those pinpointed as component parts of the goal must be ranked so that they are in logical order for instruction. For example, a goal specifying that "the student will add four-digit numbers" assumes that the student already can add three-digit numbers.
4. Evaluate the skills in the hierarchy. It is vital that evaluation take place continuously through the process. After the skills are identified and sequenced, it is important to affirm the correct placement of each in the hierarchy.

The completion of these steps should help ensure that the task to be taught is in its proper position as the first unit of the hierarchy.

Component 2: Evaluation and Activity Areas

In developing a list advancing the process, teachers in the next phase should:

1. Begin with skill no. 1 of the sequence. The lessons must be listed and skills must be taught in a logical developmental sequence. Thus, skill no. 1 not only represents the simplest one but also is a prerequisite for later acquisition of other abilities.
2. Evaluate the youth in this specific skill area. Through formal and informal classroom techniques, the student's learning style, reinforcer preferences, and material response preferences with regard to this particular skill must be identified. This will provide helpful hints for later activity selection.
3. Generate a number of activities. Resources, reference materials, activity files, textbooks, and any other available sources for activities that teach the designated skill should be identified.
4. Select appropriate activities. Some activities in this process will be more conducive to the teaching/learning process of the target skill than others. Therefore, it is important to select only those that are consistent with the student's learning modalities, do not need extensive prerequisite skills training, and are consistent with the adolescent's present level of functioning.
5. Sequence and evaluate the feasibility of activities. The order of the activities should be examined while the appropriateness, feasibility, and applicability of each are reconsidered.

A variety of instructional activities for the first and successive skills of the original hierarchy are generated in this second phase. Teachers must keep in mind that activities involving several of the sensory modalities should be included to reinforce the learning process through the student's individual strengths.

Component 3: Activities, Procedures, Evaluation, and Lesson Implementation

In this multifaceted phase, teachers should:

1. Begin with activity no. 1 of the sequence. This lesson teaches the first skill identified as necessary for attainment of the goal.
2. Analyze the skills involved in the activity. This task analysis provides a system of checks and balances to ensure that the skills are consistent with the target ability.
3. Delineate the procedures. The actual steps to be followed in the implementation of the activity must be specified and sequenced.
4. Gather materials. The specific materials for the lesson should be obtained or prepared in advance and be available at the time of instruction.
5. Alter the environment as needed. Any changes in the physical arrangement of the setting that are necessary for the effectiveness of the lesson should be made before the activity starts. Furniture or seating arrangements sometimes are imperative to control the activity.
6. Identify evaluative measures. The means of evaluation must be consistent with the objective and actually measure attainment of the skill being taught.
7. Implement the lesson. Enthusiasm and creative teaching ability can help make this activity a huge success.

In this component, the units of each activity are delineated, implementing procedures stated, materials obtained, and the classroom arranged to enhance learning. Ways to evaluate effectiveness are described, after which the lesson begins.

Component 4: The Evaluation Procedures

In this phase, the teacher follows up on the criteria just established in order to:

1. Evaluate effectiveness. If the lesson effectively taught the skill for which it was designed, the teacher should proceed to the next activity in the sequence and follow it through Component 3.
2. Call up the next skill. When all activities are completed and the skill is mastered, the teacher should return to Component 2 for the next skill identified in the hierarchy and repeat the process.
3. Return to the starting point. If the skill was not taught during the lesson, the teacher should return to Component 1 and reevaluate the entire process until the point of breakdown is identified, then alter it as necessary.

To evaluate the effectiveness in Component 4, the teacher must compare the student's performance with the criteria stated in each objective. This will indicate the achievement level of the skill being taught and the rate at which the teacher should progress to the next level skill or activity. Whether or not teachers are aware of it, this process is one that most of them think through in some fashion before starting any lesson.

This procedure for developing lessons consistent with IEP short-term goals is a continuing process. As the skills are mastered, ever newer ones are identified and sequenced. As the goals are achieved, new ones are generated. By following these procedures any teacher of handicapped students in any setting, whether it be a regular class, resource room, or self-contained classroom, can provide appropriate activities to teach the goals specified in the IEP.

Stage IV: Objective Criteria and Evaluation

P.L. 94-142 refers specifically to establishing appropriate objective criteria and evaluation procedures for determining the effectiveness of the IEP in providing a free, appropriate public education for handicapped students. Evaluation of the two major components of the IEP, the total service and individual implementation plans, is discussed next. The total service plan is more difficult to evaluate because the long-term goals are more general and not as easily measured. Exhibit 6-5 describes a system that has proved useful in evaluating the total service plan during the early stages, the interim, and the completion of the IEP year.

Through this systems approach, data are collected at various stages in the model. Feedback is provided from three directions: (1) the present status or input dimension; (2) the ease of implementation or process dimension; and (3) the learner achievement or output dimension. This procedure also provides the IEP committee with data as to the effectiveness and appropriateness of the total service plan for a particular student.

The ideal total service plan evaluation would have an "excellent" rating in all three elements. If the ratings fall in the "average" or "poor" range, specific adjustments to those particular factors must be made. If the ratings fall in the latter two when evaluating the present status and ease of implementation, this should not be viewed in a negative light but should alert the IEP committee to a possible problem situation. One of that committee's responsibilities is to identify the components necessary to truly individualize the education and meet the unique needs of the student. New and unfamiliar efforts and acquisitions may be necessary to accomplish these desired results (output). Immediate remediation must be provided to resolve any conflicts or problems that may impede the end result—a free and appropriate public education for the student.

Exhibit 6-5 Evaluation of IEP Total Service Plan

	A. Present Status Input	B. Ease of Implementation Process	C. Learner Achievement Output
Evaluation	Criteria	Criteria	Criteria
Excellent	Individualized education program objectives are appropriate Personnel available in district or school Educational facilities, materials, and equipment available in district or school	Implementing program requires little effort to influence a change in staff attitudes, in district or school policies, structure and training, or educational environment Implementing program does not suggest a radical departure from conventional district or school practices	Learner achievement and mastery of objectives excellent Placement, methods, materials, and instruction appropriate
Average	Individualized education program objectives appear complex Personnel not available in district or school but available elsewhere Educational facilities, materials, and equipment not available in district or school but available elsewhere	Moderate effort required for implementing program to effect change in staff attitudes, district or school policies, structure and training, or educational environment Implementing program requires some departure from district or school practices	Learner achievement and mastery of objectives average Placement, methods, materials, and instruction need review and modifications
Poor	Individualized education program objectives involves new or unfamiliar effort Personnel not available in district, school, or elsewhere Educational facilities, materials, and equipment not readily available	Substantial effort required to implement a program to effect a change in line with attitudes, district or school policies, structure and training, or educational environment Implementing program requires a radical departure from traditional district or school practices	Learner achievement and mastery of objectives poor Placement, methods, materials, and instruction need significant restructuring

Source: Adapted from Exhibit II Standards for feasibility evaluation. In "Cost Effectiveness Comes to the Personnel Function" by L.M. Cheek, *Harvard Business Review,* © 1973, *51*(3), 101.

IIP Evaluation

The IIP can best be evaluated through the use of a checklist. Objectives for each subject area in which the student is enrolled are written on the IIP and also should be placed on a major checklist. Appropriate criteria and performance data also should be established for each objective. The type of performance data for measuring the objective outcome could be:

1. objective met as stated
2. objective partially met
3. objective not met at all

Depending upon the status of each objective, the IEP committee then decides on the appropriate action. Some of the options available are for the committee to:

1. reinstate the objective
2. reinstate the objective with specified modifications
3. remove the objective
4. write a new objective

The teacher collects more precise data at the lesson plan level, using error analysis, task analysis, baseline data collection, and data-based instruction. These should not be confused with the IIP-level evaluation that uses the simple follow-up checkoff system to identify the degree to which the objectives have been met (Exhibit 6-6). The data collection at the lesson plan level is used by the IEP committee to determine whether or not the stated objectives have been met for the IIP. These, in turn, are used to determine whether the long-term goals of the total service plan have been achieved.

Subject Evaluation

The final type of evaluation discussed in this section relates to analyzing specific subjects (courses). For adolescents who manifest learning and/or behavior problems, there generally is a discrepancy between their performance and the standards established by a particular subject teacher. In this teacher's evaluation, this discrepancy most often is reported through the traditional grading system of A, B,

---

Exhibit 6-6 Follow-Up Checklist for the IIP

_____	1. Do instructional objectives reflect the annual goals?
_____	2. Are instructional (behavioral) objectives derived from short-term objectives (goals)?
_____	3. Are instructional objectives written in behavioral terms?
_____	4. Are instructional objectives listed in intermediate steps? Does one objective logically precede the next?
_____	5. Do the pretests and posttests assess the objectives accurately?
_____	6. Have the names of materials and publishers been included under the materials and techniques column? (If materials are teacher-made, state that fact.)
_____	7. If the student did not meet the objective, was "yes" checked on recycle? If the student did meet the objective, was "no" checked?
_____	8. If the student was recycled, was the posttest score used as a pretest score on the second attempt?
_____	9. Was the new posttest score, after recycling, recorded and dated?

C, D, and F. It therefore is imperative that the appropriate placement environment be selected carefully because the performance will be compared to that of the students in the same subject classroom and to the standards established by the teacher, usually without regard to the youths' learning or behavior difficulties. When this placement is in a regular or mainstream classroom, the student performances usually are evaluated on the basis of the subject teacher's standards and not necessarily on the criterion established in the IEP (see Chapter 8 on norm-referenced vs. criterion-referenced evaluation).

MINIMUM CREDITS FOR GRADUATION

Each state and school district has established a minimum number of credits needed for graduation from high school. These generally are referred to as "Carnegie Units," a unit of credit as the study of a subject in high school for one period a day throughout the school year. Numerous administrative systems have been devised to process handicapped students in light of these credit requirements. Whether or not students receive the standard diploma or a certificate of completion of a program of studies depends solely upon the state and/or district in which they attend secondary school. This is an issue that has not yet been completely resolved in some states and school districts. Teachers can contact their state department of education to learn the legal policy that covers their district.

Regardless of whether the students get the same diploma, someone will be teaching specific subjects in order to meet the minimum requirements the youths need to complete high school. The content will be adjusted in level of difficulty to meet student abilities. This will be contingent upon learner ability, program placement, and the teachers.

As one example, Arizona requires the following minimum credits for graduation from high school:

3 units of English, including grammar, speaking, writing, reading skills, advanced grammar, composition, American literature, literature, research methods and skills

1 unit of American and Arizona history

1 unit in American and Arizona constitution and government

4½ units of essential benefits of the free enterprise system

1 unit of mathematics

1 unit of science

8½ units of electives such as vocational education, industrial arts, physical education, driver education, foreign language, typing, or drama.

For purposes of writing IEPs at the secondary level, a program of studies should be developed to incorporate the minimum requirements of the state in which the student attends school, possibly within the range of the 11 least restrictive placement options described in Exhibit 6-1, supra. Each credit requirement should be matched with and developed around the unique needs of each student. The annual IEP should be written with these required credits in mind. A complete program of studies and a tentative master IEP, once developed, should be kept in each student's file.

SUMMARY

The formal content of the IEP document is intertwined among numerous sections of federal and state laws. The law is far reaching, spanning the nation and touching the lives of every special educator and of each adolescent identified as manifesting a learning and/or behavior problem. For the first time ever, the country has a standardized system of IEP development that is relevant to every student, whether attending school in Steubenville, Ohio; Chicago; Ajo, Arizona; or Honolulu. It is a remarkable accomplishment to see special educators around the country linked by a standard procedure dedicated to the delivery of a free and appropriate education to all handicapped children and youth. The magnitude of this venture, despite its rough edges, should be a source of deep pride to all special education teachers and educators.

Chapter 7

Instructional Approaches and Curricula for LBP Adolescents

Suzanne Lanning-Ventura, Maribeth Montgomery-Kasik, and David A. Sabatino

INTRODUCTION

This chapter presents two major premises:

1. that 10 to 12 percent of the adolescents in secondary schools are handi-capped, the majority by mild impairments that can be grouped for instructional purposes into learning and behavioral problems (LBP)
2. that the education of these youths requires a change in educator attitude and in traditional instructional practices.

Instructional programs can be viewed in terms of the process by which they are delivered to adolescents, the content, or what actually is taught, and the delivery procedures themselves. This chapter reflects the instructional focus of the text, discussing two major special educational approaches—remediation and tutoring—and their underlying instructional practices and theoretical constructs. It explores assessment procedures, objectives, and enabling steps, providing examples of several remedial practices along with materials that are useful in secondary schools. It looks at tutoring as an academic support mechanism for students learning under a special educator in a resource room or learning center.

The chapter also provides suggestions and samplings from selected material lists and reviews instructional practices, materials, and methods that special educators might consider using in self-contained classes to some degree—but most assuredly in resource rooms and learning centers. As will be seen, few materials are new; special educators have merely borrowed heavily from their colleagues in remedial education. However, the presentation here is greatly different, drawing from a well-grounded diagnosis of the learner characteristics for the youths in question. Unique to special education is the direct remedial work on learner characteristics or processes, described in some detail. The reason is that remediation of academic skills is a final objective. Failure to achieve success in that objective may be explained by the adolescents' perceptual, memory, language, academic learning, and behavioral characteristics that underlie their learning problems.

REMEDIATION AND TUTORING

For all youths, but especially those with learning and behavioral problems who have failed to achieve academically to grade level, some serious questions must be raised.

The first question could be the most difficult; it asks whether those offering the instruction know why the youths are failing to achieve as they should. The answer also is most difficult, and in recent times, those interested in operant conditioning principles with human beings have advised, "teach, not test" (Gold, 1980). They contend that valuable instructional time is wasted in attempting to diagnose adolescents through scores that do not seem to relate to instructional or behavioral management anyway.

They probably are right to some degree. Formal scores from standardized tests do not provide a basis for preparing instructional objectives. However, the scores do not provide for a diagnosis, either. They merely present comparison data on individuals. In short, they compare one person's performance on a given task to others who performed that function in a test.

Instructional diagnosis is an outgrowth of examining the intraindividual performance of students in terms of:

1. Medical history: do the students see and hear normally, is their motor performance as it should be, do they have any acute or chronic physical or mental problems that could interfere with school?
2. Psychological history: do the students relate to themselves, their peers, and significant others by displaying appropriate behavioral responses to social cues and drawing attention to favorable aspects of their behavior? Adolescents should be developing sound decision-making skills based on self-reliance, which means their value systems should be reasonably compatible with society. There is nothing wrong in teaching the importance of values as long as respect is conveyed for the values of all parties.
3. Educational history: can it be determined what is wrong through understanding how former instruction has been presented, what was taught, and when it was presented? Teaching an academic skill can begin too early in a child's development. A particular teaching method may stress a type of delivery inappropriate for a specific learning style, student characteristic, or simply the interests or preference for education that the youths choose.

4. Learning preferences: how do LBP students evidence priority for learning in one sensory-perceptual modality over another? They may show poorly developed (or, in contrast, well-developed) memories. They may display unusual language learning characteristics.
5. Learning characteristics: what are some of the hypothesized learning characteristics? A learning characteristic is a mental trait or process that permits environmental information to make sense to the person. Some youths have perceptual problems—that is, they fail to see letters or hear sounds as they really are. Others do not receive words as meaningful units, or receive words as meaningful units, but have difficulty expressing their meaning in writing or speaking.

Simply then, if youths display behaviors that interfere with learning, those behaviors should be corrected before instruction emphasizing academic skills is practiced.

Therefore, if learner characteristics can be isolated as a behavioral variable interfering in education, theoretically they should be strengthened or instructional materials (methods) should be used to avoid them (bypassing them). If there is sufficient strength in the learner characteristics to warrant teaching academic achievement skills, then remediation may be undertaken. If students respond favorably to remediation or basic skill learning, they may profit from being placed in regular educational settings and receiving support on direct instructional activities in the classroom, i.e., history, science, math, etc. Tutoring then is amelioration of a subject area curriculum where the basic skills are verified and comprehension developed.

ACADEMIC ACHIEVEMENT AND REMEDIATION

Remediation is one of the most important and widely practiced programs in the secondary schools. It often has been equated with tutoring—a great error by many regular and special educators and those dealing with special populations. What are the differences between remediation and tutoring?

Remediation includes working with a learner's cognitive processes, but frequently it focuses solely on academic skill training. Generally it involves assessment of a problem area that is interfering with a student's ability to achieve academically. Once the diagnostician has assessed the learner's deficit, specific behavioral objectives are compiled and tasks are provided to remediate the problem or help the adolescent compensate and perform better academically.

Tutoring, on the other hand, refers to academic and study skills where the tutor teaches a specific academic or vocational subject. Some educators (Scranton & Downs, 1975) believe that once a learner reaches the junior high school level, remediation is not effective, although others believe that as students grow older they still may benefit from systematic remediation. As is demonstrated next, it is possible to combine process area techniques and academic subject area remediation.

For example: incorporate the Visual, Auditory, Kinesthetic Tactile (VAKT) multisensory system for the teaching of spelling. Adapted to the secondary learner, it would be as follows:

Teacher: "Say the word 'Administrative.' "
Student: "Administrative."
Teacher: "Write each letter and say them aloud as you are writing."
Student: "A-d-m-i-n-i-s-t-r-a-t-i-v-e."
Teacher: "Say the word."
Student: "Administrative."
Teacher: "Turn your paper over and spell the word Administrative."
Student: "A-d-m-i-n-i-s-t-r-a-t-i-v-e."

The learner has utilized visual, auditory, tactile, and kinesthetic senses. To perform this task, the learner needs to use at least the following broad behavioral processes:

visual perceptual memory
auditory perceptual memory
visual perceptual discrimination
auditory perceptual discrimination
eye-hand motor coordination
visual and auditory integration
receptive language
central language
expressive language

All of these mental process areas are directly related to academic learning. One premise is that, if remedial techniques are expanded to include cognitive process at the secondary level, the students will be able to generalize from that training to their academic and vocational learning tasks as well.

The implementer of remediation could provide tasks that range on a continuum from easier to the more complex. This can provide adolescents with success and act as a reinforcer of their successive approximations in acquiring/retaining new skills. Success in remediation generally relies on two rules: (1) knowing when to initiate a program and (2) sequencing tasks into small, crucial steps, ensuring success on each.

An analogy that perhaps is too simplified that can be used with students equates the remediation process with physically exercising the body to develop strength—

lifting weights and running will tone both the upper and lower muscles of the body if built into a routine, which avoids exercising all muscle groups at the point just below the overexertion level. This holds true with learning. The more individuals practice a given task, sequenced into small enough steps to be undertaken with success, the more they learn to generalize newly acquired strengths to other achievement areas. Though very basic, this analogy has been effective in helping students rationalize the importance of both cognitive process and basic skill training. Some secondary adolescents can be informed of the mechanics of their disability as an aid in learning to compensate. Teachers must be aware that not all students can handle information about a learning or behavioral disorder with emotional maturity.

Sabatino (1981) speaks of remediation as a viable element in secondary schools in that it should occur in relationship to a student's interest and in support of meaningful academic, social, personal, and vocational goals. This section provides specialists working with academically deficient students with examples of remediation procedures with a wide range of possibilities.

The first step in remediation is assessment to obtain information about the learners, their deficit areas, and their levels of functioning. Thus, a formal or informal assessment may precede the instructional planning process.

Assessment Techniques

Formal Assessment

Formal assessment uses standardized tests and usually is part of a case study or psychological evaluation designed to find the best placement for a student. Bush and Waugh (1976, p. 101) suggest the following diagnostic battery for secondary students:

Specific Visual and Auditory Problems
  Bender Visual-Motor Gestalt Test
  Wepman ADT (Auditory Discrimination Test)

Achievement
  Key Math Diagnostic Arithmetic Test
  Woodcock-Johnson Psycho-Educational Battery

Intelligence Tests
  Stanford-Binet—Form L-M
  Draw-A-Person
  Wechsler Intelligence Scale for Children—Revised (WISC-R)
  Wechsler Adult Intelligence Scale (WAIS)
  Peabody Picture Vocabulary

Development and Communication
Purdue Perceptual Motor Survey
Detroit Tests of Learning Aptitude
Hiskey Nebraska

Sabatino, Miller, and Schmidt (1981, pp. 392-395) list other examples for assessment of secondary process deficits:

Frostig Developmental Test of Visual Motor Integration
Memory-for-Designs Test
Wechsler Memory Scale for Adults
Developmental Test of Visual-Motor Integration
Woodcock-Johnson
Specific Language Disability Test
Tests of Auditory Perception
Inventory for Language Abilities
Quick Neurological Screening Test

Any of these tests may be used to give the diagnostician an idea of where the learner may be functioning.

Informal Assessment

Usually informal assessment is done by the special educator. It consists of a criterion reference device for an assessment that should tell what the students know and do not know and where they are functioning on academic achievement learning tasks.

Remediation Techniques

Using the following hints, the team working with the secondary handicapped learner should:

1. Utilize task analysis, an important component that will aid remedial teaching. In remediation, tasks generally are designed in an instructional sequence governed by a hierarchy of behavioral objectives that state what the learner is to accomplish. A criterion for mastery and specific time expectations also should be indicated.
2. Utilize behavioral management techniques to structure the environment, such as:
   a. contingency contracting: student and teacher create an agreement spelling out the desired behavior and consequences.

b. positive reinforcement: the teacher rewards desired outcomes with positive reinforcers such as social events, activities, tokens.

c. the Premack principle, or grandma's rule: the teacher uses anything learners like to do more to reinforce any behavior they like to do less; or, "finish your work before you go out to play."

d. peer recognition and tutoring: the teacher allows students to help each other with strong and weak areas, with peers offering praise when desired outcomes are obtained.

e. modeling: the teacher provides a positive model of a desired outcome for the students to follow.

f. immediate feedback: the teacher lets the students know as soon as possible "how they did."

3. Be direct and concise when structuring the learner's task:
   a. repeat and simplify instructions
   b. use cues and/or prompts
   c. provide models
   d. be sequential

4. Use remedial materials, teacher manuals, Ditto masters:

Auditory Areas
   Perceptual Communication Skills
   Of Course I Can
   Basic Practice in Listening
   Language Master
   Tape Recorders

Visual Areas
   Michigan Tracking
   Veri Tech—Language and Math Tiles
   Developmental Learning Materials
      (DLM) Peg Patterns
   Teaching Resources—Small Mosaics
   Dubnoff Rubber Bands
   Individualized Order Tasks
   Tangrams

Games for Integration Experiences and Motivation
   Battleship
   Chess
   Trac-Four
   Psyc-Paths
   Speak and Spell
   Calculators

Expression
   Writing

Quantitative
Oral expression
Affect
Body language

Cognitive Process Remediation

"Cognitive process instruction is based on a simple premise: cognitive processes can be studied and students can benefit from the knowledge gained through such studies" (Lockhead, 1979).

It is important to gain an understanding of just what the cognitive processes are and how they relate to learning. "Perception is a cognitive process that gives meaning to sensation: perceptual motor activities are those that link the perception of events with motor-based responses. What is needed now is an earnest attempt to view perception as a functional process in the natural sequence of human development" (Sabatino, 1981, p. 219).

According to Sabatino, this requires:

1. more stable measures of perceptual traits, developed from models employing functional explanations of the processes
2. teachers who are well versed in the complex theories of perceptual and visual-auditory perceptual integration
3. teachers who can develop perceptual curricula to meet specific needs
4. elimination of motor and language contamination
5. a teaching emphasis more congruent with nature—more specifically:
   a. perceptual training based on objectives designed to improve perceptual development
   b. specific perceptual training directed at modifying either discrimination or memory processes in either an auditory or visual perceptual modality
   c. a strong emphasis on perceptual training in the preschool and early school years
   d. perceptual training when learning efficiency no longer is the question because of serious learning disability
   e. perceptual training as an alternative to persistent tutoring of academic subjects and remediations of academic skill deficits in support of language and other cognitive training
   f. perceptual learning for children with moderate learning disability and most children with severe learning disabilities as an initial objective to badly needed prevocational skills, including functional academics. (p. 219)

Valett (1974) offers a list that is helpful for remediators. Some deficit areas that are prevalent among secondary learners have been selected and modified from Valett's Psychoeducational Definition of Basic Learning Abilities:

Auditory-Perceptual Discrimination	A.	The ability to understand sounds or spoken words.
	B.	Student can follow simple verbal instructions, can indicate by gesture or words the meaning or purpose of auditory stimuli such as animal sounds, nouns, or verbs.
Auditory-Vocal Association	A.	The ability to respond verbally in a meaningful way to auditory stimuli.
	B.	Student can associate with verbal opposites, sentence completion, or analogous verbal responses.
Auditory Memory	A.	The ability to retain and recall general auditory information.
	B.	Student can act out (charades) simple plots of common stories, can verbally relate yesterday's experiences, meals, television, and story plots.
Auditory Sequencing	A.	The ability to recall in correct sequence and detail prior auditory information.
	B.	Student can imitate specific sound patterns, follow exactly complex series of directions, repeat digit and letter series.
Visual-Perceptual Discrimination	A.	The ability to visually differentiate the forms and symbols in one's environment.
	B.	Student can match identical pictures and symbols such as abstract designs, letters, numbers, and words.
Visual Memory	A.	The ability to recall accurately prior visual experiences.
	B.	Student can recall from visual cues where reading in book stopped, can match or verbally recall objects removed or changed in the environment, can match briefly exposed symbols.

When the specialist is preparing to remediate a deficit area of the secondary school learners, that professional actually is the individual with the handicapping condition—that is, unless the person is very innovative and creative at developing materials and adapting tasks to more advanced students. The problem is that little material is available for working with secondary learners' cognitive processes because in follow-up junior high classes these areas often have been discontinued as not of any importance. It was felt that the child would out-grow any perceptual problems by this developmental stage.

Just as there is a lack of assessment materials for secondary learners and adults, there also is an absence of ready-made materials. Teachers must rely on their own ingenuity.

The following suggestions are designed to give remediators a starting point. The examples include long-term and short-term behavioral objectives. The long-term goal is general—the hoped-for outcome over time; the short-term goal is what the learners should be able to do after/during a specific lesson. The goals are stated in terms of observable behaviors. These are intended to be a starting point in developing IEPs for specific students.

AUDITORY, AUDITORY SEQUENTIAL MEMORY

Long-Term Objectives

1. Auditory Memory: The students will demonstrate the ability to retain and recall information presented auditorily.
2. Auditory Sequential Memory: The students will demonstrate the ability to recall in correct sequence auditory information.

Remedial Suggestions

1. The visual approach is combined with the auditory.
2. Visual aids should be used wherever possible.
3. The students are given a sentence, then it is repeated with a word left out. The adolescents are to complete the sentence properly, inserting the missing word.
4. The students are given a short sentence and asked to repeat it. After the first repetition, more words may be added for the learner to repeat.
5. The teacher dictates several digits and asks the students to repeat them.

Sample Short-Term Objectives

In the areas of auditory and auditory sequence memory, the adolescents will demonstrate the ability to:

1. recall a given number of specific facts from a story when they previously have been given cue questions before the reading
2. recall the correct sequence of events of a story
3. repeat words spelled orally
4. relay simple messages
5. listen selectively for specific information

Exemplary Lesson: Auditory Memory

Long-Term Objectives

1. Auditory Memory: The students will demonstrate the ability to retain and recall information presented auditorily.
2. Auditory Sequential Memory: The students will demonstrate the ability to recall incorrect sequence auditory information.

Short-Term Objective

1. The students will (a) repeat orally and (b) write correctly a series of two to seven dictated digits with at least 95 percent accuracy.
2. The remediator reads the digits:
    1, pause, 2
3. The students respond:
    1, 2

Sample Digital List

2 digits	3 digits	4 digits	5 digits	6 digits	7 digits
12	219	4567	67452	654091	9000000
10	189	7623	43261	783217	4431654
32	347	2894	54672	444321	2019382
97	745	4328	67843	879000	5444432
98	220	9085	96542	998765	6107432
21	237	5357	64533	550998	7654321
43	251	4321	21126	876000	8978675
39	743	6543	45689	987013	9087231
78	761	5768	32211	986513	9198256
98	520	1239	21052	091237	6543210

Note: This same activity can be used with words, letters, syllables, sounds, and events.

AUDITORY CLOSURE

Long-Term Objectives

1. Auditory Closure: The students will integrate nonmeaningful elements of the environment into meaningful wholes and sequences.
2. The students will synthesize isolated sounds, letters, words, sentences, and stories into a whole.

Remedial Suggestions

1. The teacher institutes a sample activity: sound blending, dictating partial words.
   Example: beau___ful = beautiful
2. The teacher gives an assignment in which the initial, middle, or ending consonants or vowels may be left out of a word.
3. The teacher starts a story and the learners finish it.
4. The teacher starts an open-ended sentence, and the students fill in an appropriate word.
   Example: 1. My name is _____.
             2. I like _____.
             3. I go to _____.
             4. I see _____.
   (The difficulty should be increased progressively.)
5. The teacher asks Yes and No questions.
   Example: 1. "Does school get out at 8 o'clock?"
             2. "Do parents always have children?"
             3. "Do jets fly higher than birds?"

Sample Short-Term Objectives

In the area of auditory closure, the adolescents will demonstrate the ability to:

1. complete incomplete sentences
2. sound-blend words when they have been given in broken forms in the context of a sentence
3. sound-blend compound words broken into roots
4. avoid extra sounds when blending
5. explain how part of the word is related to the whole (roots, prefix, suffix)

Exemplary Lesson: Auditory Closure

Long-Term Objectives

1. The students will integrate nonmeaningful elements of the environment into meaningful wholes and sequences.
2. The students will synthesize isolated sounds, letters, words, sentences, and stories into a whole.

Short-Term Objective

1. The students will insert a meaningful word into a given sentence when presented with 10 sentences.

Activity

The remediator dictates each sentence, leaving out a word. The students response is to write a word that adds meaning to the sentence.

Sample: Janie is not at school today because she is home sick with a

_____.

The students' response should be: cold, fever, etc.; unacceptable: candy, dog, or any other unclear response.

1. Janie has on a _____ blazer.
2. Janie _____ visiting with her grandparents.
3. Sandy will come _____ at Christmas.
4. _____ is necessary for pasting the chart.

The remediator starts with word parts and words, moves to sentences, then stories, gradually increasing the difficulty of the task to accommodate the adolescents' progress.

AUDITORY DISCRIMINATION

Long-Term Objective

1. The students will demonstrate the ability to receive and distinguish similarities and differences in auditorily presented information.

Remedial Suggestions

1. The remediator tape-records familiar sounds, then asks the adolescents to identify them.
2. The teacher reads a story with a certain repeated sound, word, or phrase; the students raise their hands every time they hear the sound. The difficulty of this exercise may be increased by adding distracting stimuli.
3. The teacher asks the students to say whether two words are the same or different.
4. The teacher tells the students to close their eyes and listen to the sounds in and around the room and try to identify them.
5. The remediator dictates sequences of words, several beginning or ending with the same consonant except for one. The students are asked to identify the word that does not belong.

Sample Short-Term Objectives

In the area of auditory discrimination, the students will:

1. identify individual sounds
2. identify the location of sounds
3. identify (a) loud and soft sounds and (b) high and low sounds
4. identify likeness and differences in pairs of similar words
5. identify words that rhyme

Exemplary Lesson: Auditory Discrimination

Long-Term Objective

1. The students will demonstrate the ability to receive and distinguish similarities and differences in auditorily presented information.

Short-Term Objectives

1. The students will identify the different musical instruments in a given musical composition.

   Activity

   Remediator: Plays a record for the learner of the "1812 Overture."
   The teacher says: Relax and listen to the music with your eyes closed. Try to picture in your head the orchestra playing.
   The teacher starts the record over and says: This time raise your hand if you hear a clarinet, trumpet, drum, etc.
   The remediator also may instruct the students to stop the tape at that point.
2. A variation of this would be to have the students bring in their favorite rock tapes and try to write down the words to the songs. The teacher should check how many times they need to stop the tape or start over. Students should compare what they think the words are to what one of their peers or the remediator may think. The youths could prepare a songbook of their favorite tunes this way.

AUDITORY ASSOCIATION

Long-Term Objective

1. The students will demonstrate the ability to interpret and understand the information they hear and to follow verbal instructions.

Remedial Suggestions

1. The remediator should allow sufficient time for the students to respond.
2. The teacher should ask them to practice finding similarities and differences.
3. The teacher should spend time in discussion with them, tape their responses, and have them listen and comment.
4. The teacher should utilize incomplete sentences.
5. The teacher should ask the students to complete familiar analogies.

Sample Short-Term Objectives

In the area of auditory association, the students will demonstrate the ability to:

1. identify similar components of words to be placed in a category
2. complete sentences started by the remediator
3. respond correctly to a question by selecting from multiple choice clues given by the remediator
4. complete sentences using opposites
5. identify absurdities in a story

AUDITORY COMPREHENSION

Long-Term Objectives

1. The students will demonstrate the ability to understand and comprehend (get the intent of) what they hear in a meaningful way.
2. The students will respond correctly to directions.

Remedial Suggestions

1. The remediator should supply the students with words, sentences, and phrases so that they have more to draw from.
2. The teacher provides the students with the components and asks them to identify the object.

Part	*Whole Response*
spokes, gears, reflector	bicycle
ignition, carburetor, transmission	automobile
recycle, pollution, conservation	ecology
tent, propane stove, lantern	camping
referee, player, touchdown	football
keys, pedals, ivory	piano

3. The teacher supplies the learners with numerous opportunities to follow directions.
4. The students are sent on errands with verbal directions. They always should be required to repeat back what they think the teacher said. The remediator should not be afraid to repeat.
5. Directions are reinforced by asking the students not to respond until after all of the orders are given.

Sample Short-Term Objectives

In the area of auditory comprehension and following directions, the students will demonstrate the ability to:

1. answer who, what, when, how, and why questions
2. respond to verbal questions with meaningful answers
3. demonstrate understanding of stories read orally with background noises by correctly answering comprehension questions
4. follow oral directions with written responses
5. identify words with multiple meanings

Exemplary Lesson: Auditory Comprehension

Long-Term Objectives

1. The students will demonstrate the ability to understand and comprehend (get meaning from) what they hear in a meaningful way.
2. They will respond correctly to oral directions.

Short-Term Objective

1. The learner will respond correctly to oral commands.

Activity

The remediator announces to the students: "I am going to give you some directions to follow. Complete each direction immediately after it is given. Raise your hand when you are finished."

1. Write the number __9__.
2. Multiply by the number __2__.

3. Add the number __4__.
4. Multiply by the number __5__.
5. Add the number __12__.
6. Multiply by the number __10__.
7. Subtract __320__.
8. Draw a line through the tens and ones column.
9. What is your answer? (If done correctly it should be the same as the number started with. This can be done with any number from 1 to 9.)

This process can be adapted to other tasks such as map skills, crossword puzzles, and dot-to-dots.

VISUAL MEMORY

Long-Term Objective

1. The students will retain and recall accurately prior visual experiences.

Remedial Suggestions

1. The remediator should allow opportunities for tracing.
2. The students should be asked to complete unfinished figures or designs.
3. They should be allowed to use the typewriter for spelling words.
4. The teacher should utilize a tachistoscopic device, an overhead projector, or flash and other audiovisual aids.
5. The students should be allowed to work complex puzzles of a type in which they are interested.

Sample Short-Term Objectives

In the area of visual memory, the students will demonstrate the ability to:

1. return objects to their original sequence
2. reproduce a color sequence to match the stimulus presented
3. unscramble given words into appropriate spellings
4. recall a given visual sentence of events (a) visually (written, drawn) and (b) verbally
5. respond to visually presented directions

Exemplary Lesson: Visual Memory

Long-Term Objectives

1. The students will demonstrate the ability to understand and comprehend (get meaning from) what they see in a meaningful way.
2. They will respond correctly to written directions.

Short-Term Objective

1. The students will reproduce given tangram designs with 90 percent accuracy and within assigned time limits.

Activity

1. The remediator should explain that tangrams are ancient Chinese puzzles consisting of seven pieces. (See Figure 7-1.) The seven pieces can be arranged many ways to create shapes ranging from the simple to the complex.

Figure 7-1 Tangram Puzzle Basic Shape

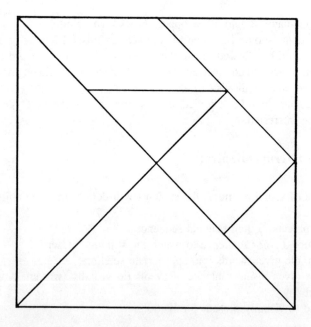

2. The students are asked to complete the first and very basic tangram shape ☐ after showing them from a distance that "yes, the seven pieces do make a square."
3. The teacher should allow 15 minutes before giving the first clue but use discretion and not cause the youths unnecessary frustration.
4. The students should be asked, after they discover the answer, to try it again from memory and time them with a stopwatch.
5. The activity should be repeated with more complex steps.

VISUAL DISCRIMINATION

Long-Term Objective

1. The students will differentiate meaningfully and accurately objects, forms, and symbols in the visual environment.

Remedial Suggestions

1. The remediator should use concrete (discriminating between colors) and then more symbolic (letters, numbers, and words) at the secondary level.
2. The teacher should present a sequence of letters and numbers:
   XGF75482
   Leave out one or two:
   _GF7_482
   Omit different ones:
   X_F75_82
   Students are to fill in the blanks.
3. The students are asked to identify familiar and unfamiliar items (people, places, and things) in photographs.
4. The teacher prepares a list of words, i.e., alligator, bureaucracy, administration and asks the students to circle each word as it is pronounced.
5. Optical illusions such as 1. $\longleftrightarrow$ 2. $\rangle\!\!\longrightarrow\!\!\langle$ which line is longer should be used.

Sample Short-Term Objectives

In the area of visual discrimination, the students will demonstrate the ability to:

1. outline hidden figures on a picture
2. outline a given visual stimulus shape located within overlapping figures
3. locate a picture that is the same as a given sample

4. select the correct path in a maze
5. identify the missing symbol when presented with a series of symbols (see No. 2 above)

Exemplary Lesson: Visual Discrimination

Long-Term Objective

1. The students will meaningfully and accurately differentiate object forms and symbols in the visual environment.

Short-Term Objective

1. The students will compile a scrapbook of photographs and/or newspaper clippings of people, places, and things with which they are familiar.

Activity

1. The remediator should ask the students to bring in pictures of people, places, and things.
2. The students should mount the photos on construction paper in book form.
3. The students are asked to label and identify all elements of the photos.

FINE MOTOR SKILLS

Long-Term Objective

1. The students will demonstrate the ability to perform detailed motor tasks.

Remedial Suggestions

1. The remediator should allow the students to use the typewriter.
2. The teacher should provide manipulatives of as many items as possible:
   plumbing pipes and wrenches
   sewing
   wood shop
   tangrams
   mosaics
3. The teacher should provide time for art activities:
   print making
   papier mâché
   string design

ceramics
crafts
painting
cartooning
4. The students should be allowed to trace.

Sample Short-Term Objectives

In the area of fine motor skills, the students will demonstrate the ability to:

1. type their names, addresses, and telephone numbers
2. construct a workable model of a hot and cold running water system
3. construct a wooden birdhouse
4. construct a tangram puzzle set out of wood
5. construct a ceramic vase
6. create a cartoon
7. manipulate small items: (a) washers, (b) nuts, (c) bolts, (d) screws
8. sew a shirt

Exemplary Lesson: Fine Motor Skills

Long-Term Objective

1. The students will demonstrate the ability to perform detailed motor tasks.

Short-Term Objective

1. The students will demonstrate dexterity when manipulating small items in an exercise such as quilling.

Activity

1. The remediator announces: "Quilling is the art of curling strips of paper, then gluing them together to form specific shapes."
2. The teacher presents the students with:
   a. strips of precut quilling paper
   b. a straight pin
   c. a pencil
   d. some glue
   e. a pattern
3. The remediator demonstrates while telling the students how to quill:
   a. take one strip of paper
   b. wrap it around the pencil as tightly as possible

c. glue the end
d. repeat until there are as many curls as are needed
e. glue them together to make shapes

TIME ORIENTATION DISABILITY

Long-Term Objective

1. The students will demonstrate the ability to judge time and time concepts.

Remedial Suggestions

1. The remediator should evaluate concepts of morning, afternoon, night, seasons, and holidays to ascertain whether the students demonstrate an understanding.
2. The teacher asks the students to estimate the time needed to complete a given task or go somewhere. They are asked to close their eyes and judge when a minute is up. They also are asked to time and record how long it takes to eat lunch, watch television, complete an assignment, etc.
3. The youths should be allowed to time themselves, using a stopwatch, then let them try to beat their past times.
4. Dance rhythms and rhythmic exercises should be taught.
5. Discussions should be conducted about time elements such as yesterday, tomorrow, last, next, this.

Sample Short-Term Objectives

In the area of time orientation and disabilities, students will demonstrate the ability to:

1. turn in assignments when due
2. arrive on time when expected to be somewhere
3. demonstrate understanding of seasons, holidays, morning, afternoon, night, today, tomorrow
4. complete a time diary for one week

Exemplary Lesson: Time Orientation Disability

Long-Term Objective

1. The students will demonstrate the ability to judge time and time concepts.

Short-Term Objective

1. The students will complete and turn in a one-week time diary.

Activity

1. The remediator should present the students with individual time charts (Figure 7-2).
2. The teacher asks them to fill out the charts as the week progresses.
3. Students are told to turn the charts in one week from that day.

Figure 7-2 Weekly Plan Sheet

Weekly Plan Sheet

Name: _____　　Week of: _____

A.M.	Sunday	Monday	Tuesday	Wednesday	Thursday	Friday	Saturday
6:00							
7:00							
8:00							
9:00							
10:00							
11:00							
P.M. 12:00							
1:00							
2:00							
3:00							
4:00							
5:00							
6:00							
7:00							
8:00							
9:00							
10:00							

4. The students discuss the week with the remediator.
5. The teacher gives the students two more time sheets, one to plan next week, the other to keep track of deviations from the plan.

A REVIEW OF REMEDIATION

Sample remedial objectives have been provided in selected process areas where cognitive remediation may be beneficial. These can serve as starting points when developing curricula for adolescents with LBPs. The remediator may adapt them to meet secondary learners' individual needs. Academic skill training has been slighted because of the volume of resources available in the form of curriculum guides and commercially available materials.

The next section differentiates between the concept of tutoring and of remediation.

TUTORING

Tutoring is the act of supporting or strengthening subject matter learning by providing structural analysis of its complexities. It assumes basic skill learning of the tool academic subjects. Aristocrats for centuries employed tutors to instruct their children in basic educational skills and the proper procedures for moral upbringing. Tutoring today could be limited to a specific task, i.e., giving a music lesson. It is supplementary to the individuals' educational processes or, more specifically, their academic lives. Tutoring is thought of as a teaching-learning circumstance in which the tutor's behavior becomes highly systematized.

Tutoring is one of the highest forms of teaching. Students become involved in a discovery form of learning. A sequence of steps is presented, the first being small in content, with successive ones altered progressively until the students function with only verbal endorsement (reinforcement). Who are tutors? Special educators frequently function as tutors, working with one or even a small group of students. To be more specific, the person willing and able to do the job is a qualified tutor. Peers, teachers, and parents all have proved to be effective.

The academic tutoring program has three goals:

1. to support the students' academic learning
2. to support the regular teachers in their work in the classroom
3. to support regular instructional goals developed in subject areas

An issue educators must be aware of is the trend toward specialization in an academic subject area. Tutors may dwell on the academic process and allow this to overshadow other problems the secondary students also might be experiencing, i.e., inner self-worth related to total self. In the education of adolescents with learning and behavioral problems, the development of their self-concept and self-esteem in conjunction with academic learning must be fostered.

Tutors can help these youths gain a feeling of success and importance by ensuring success by attaining self-confidence and a keen sense of pride in the academic sphere in which they are engaged. The feeling of self-fulfillment cannot be divorced from the motivation to achieve and, ultimately, academic success.

Homo sapiens, regardless of qualifications (age, occupation, etc.) has a need for success before taking the next step forward. LBP students, who may be failing to learn academically and socially to their own expectancies, are no exception to this rule. The following diagram and formula may help explain this:

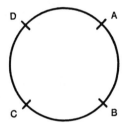

A. Success

B. Pride

C. Interest

D. Study

Formula: $A = B + C + D = A$

Success results in *Pride* which stimulates *Interest* which instigates *Study* which culminates in *Success*.

This is a never-ending cycle in the process of tutoring since one student success mandates another, and so on. The starting point for the tutor should be A. If B or C begins the process, then limits are imposed, although it can be, has been, and will be done any of these ways.

Example: A class of secondary students has just begun a lesson with a tutor. Rather than starting with a boring and detailed explanation of the structure of the library, the tutor should begin immediately by telling them to find a book. This can result in (A) instant success, (B) pride in their efforts, and can lead to C and D.

Example: The tutor, rather than having the students start by memorizing and repeating the alphabet, should have them learn by copying the letters in their names. From this A beginning, they will proceed naturally to B, C, and D.

Good, bad, or indifferent, this process should be implemented by tutors for use with LBP secondary students. There appear to be so few absolutes in this world that no one has the right to reject this process. Opinionated disagreement is another matter, of course.

Tutoring by Adapting

Accommodating the students with learning and behavioral problems implies "a variety of methods of adapting the school system's organization, curriculum, or instructional methods to the learner" (Marsh, Gearheart, & Gearheart, 1978, p. 87). Generally, secondary handicapped students are able to comprehend the content and concepts of a subject as do other youths if their reading levels are adjusted to the material they use.

Tutoring to Student Learning Preferences

Tutoring to the students' learning preferences—teaching only what they are most interested in, not what they need to know—can hinder their acquiring the ability to respond to, or complete, an assigned task.

Tutoring as a Curricular Support System

Tutoring augments the instruction of the classroom teacher. Tutoring programs can provide students with a model and give teachers the extra help and support they need to maintain the teenagers' interest and their progress in both basic skill and key subject academic achievement. The principle feature by which LBP students are measured is their ability to complete academic subjects successfully. If they fail, some adjustment in teaching delivery or testing procedure must be developed.

General Recommendations

When preparing their lessons, tutors should:

- Keep the lesson as practical as possible.
- Provide ideas to implement what the students want or need
- Use handouts if at all appropriate; students need to have something they can refer to later to refresh their memories.

- Try to utilize a variety of styles in the lessons.
- Do not overwhelm the students with any part of the lesson.
- Use audiovisual equipment, student participation, and interaction between tutor and youths to add variety to the program.
- Consider giving the students the opportunity for "hands-on" interaction with the materials if appropriate for the lesson; this can greatly increase the lesson's effectiveness.
- Know the lesson well; there is nothing as boring for secondary students as merely putting in time in a tutoring session.
- Be sure to time the lesson in preparing it because it is important to fully utilize the allotted time.
- Do not stop the session before the lesson has been completed as this could be disruptive for the students; this is an example of why it is essential to time the lesson.
- Allow time at the end of the lesson for questions and answers; it is frustrating for the students to have no opportunity to ask questions because the class lasted the entire hour.

Tutors want to structure their assistance in ways that will furnish LBP students with information in subjects that will be helpful in their daily academic lives. If the tutors know how to make their lessons interesting, they will be useful for the teenagers. Most innovative tutors strive to encourage the students' imaginations to flourish. Since those imaginations essentially are undisciplined, stifling them for the sake of a lesson plan is nonproductive.

If that premise is correct, however, the problem is that imagination is finally meaningless, even to the imaginer, if it is not given some form. Therefore, the more innovatively the tutors translate the lessons into meaningful form, the more they express. Whether it is for the sake of students who imagine something or for the benefit of the tutors who might see or hear or touch or sense it, that expression is the end, the fulfillment, of what is imagined.

Students generally seek desperately to communicate to others the feelings that overtake them. If they are to do that, tutors must help them to better understand their thoughts and feelings through individual counseling.

Tutors must always provide relevant tasks worthy of being learned. Their perceptions of the academic task—and the perceptions of the learners—must be real and treated as such.

Tutoring has been referred to as help within the academic areas. To enable tutors to approach the problem of analyzing the student, task, and environment, the following sample objectives and exemplary lessons will aid them in meeting the needs of their students.

EXEMPLARY LESSON 1

The students are unable to write a coherent collection of appropriate sentences to express a thought unless they have a grasp of grammar. Tutors may use the following lesson in conjunction with commercially prepared materials.

Long-Term Objective

1. The students will demonstrate the ability to outline.

Short-Term Objective

1. The students will demonstrate the ability to read an article of interest to them and to construct a topic outline.

Suggested Materials

Title/Publisher	Area	Level	Input	Output	Cost
Steck-Vaughan Company Publishers, Austin, Texas					
English Mastery	Language		Visual (text)	Verbal	$2.05 each
Book 1		9			
Book 2		10			
Book 3		11			
Book 4		12			

Activity

1. Outline: the topic outline—a list of the points a theme will discuss, arranged to show their equal or unequal importance.

EXAMPLE: Topic: Interscholastic football is not the sport for four classes of boys.
Introduction: This article is necessary though unpopular.
I.   Some boys occupied with more important things
II. Some boys unfit physically
III. Some boys unfit intellectually
IV. Some boys unfit emotionally
Conclusion: This article intended to help, not to stir controversy.

DO'S AND DONT'S FOR TOPIC OUTLINES:
1. Do not use letters or figures in front of "introduction" and "conclusion."
2. Use Roman numerals to set off the body of the outline.
3. Begin each heading of an outline with a capital.
4. Do not use a period after the headings of a topic outline unless they make a complete sentence; a question mark or an exclamation point may be used if either is needed for clarity.
5. Label the head and subheads with alternating figures and letters in this order: I. II. III.; A. B. C.; 1. 2. 3.; a) b) c); (1) (2) (3); (a) (b) (c); i. ii. iii.
6. Put a period after all the letters and figures in Rule 5 that are not followed by a parenthesis mark.
7. Do not put a period after the letters and figures in Rule 5 that are followed by a parenthesis.
8. Begin each head in the same series with the same or an equivalent part of speech if at all possible (and it usually is).

EXAMPLE: I. Noun
          A. Verb
             1. Preposition
             2. Preposition
          B. Verb
       II. Noun
          A. Adverb
          B. Adverb
             1. Verb
             2. Verb

9. Line up vertically all heads that have the same kind of numbers or letters. Indent heads labeled A,B,C ; indent 1,2,3 more deeply than A,B,C ; and so on.

EXAMPLE: I.
          A.
          B.
             1.
             2.
                a)
                b)
                    (1)
                    (2)
                        (a)
                        (b)
                          i.
                          ii.

10. Make each head and subhead as definite as possible without being wordy; use statements more often than questions:

Wrong	*Right*
I. The attack on Pearl Harbor	I. The attack on Pearl Harbor
A. When?	A. December 7, 1941
B. How?	B. By air and by sea
C. By whom?	C. The Japanese naval air and navy forces.

The following regulations will produce a neat, legible outline that will help in studying. The do's and dont's apply for typewritten and handwritten outlines for adolescent students with learning and behavioral problems.

SKILL: Outlining

ACTIVITY WORKSHEET 1

DIRECTIONS: 1. Read the following article.
2. Outline the article appropriately.
3. Hand in a completed outline.

Story

Introduction.
I.
II.
III.
IV.
Conclusion.

SKILL: Outlining

ACTIVITY WORKSHEET 2

DIRECTIONS: 1. Read the following article.
2. Choose the correct outlining procedure.
3. Hand in a completed outline.

Story

Introduction.
I.
 A.
 B.
 C.
II.
 A.
 B.
III.
 A.
 B.
  1.
  2.
Conclusion.

SKILL: Outlining

ACTIVITY WORKSHEET 3

DIRECTIONS: 1. Read the following article.
 2. Choose the correct outlining procedure.
 3. Hand in a completed outline.

Introduction.
I.
 A.
 B.
II.
 A.
 B.
III.
 A.
 B.
  1.
   a)
   b)
   c)
  2.
  3.
Conclusion.

EXEMPLARY LESSON 2

Long-Term Objective

1. The students will demonstrate the ability to understand and communicate through mass media.

Short-Term Objective

1. The students will demonstrate their ability to understand oral communication through mass media.

Suggested Materials

Title/Publisher	Area	Level	Input	Output	Cost
Steck-Vaughan Company Publishers, Austin, Texas					
Language in Daily Living	Conceptual Language (Functional)	10-12	Visual (text)	Written/ Verbal	$1.60 each
Book 1: Verbs and Subjects					
Book 2: Phrases, Clauses, and Sentences					
Book 3: Pronouns, Modifiers, and Verbals					
Book 4: Punctuation and Capitalization					

Activity

1. Use complete sentences
2. Use various types of sentences
3. Use pronouns correctly (I, me, she, he, we, you, they, them)
4. Use correct verb-noun agreement (she, was, they, were)
5. Use oral communication:
   1. speaking in front of group
   2. retelling events
   3. conveying emotions through oral language

EXEMPLARY LESSON 3

Long-Term Objective

1. The students will demonstrate the ability to read a card catalogue.

Short-Term Objective

1. The students will listen for directions given by the librarian.

Suggested Materials

Title/Publisher	Area	Level	Input	Output	Cost
Frank E. Richards Publishing Company, Phoenix, N.Y.					
Learning Functional Words and Phrases for Everyday Living	Conceptual Language (Functional)	10-12	Visual (text)	Verbal	$2.00

Activity

1. Check which rules students follow (work quietly, check with librarians to locate items, put materials back in correct place, follow directions for checking out books).
2. Have students demonstrate the ability to locate books and information in the library.
3. Have students practice locating books with information on title, author, or subject.
4. Prepare a treasure hunt for students to locate books with clues such as title, author, or subject.

EXEMPLARY LESSON 4

Long-Term Objective

1. The students will demonstrate the ability to use dictionary guide words.

Short-Term Objective

1. The students are given a list of pairs of guide words and will write a word that could be found under each pair.

Suggested Materials

> Dictionary
> Word lists (see following example)

Activity

1. Look at a dictionary with the students.
2. Examine the two guide words at the top of each page and the entry words listed under them.
3. Give the students a list of words headed by two guide words.
4. Ask the students to identify which particular words would be found under those guide words and which would not.

marksman   marvelous

> martin
> markings
> martini
> marlin
> marshal
> marvel
> marvelous
> marshmallow
> maroon

EXEMPLARY LESSON 5

Long-Term Objective

1. The students will demonstrate their ability to use an encyclopedia index.

Short-Term Objective

1. The students, given an encyclopedia index, will locate specific topics in it.

Suggested Material

Title/Publisher	Area	Level	Input	Output	Cost
Communication Skill Builders, Inc., Tucson, Arizona					
Concept Box	Conceptual	Ages	Visual/	Verbal/	
	Language		Auditory	Motor	
#3082-H		3-8			$6.00

Activity

1. Look at an encyclopedia index with the students.
2. Aid the students in identifying words under which specific topics might be located:

Specific Topic	Volume	Letter	Page
Abraham Lincoln	_____	_____	_____
Revolutionary War	_____	_____	_____
Strip Mining	_____	_____	_____
Springfield, Illinois	_____	_____	_____
Arabian Horse	_____	_____	_____

Questions tutors may want to list in their lesson preparation file are as follows:

1. What strategies were most successful with this LBP adolescent?
2. Can this tutoring academic skill be generalized to other skill areas?

Tutors may wish to keep management profiles (Figure 7-3) on these students in their files. The profiles may be developed or modified at the tutors' convenience.

Figure 7-3 Tutoring Program Management Profile

Student _____

Age _____

Academic Achievement _____

Vocational Performance _____

Social Development _____

Personal Development _____

	Long-Term Objectives	Short-Term Objectives	Activities	Materials Resources	Supportive Services	Performance
Academic						
Vocational						
Social						
Personal						

A REVIEW OF TUTORING

This section has provided sample suggestions for tutors of secondary LBP students. As with remediation, these examples can serve as starting points when developing curriculum and locating commercial materials.

Tutoring and remediation both are viable educational tools and can be utilized either independently of, or in conjunction with, each other.

SUMMARY

This chapter has analyzed two major special education approaches— remediation and tutoring:

1. Remediation: working with learners' cognitive processes; assessment and programming to ameliorate a process area deficit that is interfering with their ability to achieve academically.
2. Tutoring: working with learners' academic tool skills; the act of supporting or strengthening subject matter learning.

This chapter organizes instructional practice assessment procedures, long-term and short-term objectives, suggestions for remediation, and exemplary lessons for developing individualized education programs for LBP students.

Chapter 8

Methods of Instruction: A Process-Task Approach for LBP Adolescents

Kathleen M. McCoy and Nancy Ralph Watson

INTRODUCTION

Secondary students with learning and behavior problems often experience academic frustration in mainstream settings. This chapter focuses on an educational evaluation model that assumes a shared responsibility between a content specialist and a resource teacher for the education of the mildly handicapped student who spends part or all of a day in a regular class setting.

The nature of the academic problems these students experience varies with the emphasis of the course. Content courses, such as the humanities, social sciences, and natural sciences, demand proficiency in reading-related skills. Mathematics courses demand skills in arithmetic and logic.

Most mainstream secondary students are required to take specific courses in order to graduate. Many of these courses may be impossible for mainstreamed LBP adolescents to complete unless the content specialist and resource teacher take joint responsibility for helping them.

EVALUATION MODEL

A commonly expressed but rarely implemented intervention is individualization. Individualized instruction for 30 students for five periods a day can be an awesome task. It should be noted, however, that individualized teaching is a matter of degree. The evaluation model in this chapter provides a procedure whereby the content specialist and the resource teacher can individualize in content and mathematics courses.

Evaluation of the Content

Designing an individualized program in a content area requires a two-part evaluation procedure. The practitioners responsible for mainstreamed students, whether the resource teacher or content specialist, must work with each other to evaluate the content and the students' knowledge of it. On the left of the model in Figure 8-1 is the Evaluation of Content.

Evaluation of the content or subject matter must begin with a definition of the actual scope and sequence of the material. Generally this sequence is in the form of a content outline. The outline then needs to be put into topical units, which in turn can be developed into objectives for the course.

It could be argued that the objectives should be established first and the content then specified. For the sake of expediency, however, it is simpler to use the scope and sequence of the available school district materials. Most texts are well written and well organized. Should the need arise, the teachers probably would find it simpler to augment or rearrange existing texts than to supply an original set of objectives.

Figure 8-1 Evaluation Model for Content Areas

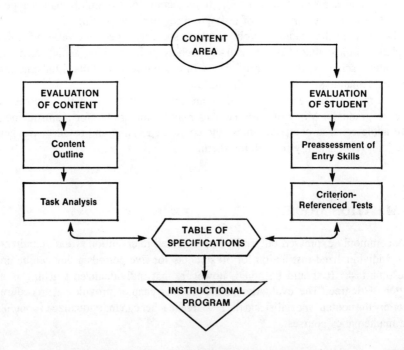

A task analysis of the objectives helps both the content specialist and the resource teacher develop testable and thereby more easily teachable units of instruction.

One organizational system for the task analysis is the Table of Specifications (Table 8-1). A Table of Specifications is simply a matrix of content and behaviors. The behaviors are those that the students are expected to demonstrate at the end of the unit.

Evaluation of the Student

On the right side of Figure 8-1 is Evaluation of Student. Secondary students have been in school for at least eight years. They have been introduced at the elementary level to the beginning concepts of many of the required high school courses. For mainstreamed mildly handicapped students, there often are gaps in their foundation knowledge that can cause failure at the secondary level.

To establish the students' immediate skill level, a preassessment of entry abilities is vital. Based on the skill level of knowledge, the teacher can then determine whether to return to a more basic level of instruction or to introduce advanced material.

Table 8-1 Table of Specifications—General Model

	A. First major behavior	*A.1 Subbehavior 1*	*A.2 Subbehavior 2*	*B. Second major behavior*	*B.1 Subbehavior 1*	*B.2 Subbehavior 2*
Content I. Major Category from content outline	Goal			Goal		
I.1 Subcategory 1	Sub- goal	obj	obj	Sub- goal	obj	obj
I.2 Subcategory 2	Sub- goal	obj	obj	Sub- goal	obj	obj
I.3 Subcategory 3	Sub- goal	obj	obj	Sub- goal	obj	obj

IA and IB are goals
I.1/A.1 and I.3/B.1 are behavior objectives
I.2/B and I.3/A are subgoals

Criterion-referenced testing measures the extent to which students possess particular skills. Applied to entry level skills, this is one of the most appropriate evaluation techniques for subject materials. In criterion-referenced testing, items can be developed from a Table of Specifications. Errors reflect the students' instructional deficits. Each student is likely to have unique (as well as common) needs with others. Instructional programming can be adjusted to fit the needs of the group as well as the individual.

ORGANIZING/ANALYZING CONTENT MATERIAL

There is a great deal of information in any content area, some of it more critical than others. For typical secondary students, basic concepts can be augmented and embellished with interesting facts, vignettes, and activities. These extra activities require time to complete, and typical high school students can use this time to enrich the basic concepts. However, mainstreamed LBP students typically have not learned the basic concepts of the course. They need to focus more on learning the basic content and cannot afford to spend time on enrichment activities. The content specialist is trained in a particular subject matter—training that provides expert judgment for evaluating the merits of the material.

Content Outline

Content can be divided into basic information and enrichment activities more easily by the content specialist than by the special education teacher. Since the emphasis at the secondary level is directed toward content, the specialist can prioritize objectives. If objectives are put into order, direct instruction can focus on the most basic areas. A unit outline of the subject matter can be constructed from the objectives. Ideally, the resource teacher and the content area specialist would outline the material jointly. Sometimes, however, because of time constraints and scheduling conflicts, this joint effort may not be possible. In such cases, the resource teacher need not despair. Most textbooks already outline major points and subtopics.

Task Analysis

Task analysis is the systematic, step-by-step breakdown of major units of instruction into smaller subunits or short-term objectives. With content broken into small units, the teacher can focus on students' specific needs. A task analysis can be used to organize the content objectives into a series of easily mastered short-term objectives that are arranged so the simplest and most easily learned information is presented first. Each objective builds from the previous one—as objectives are learned, the complexity of the information increases.

Task analysis is essential in planning the assessment and teaching program. Both content and expected behaviors should be outlined in a task analysis. The analysis orders the material so that the subtasks, which lead to the goals and long-term objective, are mastered in short, logical steps. Both the overall presentation and subtasks are presented sequentially. The focus in analyzing the task is only on skills that are a direct part of the content being taught. These content skills are critical for fundamental mastery of the material. An alternate way to specify content is to construct a Table of Specifications.

Table of Specifications

A Table of Specifications (Table 8-1, supra) provides a framework for behavioral objectives and for separating the content material and the expected behaviors. The content material generally is listed down the left side of the table in the form of a sequenced content outline. The conditions or behaviors are listed across the top and also are sequenced. By arranging the objectives in a Table of Specifications format, both goals and objectives can be stated efficiently and economically. An intersection of content material with behavior becomes either a goal or an objective. Each major cell intersection is a desired goal. An example in Table 8-1 would be combining I with A, and I with B.

Objectives, on the other hand, are much more specific. They require observable behaviors. Combining subcells creates the objective. Mastering of objectives ensures the achievement of the goals and subgoals. For example, mastering objective I.1/A.1 means that the student has achieved subgoal I.1/A.

This Table of Specifications provides for two goals, six subgoals, and 12 behavior objectives. It is from tables like this that criteria measures directly related to the content being taught can be developed. Both pretests and posttests based on the objectives can be developed from the tables. In addition, individualization can take place in a fairly simple and time-efficient manner.

EVALUATING THE STUDENT

Evaluation of secondary students for the purpose of individualizing programs may be a joint project involving both classroom teachers and the special educator, or one teacher may have this responsibility. As discussed earlier, it is necessary to have content outlines, objectives, and a list of prerequisite behaviors for the content area being individualized. Then the evaluation of the student may begin.

Student Skill Level

The first step in the process is for the teacher to identify the basic skill strengths and weaknesses of the students so as to determine the skill level at which the evaluation materials must be developed. Evaluation materials may need to be altered or modified, depending on the individual, in order to test knowledge of the content accurately. If secondary students cannot read material or follow a certain format, then the resulting scores may be difficult to interpret. They may reflect the students' inability to read the material rather than their actual knowledge of it.

The modification of materials designed to evaluate individuals' knowledge in a given content area can take place on two levels: (1) difficulty of skill and (2) difficulty of format. The difficulty of the material must not surpass the students' tool skill level, i.e., their basic abilities in word recognition or language comprehension. If the youths are expected to read the majority of the test items, then they must be able to read the vocabulary at an independent level. They also must have instant recognition of the key words in the test directions in order to know what is expected. The reading level of the test material must be matched with the students' reading ability.

The other area of adjustment can be in format of presentation. Simple problems such as teaching a student how to use a computer answer sheet or eliminating the answer sheet altogether can lead to more accurate assessments. Response modes for testing can be adjusted a number of ways. Oral responses can be substituted for written ones. Cassette tape recordings can provide permanent records of the responses.

Preassessment of Entry Skills

Once the format and difficulty level of the evaluation material are established, the teacher can assess the students' content needs. The first step in this process is to administer a preassessment of entry behaviors. Entry level behaviors are skills that must be acquired before students begin the next unit of instruction. To determine whether or not the students have sufficient background knowledge for the new task, they must be tested on these behaviors. The preassessment is designed to evaluate the learners' capabilities relevant to the instructional objectives.

The major reasons for assessment prior to beginning instruction are to determine (1) how much related materials the students already know, and (2) which aspects they still need to learn.

The mainstreamed LBP or low-achieving secondary student often lacks basic information in content areas. To teach the prespecified objectives in a subject, the teacher needs to be sure that the students have the foundation or background knowledge necessary for the acquisition of the higher level behaviors. Before attempting to learn how to multiply fractions, for example, they first must know how to multiply whole numbers.

For each special student enrolled in a content area course, entering capabilities need to be delineated. In most subjects, the preassessment test also should include evaluation of the students' understanding of key vocabulary terms and basic concepts.

Criterion-Referenced Testing

One evaluation procedure commonly used to measure the attainment of each instructional objective is the criterion-referenced test (CRT). CRTs are composed of instructional objectives and subobjectives. If a task analysis has been done, it can be used to write the CRTs. Each item on a CRT specifies a measurable behavior the teacher wants the student to learn during the semester or academic unit.

CRTs tell the educator specifically what the student has learned and still needs to acquire. For example, one set of objectives may cover one chapter or one learning unit of the entire content material. In criterion testing, the results are described in behavior or performance terms. The criterion behavior provides a standard against which to compare an individual student's achievement (Gronlund, 1973). Criterion-referenced testing can be used for both preassessment and postassessment. It also can be written in the form of an IIP (individualized instructional program) if the student is in a resource situation.

Pretests should be conducted on the material the students are expected to learn. This type of assessment sometimes is referred to as preassessment of terminal behavior (Kibler, Barker, & Miles, 1974). It is a direct measure of the objectives the students are to complete for specific academic units. Pretests should be used throughout a unit as new material is taught.

Once the students have completed the academic unit, an evaluation tool identical or similar to the pretest is administered. If CRTs (pretests) have been used periodically during the teaching unit, the youths' achievements on the posttest should be predictable. If the format and difficulty level of the assessment materials are developed according to the students' strengths and weaknesses, they should do as well on the posttest as throughout the individualized program of study.

Criterion-referenced testing has two major components: (1) content material and (2) behaviors the students will demonstrate regarding that content.

Content Material

The development of a content outline was discussed earlier. Having established the content to be covered and having delineated it by topic, the teacher now is ready to develop the behavioral component of the criterion test.

Expected Student Behaviors

The behavioral component of the CRT is a statement composed of three parts: (1) what the students are to do, (2) the conditions under which they are to act, and (3) a standard of accuracy or rate (where appropriate).

What Students Are To Do. There are many different types of behavior students might be asked to demonstrate, such as to explain, discuss, solve, or analyze some aspect of the content. Bloom, Engelhart, Furst, Hill, and Krathwohl (1956); Harrow (1972); and Krathwohl, Bloom, and Masia (1964) provide a taxonomy of educational objectives for the cognitive, affective, and psychomotor domains. Most resource teachers will be interested primarily in the cognitive domain, which is most appropriate with respect to the acquisition of content material at the secondary level.

Bloom et al.'s (1956) categories have been condensed (Sanders, 1966) to allow for ease in writing test questions:

1. Memory: The student recalls or recognizes information in a different symbolic form or language.
2. Translation: The student changes information into a different symbolic form or language.
3. Interpretation: The student discovers relationships among facts, generalizations, definitions, values, and skills.
4. Application: The student solves a lifelike problem that requires the identification of the issue and selection and use of appropriate generalizations and skills.
5. Analysis: The student solves a problem in the light of conscious knowledge of the parts and forms of thinking.
6. Synthesis: The student solves a problem that requires original, creative thinking.
7. Evaluation: The student makes a judgment of good or bad, right or wrong, according to designated standards.

It should be noted that the behaviors are specified by two types of verbs. General topic verbs, such as "knows," are broad and encompassing. These types of global behaviors in conjunction with content material can be translated easily into goal statements or objectives. Subtopic verbs are more specific. They describe measurable behavior, e.g., define or select. These observable behaviors, coupled with content material, convert easily into specific short-term objectives.

Researchers in the Classroom Learning Laboratory at Arizona State University and in the Southwest Regional Laboratory (Gerlach & Ely, 1971) have produced their own list of words to help teachers describe objectives in their field: (1) identify, (2) name, (3) describe, (4) order, and (5) construct.

1. Identify: Synonyms for identify include words such as match, locate, recognize, and select. In identification, students indicate in some manner an object or event and may underline answers, point, touch, or verbally indicate the desired response.

2. Name: In naming, the students supply a label, which can be oral or written. Synonyms for label are designate or term.
3. Describe: Describing is a more complex behavior, involving such actions as defining, telling why, explaining, and giving examples. In a describing activity, the students must be able to identify salient characteristics of the event or object. The description may be either oral or written, depending on the youths' skills.
4. Order: Ordering is synonymous with ranking and sequencing. Ordering can take place on two different levels—chronological or step sequencing. Students can be asked to order chronologically: "List in sequence the admission of the following states into the United States: Virginia, Rhode Island, Delaware, and New York." An example of delineating steps would be "Tell, in order, the steps by which a territory becomes a state." Or, in industrial arts, "Order the steps that must be followed in constructing a sequence of service operations designed to develop skills in brake service and repair."
5. Construct: Some of the many synonyms for construct are draw, build, create, or make. In an objective requiring construction, the students are expected to meet prior specifications in order to produce a given piece of work. In biology, they may be asked to construct a model of a tree. This assumes that they already know the basic components of a tree's system, i.e., roots, tap root, trunk, branches, etc.

While these five words are not all-encompassing, they certainly can be an aid in defining what behaviors are expected of students. Their simplicity also becomes an aid to communication between the content specialist and the resource teacher.

Conditions. Conditions refer to the situations or circumstances (when, what, where, and how) under which the behavior stated in the objective is to occur (Designing Effective Instruction, 1970). Conditions especially need to be specified when the students are completing the behavior under a special education program. For example, if a slow student is using taped lectures or peer tutoring, this needs to be made clear. By knowing the particular conditions for the students, the content specialist will have a more accurate understanding of how they perform.

The conditions of the behavior must be parallel to the teaching and testing situation. Watching films and listening to tapes of key moments in history is quite different from reading a list of printed facts. Yet, for some high school students who have very low (or poor) reading skills, the informational input of films and audio tapes bears a critical relationship to the ultimate outcome—the acquisition and retention of historical facts and definitions. Caution must be taken, however, when specifying conditions. It is critical that the objective not be confused with a media-related activity.

Standard of Accuracy. The degree to which students must demonstrate knowledge needs to be agreed upon by the teachers involved in the individualization process. Some content material may be sufficiently covered at the memory level. It may be enough for the students to define a special term. Other concepts may need to be tested at an application level (next). In such cases, the adolescents may be asked to explain how a specific term applies to them.

APPLICATION OF THE EVALUATION MODEL

The evaluation model presented thus far has provided general guidelines. The following section discusses its application to a content area subject. Examples of a content outline, task analysis, and a table of specifications for United States history are presented.

Content

At the secondary level the subject areas draw primarily from the social sciences, humanities, and natural sciences. These then are transformed into narrower topics such as American history, biology, English literature, etc. Since each topic area is concerned with a particular set of facts, ideas, and terms, the majority of the coursework relies heavily on literal comprehension and vocabulary skills (Wallace & Kauffman, 1978) (Figure 8-2).

For mainstreamed LBP students, the following content comprehension behaviors are necessary to meet minimum course requirements at the secondary level:

A. Know vocabulary
    A.1 Define word literally
    A.2 Define word in own terms
B. Comprehend on literal level
    B.1 Select detail taken directly from passage
    B.2 Select main idea

Vocabulary Development

Vocabulary development consists of word recognition and word meaning. Word recognition refers to students' ability to read a word orally within one second of seeing it. It implies an automatic response (naming a word) to a stimulus (the printed word). Immediate recognition of key vocabulary terms increases reading rate as well as reading comprehension (Spache, 1976). Immediate recognition of words allows students to direct their energy toward the meaning of the content.

Meaning should be developed along with word recognition. Slower students often memorize word meanings. To circumvent meaningless memorization, the teacher needs to have the students define important terms in their own words.

Figure 8-2 Evaluation Model for Academic Areas

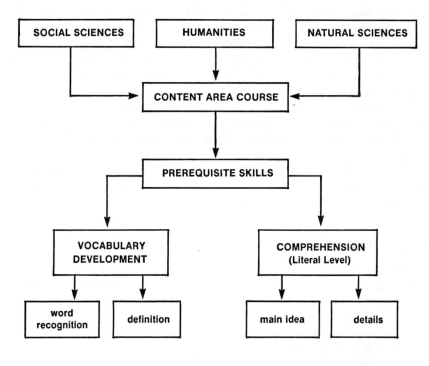

Literal Comprehension

Literal comprehension and vocabulary development occur simultaneously. One main skill of comprehension is selecting details from the reading material. Students must learn how to choose important details from what they are studying such as names, dates, and events. The ability to determine the most important point or theme of a passage also must be taught. However, to find a main idea or select details, the student also must know the vocabulary of the content material. Therefore, all of these skills must be included when preparing the individual course programs.

Developing a Content Outline

Content outlines provide the scope and sequence of course material. Course material ideally is arranged in a sequential manner, which provides a natural guide for individualizing a program.

Sources

The first step toward developing and individualizing a program for a subject area is to write a content outline. There are three major sources for finding a content outline: (1) teacher's manual, (2) table of contents of the text, and (3) chapter outlines in the text. Most teachers' manuals contain content outlines and *should* be used by resource teachers to develop programs. The resource teacher does have copies of the student textbook and can inspect the table of contents, which in some texts is complete enough by itself for use as a content outline. Each chapter is analogous to a teaching unit. The students may need additional help in only one aspect of a content area. In such a case the teacher would need to use only one topic on which to base the content outline.

In cases where the table of contents is very general, the teacher still can use the student text effectively. Major topics usually are in large boldface type, with subtopics set apart by different type styles.

Example of a Content Outline

An instructional unit can be developed for a basic course in U.S. history by following the evaluation model step by step, using the paragraphs in Exhibit 8-1. The following outline can be written for these paragraphs:

I. Legal and Social Changes
   A. End of Primogeniture
   B. Limited Abolition of Slavery
   C. Distribution of Loyalist Property
   D. Disestablishment of Religion
   E. Westward Thrust

This now can serve as the basis for the Task Analysis.

Example of a Task Analysis

The following are examples of a task analysis leading up to mastery of a long-term objective or goal:

GOAL IA: The students will know the vocabulary dealing with legal and social changes occurring in the post-Revolutionary years.
   Objective 1: The students will literally define vocabulary dealing with the End of Primogeniture. (terms: primogeniture, inherit)
   Objective 2: The students will literally define vocabulary on the topic of Limited Abolition of Slavery. (terms: plantation, abolished)

Exhibit 8-1 Textual Basis for a Content Outline

Legal and Social Changes of the Post-Revolutionary Period

End of Primogeniture

In many colonies there was a practice called primogeniture. This was when, upon a father's death, all of his property was given to the first-born son. This European custom of the first son's inheriting his father's estate was found most frequently in the Southern colonies. As the states adopted their individual laws, primogeniture was found to be unconstitutional and was no longer practiced.

Limited Abolition of Slavery

Slavery was found in all the colonies but was more prevalent in the South. Gradually, laws were passed to abolish slavery, beginning with Pennsylvania in 1780, and soon other Northern colonies abolished slavery. However, this did not occur in the Southern colonies because of the severe need for labor on the large plantations. Seventy-six years passed before slavery was abolished in all the United States.

Distribution of Loyalist Property

Many Loyalists still owned property in the colonies. Some of it was taken by the states and sold in small parcels to colonists without land. More often, however, opportunists and speculators gained possession of the large land holdings of the Loyalists, taking advantage of the chance to become wealthy as the Loyalists were stripped of their possessions.

Disestablishment of Religion

By law colonists paid taxes to maintain the established church, the church which the colony accepted as the state religion. Churches associated with England were also supported by taxes, especially in the South. Gradually, the Southern colonies withdrew government support or disestablished themselves from these churches.

An argument ensued because some believed there should not be one established church receiving government funds but that all churches should share in the tax monies. Others felt that all government aid to churches should be cut off, thereby causing a separation of church and state. This is what was finally done and was written into our Constitution, and this continues to be one of our country's basic principles today.

Westward Thrust

After 1789 the acquisition by the United States of areas to the west increased the amount of land available for settling. Many colonists were anxious to relocate, hoping to find new opportunities and freedoms. Lands west of the Appalachians were fertile and did not disappoint those who chose to begin their new lives in these unknown places.

Objective 3: The students will literally define vocabulary on the Distribution of Loyalist Property. (terms: Loyalists, speculators, opportunists)

Objective 4: The students will literally define vocabulary associated with the Disestablishment of Religion. (terms: established church, disestablish, separation of church and state)

Objective 5: The students will literally define vocabulary involving the Westward Thrust. (terms: acquisition, relocate, Appalachians)

Objective 6: The students will define vocabulary on the End of Primogeniture in their own words. (terms: primogeniture, inherit)

Objective 7: The students will define vocabulary dealing with Limited Abolition of Slavery in their own words. (terms: plantation, abolished)

Objective 8: The students will define vocabulary on the topic of Distribution of Loyalist Property in their own words. (terms: Loyalists, speculators, opportunists)

Objective 9: The students will define vocabulary on the Disestablishment of Religion in their own words. (terms: established church, disestablish, separation of church and state)

Objective 10: The students will define vocabulary for the Westward Thrust in their own words. (terms: acquisition, relocate, Appalachians)

In this task analytic format, students must first define each term literally (Objectives 1-5) and then in their own words (Objectives 6-10). When these ten objectives are successfully mastered, the teacher can be confident that the students have reached Goal IA: knowing the vocabulary dealing with legal and social changes occurring in the post-Revolutionary years.

Continuing the task analysis format, a second goal (IB), relating to the literal level of the material, is specified:

GOAL IB: The students will understand the literal (actual or factual) level dealing with legal and social changes occurring in the post-Revolutionary years.

Objective 1: The students will select details taken from passage in text on the End of Primogeniture.

Objective 2: The students will select details from text on Limited Abolition of Slavery.

Objective 3: The students will select details from text on Distribution of Loyalist Property.

Objective 4: The students will select details from text on the Disestablishment of Religion.

Objective 5: The students will select details from text on the Westward Thrust.

Objective 6: The students will select the main idea from passage in text on the End of Primogeniture.

Objective 7: The students will select the main idea from text on Limited Abolition of Slavery.

Objective 8: The students will select the main idea from text on Distribution of Loyalist Property.

Objective 9: The students will select the main idea from text on the Disestablishment of Religion.

Objective 10: The students will select the main idea from text on the Westward Thrust.

Specifying these short-term objectives is important to guide and evaluate instruction. The format, however, is redundant, e.g., the phrase, "the student will literally define vocabulary dealing with . . . ," is repeated in Objectives A1-5. There also are repetitions in Objectives A6-10, B1-5, and B6-10. Writing out every objective in this format is time consuming and somewhat tedious. An alternate way to specify content is to construct a Table of Specifications.

Table of Specifications

The essential ingredients now are available to construct a Table of Specifications (Table 8-2). Using the task analysis is a simple process. The conditions or behaviors are listed across the top of the table in the sequential form followed in the task analysis. Content material is listed down the left side, following the order in the text passage. The intersection of I and A combines content and behavior to form GOAL IA from the task analysis in Table 8-1, supra. The intersection of I and B combine to form GOAL IB from the task analysis.

Following further in Table 8-2, Objective 1 under GOAL IA is merely a combination of the content and behavior into their common cell or objective I.1/A.1. Each task analysis objective written for this learning unit is now placed on a matrix that is compact and easy to follow. In addition, it can be used easily as a recordkeeping system by enlarging the matrix so that the cells have space for writing in progress notes and grades.

Preassessment of Students

In the initial step in actual instruction—determining whether or not the students have the prerequisite skills for the content materials—the teacher conducts a

Table 8-2 Sample Table of Specifications

Content: U.S. History; Legal and Social Change of the Post-Revolutionary Period	Behavior A. Knows Vocabulary	A.1 Defines word literally	A.2 Defines word in own terms	Comprehension of Literal Level B.	B.1 Selects detail taken from passage	B.2 Selects main idea
I. Legal and Social Changes	IA			IB		
I.1 End of Primogeniture Terms: Primogeniture, inherit		I.1 A.1	I.1 A.2			
I.2 Limited abolition of Slavery Terms: plantation, abolished						
I.3 Distribution of Loyalist Property Terms: Loyalists, speculators, opportunists						
I.4 Disestablishment of Religion Terms: established, church, disestablish, separation of church and state						
I.5 Westward Thrust Terms: relocate, acquisition, Appalachians						

preassessment of entry skills. Many low-functioning LBP adolescents need to acquire basic vocabulary before they can be introduced to more advanced content. A common procedure is to review prior related coursework. Generally, a multiple-choice test can be administered on the basic content of a course, with the results serving as a guide for review.

In the case of a history class, the preassessment may include having the students define such words as Constitution, government, United States, George Washington, president, etc. The prerequisite materials also can be organized into a Table of Specifications, and coded learning aids can be included in the course objective file. Main ideas and vocabulary can be reintroduced in this way. Given a solid background, the students then can proceed to new learning situations.

Using the Table of Specifications, a comprehensive CRT can be written for the history unit with test questions in four basic forms: (1) true-false, (2) multiple choice, (3) matching, and (4) short-answer or fill-in (Gronlund, 1973). Exhibit 8-2 is a partial CRT based on objectives for Goal I.3 from the Table of Specifications in Table 8-2. Once the evaluation materials are prepared, the instructional program can be administered.

Exhibit 8-2 Coded Test for a Table of Specifications

(I.3/A.1)
1. Match the term with the correct definition:

    a. Loyalists   a. those who took advantage of the situation to buy property cheaply

    b. speculators   b. those living in the colonies who still supported England

    c. opportunists   c. those who bought a lot of property from the government hoping to make a profit

(I.3/A.2)
2. Define the following terms in your own words and use each one in a sentence:
    a. Loyalist: _____
    b. speculator: _____
    c. opportunist: _____

(I.3/B.1)
3. Circle the answers that are correct:
    a. The colonies seized property from the Loyalists.
    b. The colonies gave Loyalist property to poor colonists.
    c. Many people took advantage of the property that was taken from the Loyalists.

(I.3/B.2)
4. Put true or false next to each of these statements:
    _____ a. Loyalists were not allowed to own property in the colonies.
    _____ b. All of the Loyalist property was sold to the poor.

The Instructional Program

Once the evaluation model for a course has been written to include a preassessment, CRT, content outline, task analysis, and/or Table of Specifications, the instructional program can be administered. A filing system can facilitate this.

Teaching aids, e.g., work sheets, textbook passages, etc., can be placed in a folder and filed by objective number. In history, for example, all material related to the students' ability to literally define the terms primogeniture and inherit can be placed in a file coded I.1/A.1. This also can be done in mathematics. Material for each objective can be coded and filed sequentially according to the original task analysis or Table of Specifications.

Students who enter with different skills as indicated by the results of their criterion-referenced tests can be supplied with the appropriate materials. They or the teacher can go to the file for the needed area for materials specific to the content deficit (Exhibit 8-3). In this way the teacher has written one basic program but can individualize it for each student.

Exhibit 8-3 Example of a Coded Work Sheet

I.1/A.1,2
Vocabulary: End of Primogeniture
    1. Read pp. _____ in the text.
    2. Write down the definition of *primogeniture* found in the text.
    3. Read pp. _____ in the text.
    4. Write down the definition of *inherit* found in the dictionary.
    5. Do the work sheet in this folder.

WORK SHEET I.1/A.1,2
Make a list of ten things you might get if you had lived in 1780, were you the oldest son in your family and your father died:

    1.   6.
    2.   7.
    3.   8.
    4.   9.
    5.   10.
What you have just written has to do with _____.
Fill in each blank below with one of these words:
            primogeniture   inherit
1. I wish I would _____ a lot of money.
2. _____ used to be a law in 1780.
3. Did you _____ your mother's blue eyes?
4. Today, _____ does not occur often because when a father dies he usually leaves his property to his wife and kids.
5. If _____ were a law today, would you _____ all your father's property?

MATHEMATICS INSTRUCTION

For the mainstreamed LBP high school student, the majority of mathematics instruction will be in general skills in this field. Application of these skills is necessary in practical or vocational classes such as home economics, business math, typing, shop, etc. Mathematics instruction at the secondary level, however, is simultaneously one of the most rewarding and frustrating topics to teach.

Many mainstreamed high school youths resent covering material they have seen throughout their elementary school years. Other low-achieving students are afraid to work with numbers because they have a history of failure with mathematics (Otto, McMenemy, & Smith, 1973; Rusman, 1972). Yet, given the sequential nature of mathematics, skill deficits are located quickly and often are remediated easily.

Number Systems

General math skills deal primarily with two number systems: whole numbers and rational numbers. Whole numbers are 0, 1, 2, 3, and on to infinity. Rational numbers include fractions, negative numbers, and all quotients of these numbers (excluding division by zero).

Both the whole number and rational number systems have foundation level skills (Figure 8-3). Sometimes the failure in mathematics performance for mainstreamed secondary students can be traced to deficits in these skills (Wallace & McLoughlin, 1975; Wallace & Larsen, 1978).

Figure 8-3 Relation of Foundation Skill to Problem Solving

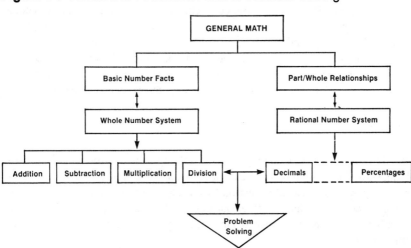

Problems in Rational Number System

In the rational number system, low-achieving students often are unsure of basic identification of commonly used fractions. Before proceeding with any areas of instruction in the rational number system, it is imperative that students understand part-whole relationships. Decimals, percentages, and money all are areas in which understanding is dependent upon part-whole relationships.

Problems in Whole Number System

One of the most common deficit areas in the whole number system is a lack of knowledge of the basic number facts. Number facts are represented in addition, subtraction, multiplication, and division tables. Number facts are automatic responses to stimuli. Often, errors in mathematics result from faulty memorization of combinations. Lack of familiarity and slowness in recalling number facts also can interfere with basic processes. Energy expended on searches for number facts is diverted from the basic process and problem solving.

Pretesting on number facts or prerequisite skills allows both the content specialist and the special educator to share a common understanding of the secondary students' skills. From analysis of the prerequisite skills, a mutual program decision can be made. The goals and objectives for the students may be concentrated in prerequisite skill areas or in basic process areas.

Basic Processes

Basic processes refer to calculations that require more than a simple stimulus-response learning. They need several consecutive steps to complete. In essence, a basic process problem is solved by a series of chained stimulus-response pairs. Carrying, borrowing, and long division all are examples of basic processes.

Testing basic processes in both the whole and rational number systems is sequential. Sequences of these systems can be found in almost any teacher's manual. The table of contents in most math books generally is sequenced as well.

Problem Solving

As skill deficits are remediated, problem solving can be introduced. Problem-solving skills enable high school LBP adolescents to use basic processes to clarify some component of a real-life situation. Basic addition and subtraction skills give them the freedom to balance a checkbook or budget toward a new car or stereo. It is the application of the basic processes in problem solving that provides meaning to mathematics.

Developing a Content Outline in Mathematics

Content Outlines

Writing a content outline for developing an individualized mathematics program can be done quickly. The sequential nature of mathematics makes the material easy to organize. Most math texts provide a content outline in the form of a table of contents. The teacher's manual is a source for an outline from which a task analysis can be written.

Here is an example of a content outline written for a math unit on money:

I. Money Values
   A. Coins
   B. Currency

Content outlines in math generally are complete, but the behavior outline is nonexistent. Mathematics is an area in which students must perform many different types of behavior within essentially one or two number systems.

Goals can be identified parallelling each topic and a step-by-step analysis developed. A partial task analysis of the Goal IA from the outline above follows:

GOAL IA The students will be able to recognize each coin denomination on sight according to its name and monetary value.

Objective 1: The students, on being shown a penny, will say its name.

Objective 2: The students, on being shown a nickel, will say its name.

Objective 3: The students, on being shown a dime, will say its name.

Objective 4: The students, on being shown a quarter, will say its name.

Objective 5: The students, on being shown a half-dollar, will say its name.

Objective 6: The students, on being shown a penny, will indicate its monetary value.

Objective 7: The students, on being shown a nickel, will indicate its monetary value.

Objective 8: The students, on being shown a dime, will indicate its monetary value.

Objective 9: The students, on being shown a quarter, will indicate its monetary value.

Objective 10: The students, on being shown a half-dollar, will indicate its monetary value.

There are many lists of math objectives available to aid in writing a task analysis. State departments of education, individual school districts, or university education departments are excellent sources. Lists of objectives also accompany diagnostic tools, e.g., the Key Math Diagnostic Arithmetic Test (Connolly, Nachtman, & Pritchett, 1971).

Objectives A1-5 and A6-10 differ from each other only in terms of the coin mentioned. Repetition of the conditions in each objective can be dropped if a Table of Specifications is created.

Table of Specification in Mathematics

Table 8-3 is a Table of Specifications that has been constructed for the math outline shown in Figure 8-3, supra. Content material is listed down the left side and behaviors across the top. Goal IA corresponds to the one on which the task analysis was done. However, the table has eliminated the need for writing out each objective separately. Use of the Table of Specifications instead of a lengthy list of objectives combines an entire unit of study on one page, decreases paper work, and facilitates recordkeeping on individual students (Bloom, Hastings, & Madaus, 1971).

Preassessment of Students in Mathematics

As in the content areas, the initial step in instruction is to determine student entry level skills. A common procedure is to sample problems from the beginning, middle, and end of a math text. A survey of the students' abilities with tables in addition, subtraction, multiplication, and division can provide valuable instructional information.

Preassessment tests usually are found in every math text resource teacher's files and/or district math centers. By means of an error analysis, it can be determined exactly in what skill areas an individual student has deficiencies (Ashlock, 1976).

A test with one problem per skill level, increasing in difficulty, provides much information concerning specific needs. For example, a preassessment on addition might begin with problems like these:

4	2	4	8	12	55	15	74	17,583
+0	+3	1	+7	+ 5	+43	+ 6	+18	+79,275
		5						
		+9						

Information on student progress can be provided by the previous teacher to help determine a specific placement.

Table 8-3 Table of Specifications in Mathematics

Content: Mathematics Money Value	BEHAVIORS A. Identification	1. Knows name	2. Knows value	B. Equivalency	1. Combines equivalent and values	2. Combines money to get totals under $1	3. Combines money to get totals over $1	4. Uses both coins and currency	C. Making Change	1. Computes written word problems on paper	2. Computes realistic verbal problems using manipulatives
I. Value of Coins											
A. Penny											
B. Nickel											
C. Dime											
D. Quarter											
E. Half-dollar											
II. Value of Currency											
A. One-dollar bill											
B. Two-dollar bill											
C. Five-dollar bill											
D. Ten-dollar bill											
E. Twenty-dollar bill											
F. Fifty-dollar bill											
G. Hundred-dollar bill											

A set of CRTs may be included in the file together with each Table of Specifications from which they are generated (Gronlund, 1973). One or more criterion tests can be developed from each table. Their specificity is related to the difficulty of the concepts and the test tolerance level of the high school LBP student.

With respect to the Table of Specifications in Table 8-3, the basis for three CRT tests could be found by combining the content with (1) Identification behaviors, (2) Equivalency behaviors, and (3) Making Change behaviors. As each objective is learned, a CRT can be administered to evaluate whether mastery has occurred. If it has, this can be indicated in the appropriate cell of the table. If not, this also can be noted and further assignments can be given to aid mastery.

The Instructional Program

Once the evaluation model for a course has been written to include a preassessment, CRTs, a content outline, task analysis, and/or Table of Specifications, the instructional program can be administered. A filing system can facilitate this.

Material Organization

Teaching aids, e.g., work sheets, textbook passages, etc., can be placed in a folder and filed by objective number. In general mathematics courses, for example, all material related to a student's ability to perform long division problems can be placed in a coded file. Material for each objective can be coded and filed sequentially according to the original analysis or Table of Specifications. Students who enter with different skills as indicated by the result of their CRTs can be supplied with the appropriate materials. The teacher or student can go to the file for needed materials that are specific to the content deficit. In this way the teacher has written one basic program but can individualize for each student (Figure 8-4).

Contracts

The Table of Specifications also can be used to motivate and encourage students to assume a more responsible role in learning mathematics. By using all or part of the table, students and teacher can keep a daily record of class performance. With minor modifications, the tables can be altered into learning contracts. By setting specified timelines or proficiency levels, high school LBP students can take an active part in determining their own objectives.

A term contract can be set up to determine credits and grades. The materials can be broken into units, with a specified teaching mechanism and a specified response requirement for the student. Contracts also can allow for performance practice, contingent grades, and a performance criterion.

Some mainstreamed LBP students would be overwhelmed at contracting to learn all the material in a unit. A single contract over an entire unit would not allow for immediate or short-term reinforcement. It also assumes that the youth has pacing skills, i.e., the ability to judge how much and how often work must be done in order to meet the contract requirements. Many mainstream students do not appear to have appropriate pacing skills.

In the contract in Figure 8-5 are performance requirements and consequences. Performance requirements include: (1) doing all assignments, (2) completing them within two weeks, (3) showing all work, and (4) having a chance to redo (practice). The performance consequences include: (1) definition of grades (A, B, C, D), and (2) delineating a performance criterion (e.g., nine out of ten problems correct). Contracting in this manner has proved to be more effective than traditional lecture methods (Becker, Englemann, & Thomas, 1975).

Figure 8-4 Individual Performance Chart

Name _____ Long Division										
Content Whole Number System	A. Divides into numbers without a remainder	A.1 Single digit dividends	A.2 Two digit dividends	A.3 Three digit dividends	A.4 Four digit dividends	B. Divides into number with a remainder	B.1 Single digit dividends	B.2 Two digit dividends	B.3 Three digit dividends	B.4 Four digit dividends.
I. 0-9										
II. 10-99	M									
III. 100-999	M									
IV. 1.000-9.999	1/8/									
V. Any number 10.000										

M — Mastered at initial testing
1/8 — Began work on objective January 8
1/8 — Began work on January 8;
-1/20 mastered work on January 30

Figure 8-5 Two-Week Contract Based on Table of Specifications

Performance Requirements

I, _____ agree to complete Objectives I/A.1, I/A.2, I/A.3,
(student name)
and I/A.4 by doing all assignments related to these objectives in two
weeks. I must show all work. I may redo assignments.

Performance Consequences

To receive an A, I must answer 9 out of 10 problems correctly on
each assignment.

To receive a B, I must answer 8 out of 10 problems correctly on each
assignment.

To receive a C, I must answer 7 out of 10 problems correctly on each
assignment.

To receive a D, I must answer 6 out of 10 problems correctly on each
assignment.

LONG DIVISION		A. Divides into numbers without a remainder	A.1 Single-digit dividends	A.2 Two-digit dividends	A.3 Three-digit dividends	A.4 Four-digit dividends	B. Divides into number with a remainder	B.1 Single-digit dividends	B.2 Two-digit dividends	B.3 Three-digit dividends	B.4 Four-digit dividends
CONTENT: Whole Number System	I. 0-9		(contract)								
	II. 10-99										
	III. 100-999										
	IV. 1,000-9,999										
	V. Any number 10,000										

SUMMARY

The process for individualized content material and mathematics discussed here may seem time consuming. However, the process is one that either a content specialist or resource teacher can guide an aide, volunteer, or cross-age tutor to set up with minimal supervision. It is not critical that all material be gathered for every unit in the course before initiating the system. During the first year, materials can be assembled and coded as the LBP students progress through the program.

When the materials have been completed for one course, they can be used for individualized instruction as long as the same course is taught. Modification may be necessary periodically as the teacher improves the study materials by adding to them or deleting certain parts. It also is possible that more than one teacher will be using this same evaluation model, thereby reducing the load on one teacher for developing the course.

The model presented here can aid in the successful education of mainstreamed LBP students. Built into this model is a common source of information that can aid in the communication between a content specialist and resource teacher. Students' problems can be identified objectively. Material specific to the needs of the students can be provided in a systematic fashion and the teenagers can receive a successful learning experience.

Chapter 9

Formative Evaluation and Data Management Systems for LBP Adolescents

Michael J. Fimian and Stuart A. Goldstein

INTRODUCTION

Today's is an information-conscious society. Millions are spent annually for data management activities that include assessing information via computer; electronically monitoring the performance of sports teams; and recording not only the price of that pair of socks bought last weekend but also the item's inventory number, the date, hour, and minute of purchase, the teller's identification number, and possibly the current phase of the moon.

A decade ago hand calculators were unheard of and prohibitively expensive. Now, third graders purchase them with allowance money to help them complete their math homework. And anything larger than a credit card is considered cumbersome. Similarly, home computers have ceased to be the playthings of the affluent and have become integral selling items in electronic supply stores. Indeed, a multipaged advertisement in a comics magazine outlined the benefits of using home computers to children of elementary school age.

In light of the growing sophistication about and adaptation to this hardware and data-conscious technology, questions should be asked regarding the application to educational practices.

Should teachers spend at least as much time monitoring the specifics of students' classroom and instructional performance as on hallway, playground, and lunchroom duty; monitoring the restrooms; organizing the breakfast and lunch tickets; organizing PTA meetings; planning for holiday parties, plays, and other festivities; shooting the breeze in the breakroom, and any other of the various noninstructional activities in which they often find themselves involved?

The stance of this chapter is an unequivocal "Yes, teachers should be spending the time." "Will monitoring pupil progress take a bit of extra time? Probably yes." "Will it increase the teachers' load of paper work somewhat? Very probably yes." "Will these procedures and techniques make teachers more responsive to the learning rates and styles of the students? Most definitely yes."

EVALUATION AND EXCEPTIONAL LEARNERS

This chapter addresses a variety of pragmatic concerns related to the role of instructional evaluation and presents a number of methods of and management systems for monitoring progress-related data on students. Three major topics are discussed: (1) a general overview of evaluation of the handicapped, (2) formative evaluation, and (3) a procedural analysis combining both formative evaluation and data management for the classroom.

The choice and use of data-monitoring techniques and systems in classrooms for adolescents with learning and behavioral problems are best left to the discretion of the individual teacher, as not all of the techniques will be used with all students in each class. For this reason, it is important to note not only the conditions under which each technique can be used but also what type of information each will provide.

What Are Evaluation and Assessment?

At the outset, terms such as evaluation, assessment, and testing should be defined. In a general sense, evaluation is a comparison activity designed to determine individual functional levels, rate of acquisition or performance, and techniques for dealing with the environment (Smith & Neisworth, 1975). More specifically, it is composed of the activities of information gathering, organizing, synthesizing, and comparing that aid the teacher in making effective decisions about the status of each student's program. Evaluation can take various forms, two of the most common of which are termed summative and formative.

Summative evaluation can be used synonymously with the phrase "determining the present functioning level of the students." Based on information derived almost exclusively from normative measures, it usually yields performance facts such as mental age and grade norms that may prove inappropriate for many LBP adolescents. Typically, summative evaluation is a one-shot deal, consisting of testing and diagnosis at the beginning and end of the school year. Although this type of testing can be valuable, it nonetheless poses two major drawbacks:

1. the task of determining at the end of the school terms what the students did and did not learn during the year may leave little or no time for teachers to act on the information
2. the information generated from such testing probably is not detailed enough to enable the teachers to determine what the specific learning problem may be.

Formative evaluation, on the other hand, is used interchangeably with the phrases "continuing evaluation" or "periodically and repeatedly determining the present functioning level of the students.'' This involves the use of frequent evaluation of or progress checks on predetermined instructional objectives and the provision of feedback that will enable the teachers to effect continual modifications of the students' programs. In short, the instruction is formulated and reformulated, based on feedback concerning the youths' performance.

Assessment, which often is used in lieu of the terms diagnosis and evaluation, is a basic component of formative evaluation. It implies direct and frequent observation of each student's behavior and ''is clearly and simply the process of collecting data for the purpose of making decisions about pupils and their instructional programs'' (Ysseldyke & Regan, 1980, p. 465). Since the concepts of assessment and formative evaluation are closely allied in this chapter, they are used interchangeably.

However, neither assessment nor evaluation is used synonymously with the term testing. Testing, or what teachers do when they do not know ''where the child is at'' in terms of some predetermined skill sequence or body of concepts, is only one component of either assessment or evaluation—an important part, yet not the whole picture. Formative evaluation, in this sense, is not testing, per se. As indicated in Figure 9-1, it is any frequent and systematic means of observing, recording, analyzing, and displaying instructional data.

Why Evaluate Exceptional Learners?

The reasons for evaluating secondary students with learning and behavior problems are numerous. Three categories, based on (1) logistical or administrative, (2) programmatic, and (3) instructional reasons are most prominent.

Logistical Reasons for Evaluation

From an administrative viewpoint, exceptional students must be evaluated so that they first may be categorized according to impairment, disability, and/or handicap, and then placed in appropriate educational settings. The reason for this is simple—no selection, categorization, and placement of students, no federal or state money for program development and maintenance; no money, no special education programs; no programs, no special services to needy children.

Despite the advantages and disadvantages of using a categorical or taxonomic system reflecting either federal or state funding frameworks, the financial Zeitgeist of the early 1980s dictates that special students be categorized and labeled on at least an administrative level. The important distinction between the logistical and programmatic or instructional types of evaluation lies in the fact that whereas the latter procedures demand extensive and specific data, the former depend only on a minimum of two or more general types of norm-based data derived from the process.

Figure 9-1 The Generic Formative Evaluation Model

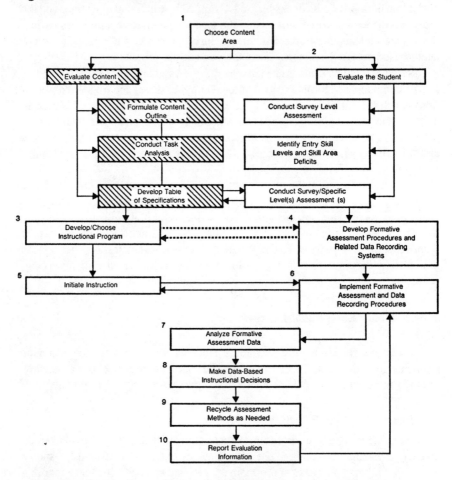

Note: Shaded areas denote procedural components discussed in Chapter 8.

Programmatic Reasons for Evaluation

Programmatic, as the term implies, links pupils' performance evaluation to the relative worth and validity of their programs. In at least some cases, the appropriateness of the special education program—i.e., the overall classroom program to which the students are assigned—is evaluated in light of how well it meets the youths' abilities and needs (DuBose, Langley, & Stagg, 1977). In most cases, however, program evaluation refers to the continuing critical analysis of the assigned instructional programs.

The evaluative focus in programmatic assessment, therefore, is not so much on the students as it is on the program or services offered. The teacher may ask such program evaluation questions as, "How do I improve the student's program?" "How do I maintain and improve upon the quality of the instructional programs already in progress?" "How can I validate the student's progress and establish a clearly defined link between that progress and my instructional decisions?"

Programmatic reasons are discussed here in a somewhat peripheral fashion because of similarities between these and the following instructionally based reasons for evaluating students.

Instructional Reasons for Evaluation

The third category of reasons for evaluating students pertains directly to those of an instructional nature. As a category, the information needed to effect precise and data-based instructional decisions is much more specific than that required by either the logistical or programmatic evaluation categories (Howell et al., 1979). The data derived from the evaluation should allow the teacher to determine: (1) students' present functioning level; (2) which skills they do and do not know; and (3) how rapidly they are learning what they do not know (Alper, Newlin, Lemoine, Perrine, & Bettencourt, 1973).

In terms of the students' individualized education plans (IEPs) and the teacher's compliance with P.L. 94-142, instructional evaluation determines: (1) the present level of the adolescents' educational performance; (2) annual goals and related short-term objectives; (3) the educational services to be provided; and (4) objective criteria and a variety of evaluation procedures that identify instructional success.

In short, instructional evaluation should be specific enough to allow for teacher decisions about the effectiveness of day-to-day instructional procedures followed and decisions made in the classroom.

FORMATIVE EVALUATION

Simplified Evaluation Models

When evaluating exceptional learners on either a summative (one-shot) or formative (continuing) basis, the same basic type of information is sought. That is, the evaluator seeks to measure the discrepancy between the LBP student's real, actual, or current performance and some preestablished goal or set of goals. The manner in which this information is accumulated is set out in some sequence of procedures—through testing and observation. This sequence of procedures is termed an evaluation model.

An example of a traditional summative model of evaluation is that presented by Smith (1974):

LEVEL 1 Referral
LEVEL 2 Evaluation
LEVEL 3 Educational plan development
LEVEL 4 Assignment of a suitable educational environment

Such models tend to be very general and represent logistical, programmatic, and instructional reasons for evaluation. They often are concerned with where the youth will be placed as opposed to what should be taught. It was not until the 1970s and the advent of the team approach or multidisciplinary staffing model mandated by P.L. 94-142 that the evaluation emphasis was expanded from only placement to include instructional goals and objectives derived from evaluation. This shift toward continuing instructional evaluation is best represented by two simplified models of formative evaluation—the DASIE and OTTER paradigms (Bateman, 1971). Each word is an acronym, each letter of which represents one step in the evaluation/teaching cycle.

D - *D*etermine objectives
A   - *A*ssess student and program
S   - *S*pecify instructional objectives
I   - *I*ntervene with instruction
E   - *E*valuate student progress (while reassigning objectives as needed)

O   - *O*bjectify
T   - *T*est
T   - *T*each
E   - *E*valuate
R   - *R*ecycle

In either case, the last or recycle step of each model differentiates it from those of a summative nature. Whereas summative evaluation tends to stress the first four steps in each of these models, formative evaluation emphasizes all five and particularly the last, or recycle, step. Although the two models enjoy widespread use, they still do not specifically address the transition procedures used in moving from the assessment/testing to the intervention/instruction and back to the assessment/testing stages. This rather complex transition is the focus for the balance of the chapter.

Formative Assessment in the Classroom

Formative assessment, which consists of a series of continuing procedures to define and gather the instructional information upon which decisions about pupils are made, is a prerequisite to effective and responsive education. It serves as a means both to diagnose and to monitor pupil learning problems and progress across instructional time.

Aside from the DASIE and OTTER paradigms, numerous theoretical models are used in the formative evaluation of instructional progress. Their characteristics tend to vary, but there is one attribute common to all: the recording of data in some continuing and systematic fashion. This has a number of advantages, among the most important being: (1) the rapid detection of potential problems; (2) the variety of techniques used in evaluating student growth and learning as it occurs; (3) the frequent and up-to-date feedback on instructional performance; (4) the earlier-than-usual changes in program procedures, if needed; and (5) more rapid student growth and learning.

To provide such responsive individual programming, the teacher must be able to accurately measure across and within content areas the skills that the students may or may not have acquired as yet. The teacher also must be able to monitor student progress through each curricular area. This entails gathering data, information, or facts regarding pupil performance. Collecting and analyzing data is not a recent or novel concept in educational circles. For years teachers routinely have monitored performance using grades and report cards or including anecdotal entries in students' files.

More recently, the concern for and views of instructional performance have become more refined in scope and more exacting in specificity. Accordingly, so too have the procedures for collecting, storing, and analyzing data. No longer are teachers concerned solely with global curricular areas such as reading. Rather, they need to know specific facts about which of the numerous decoding and comprehension skills and subskills their students may or may not know (Anderson, Hudson, & Jones, 1975).

The concept of evaluation, therefore, has been extended to include much more than testing and reporting scores. Testing may play an important role in the assessment of most handicapped adolescents, but it no longer is the only or the most important factor.

The Generic Evaluation Model

A generic evaluation model that outlines a number of important steps in evaluating student progress is presented next. Because it is generic, it does not state which norm-referenced and criterion-referenced tests, probes, quizzes, programs, and instructional sequences should be used with particular students. Such concerns are better left to the discretion of the teacher. It does, however, describe an evaluation procedure that not only increases the quantity and quality of instructionally relevant information in the classroom but also improves the effectiveness with which this material can be used in prescriptive programming.

Before discussing the generic model of formative evaluation, a number of already marketed and/or published models bear mentioning. These range from informal and anecdotal recordkeeping to the more formal structure of precision teaching. Although most or all models collect and utilize data, the types of materials amassed and the methods for interpreting them vary from model to model. The following represent some of the models used most frequently.

The Diagnostic-Prescriptive Teaching Model

The Diagnostic-Prescriptive Teaching Model consists of a number of methods using diagnostic information in the modification of educational programs (Peter, 1965). It is intended to modify instructional and environmental factors in order to offset students' process deficits. A prescriptive educational program is designed using a multidisciplinary approach with a strong emphasis on students' medical and psychomedical disorders. Both instructional and noninstructional data such as medical information, family histories, social and psychological reports, and norm-referenced and other standardized test scores are collected and presented in a case study format. Data are recorded infrequently as few direct measures of student progress are obtained. (Direct and indirect measures are discussed in more detail later in this chapter.) Because of definition problems with a number of the measured constructs, difficulties also occur often in interpretation.

The Diagnostic-Teaching Model

Kirk's (1972) Diagnostic Teaching Model shares many of the same features and techniques of the previous model because both are primarily process oriented. The major difference, however, is that the Diagnostic Teaching Model places less emphasis on the use of case histories and greater stress on the identification of the student's learning style preference. Once the latter has been determined, instruction is tailored to that learning style.

The model also uses data derived from global tests such as the Illinois Test of Psycholinguistic Abilities (ITPA), other standardized and norm-referenced tests, and informal observation. However, data frequently are recorded and derived more from the process-oriented assessment instruments than from direct measures such as observation and probe testing. As in the previous model, occasional difficulties in interpretation are encountered because the system's process-based terminology and proficiency are determined by comparing students' test scores in relation to preestablished levels found in norm-referenced instruments.

The Narrative Log

The Narrative Log and its use are described at some length by Howell et al. (1979). The Log is simply a written record of teachers' observations to increase their awareness of student gains by providing feedback to and structuring observations for them. Data are collected daily in anecdotal and longhand form—a tedious procedure at best. The most effective type of information to include in the Narrative Log is a written account of student performance and task results, in addition to other general instructional observations.

The Precision Teaching Model

The Precision Teaching Model employs a highly structured and standardized procedure to plan, monitor, and evaluate growth and changes in student performance through the direct, continuing, and daily measurement of academic behavior. Its strategies are based on the task analyses and behavioral models of teaching as they monitor and direct students' academic growth in terms of the discrete skills the adolescents may or may not know. Although the type of data collected and plotted is exclusively in rate form, percentages can be determined quickly (White & Haring, 1976). Skill-specific data are recorded very frequently—as often as every day—and usually in terms of the direct measures of one correct rate and one error rate per task per day.

The Directive Teaching Model

The Directive Teaching Model developed and later revised by Stephens (1970, 1977) is a "system of instruction that aids those who teach children with learning and behavioral difficulties to be effective in academic instruction" (Stephens, 1977, p. 109). Based on a behavioral and task analysis format, a hierarchy of component skills is taught in such a way that the acquisition of a number of complex terminal behaviors results. Mastery criteria are defined in measurable terms. The revised evaluation model—the Directive Teaching Instructional Management System, or DTIMS—contains curriculum and social skills assessment instructions. The direct measures of observation and probe testing produce data that are recorded and easily interpreted.

The Criterion-Referenced Testing Model

Criterion-referenced skill testing, which is outlined by Gronlund (1973) and discussed at length by Howell et al. (1979) and Howell and Kaplan (1980), represents a general approach to the use of teacher-developed and teacher-adopted CRTs. Commonly referred to as informal testing, criterion-referenced models allow student populations to be directly evaluated across a broad range and variety of instructional continua. (Chapter 8 and the material later in this section provide a more detailed discussion of the characteristics and uses of CRTs.) The goal of the CRT Model is to determine entry level skills that are based on the mastery of specific subtasks of the terminal objective.

Essentially, what is pretested . . . is what is taught . . . is what is post-tested . . ., ad infinitum. Data are behaviorally based, specific, observable, and measurable and are presented in a task format. Both speed and accuracy criteria are determined by the teacher on either an a priori basis or from research that has determined accuracy, mastery, and automatic criteria for various tool skill areas such as reading and mathematics. The teacher can record easily understood data from direct measures such as observation, probe testing, and the use of true trials and short CRTs.

Task Analysis Evaluation

Task Analysis Evaluation, as proposed by Howell et al. (1979) and Howell and Kaplan (1980), is very similar to the previous model. Being skill based, evaluation is conducted to determine which skills a student may or may not know. Accuracy, mastery, and automatic criteria levels across major skill areas are outlined. Data can be recorded through the use of direct measures and generally are easily interpreted.

Miscellaneous Models

Numerous other formative assessment models exist.

Individually Prescribed Instruction. Closely related to the previous two models, this is an evaluation system in which the content material is "sequentially ordered into tracks of skills . . . that build upon one another. Placement tests and pretests determine what lesson would be worked on or skipped . . . [and when] it is time to move to the next unit" (Becker, Englemann, & Thomas, 1975, p. 8). Data are recorded frequently to ensure rapid progress through predetermined skill continua.

Management by Objectives. This model is a "strategy of planning and getting results in the direction that management [or the teacher] wishes . . . while meeting the goals and satisfaction of its participants [or students]" (Mali, 1977, p. 1). By setting projected goal dates, teachers automatically increase their efficiency in future teaching and learning activities. Data collected on task proficiency usually are behavioral and task specific.

Clinical Teaching Model. This method (Lerner, 1971) is based on the behavioral model in which both instruction and assessment are continuous and interrelated. The model incorporates an alternating test-teach-test-teach methodology to accumulate a reliable data base from which effective and responsive instructional decisions may be made. Data are gathered by compiling case histories, clinical observations, informal test results, and standardized and normed test scores.

Classroom Communications System. Proposed by McCormack and Chalmers (1978), this is similar to the previous three models in that it is based on a skills testing and teaching format that provides for continuous assessment of pupil growth across time. Its major strength is its systematic and easily used data recordkeeping system (described at length later in this chapter).

Decision Model for Diagnostic Teaching. This model, proposed by Cartwright, Cartwright, and Ysseldyke (1973) and discussed by Ysseldyke and Regan (1980), stresses the role or hypothesis formation and testing in teacher and psychologist decision making. It also involves the systematic alteration of objectives, materials, methods, and instructional techniques that occurs until procedures that accelerate pupil progress are identified.

In summary, these formative assessment models include, in varying degrees, the following characteristics: (a) the procedures are continuous, (b) instructional data are collected with varying frequencies, (c) potential problems are detected rapidly, (d) programs and program modifications stem from the data base, (e) student instructional gains across time are monitored, and (f) frequent and updated feedback is available to both teachers and students.

THE INSTRUCTIONALLY BASED MODEL

The generic and instructionally based model of formative evaluation typifies a number of previously outlined characteristics and therefore is similar to a number of these models. In short, it incorporates a number of attributes common to all models, thus making it a model in the generic sense. This section views the model conceptually in terms of its component parts; the next section discusses its evaluation activities, including norm-referenced and criterion-referenced tests.

The Trilevel Evaluation Model in Figure 9-2 has its roots in the task analysis and instructional objectives traditions. It is an extension of the model in Figure 9-1, supra. Instead of more traditional models that specify only a chronological sequence of evaluation activities or that propose or oppose the use of only CRTs or NRTs, the generic model is premised on three levels of evaluation: survey, specific, and intensive.

Levels of evaluation are defined in terms of the specificity of test questions, the resultant data, and the level of analysis needed to effect programming decisions. On the survey level of evaluation, general ability or achievement tests—typically NRTs—are used to collect data. These data are of a general nature and are used in formulating hypotheses about groups or categories of errors that the students may exhibit. These hypotheses are accepted or rejected by proceeding to the next, more specific, level of evaluation.

The more specific test items should yield additional specific data that may validate or invalidate the original hypothesis(es) and/or more clearly define error

Figure 9-2 Three Levels of Evaluation

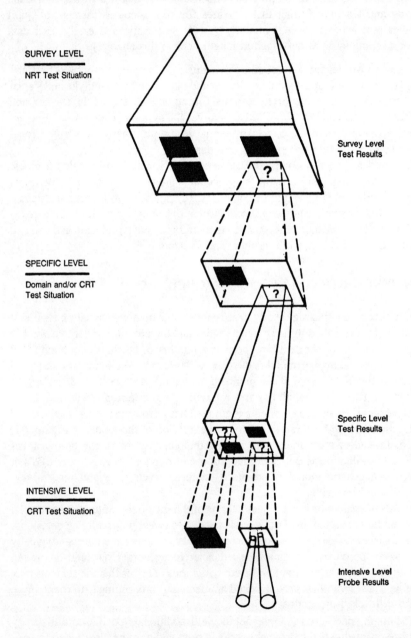

SURVEY LEVEL

NRT Test Situation

Survey Level
Test Results

SPECIFIC LEVEL

Domain and/or CRT
Test Situation

Specific Level
Test Results

INTENSIVE LEVEL

CRT Test Situation

Intensive Level
Probe Results

patterns that the students may exhibit in either test or observation situations. If even more specific information is needed to validate this or subsequent hypotheses, the teacher may have to proceed directly to the third (intensive) level of evaluation.

Although some models such as Howell et al. (1979) stipulate a two-level model very similar to the one proposed here, it has been these authors' experience that a third and intensive level of evaluation may sometimes be needed when evaluating more seriously involved students. What follows is a summary of each of the levels in the Trilevel Evaluation Model, and a description of the activities at each level.

Survey Level Evaluation

Survey level evaluation is the first step in assessing adolescents with learning and behavioral problems. Initially, most students are evaluated on this level. Some learners—younger or seriously involved ones, for instance—may enter the sequence by being evaluated on the second (specific) or third (intensive) level.

Survey level evaluation usually is conducted by the special education teacher, school psychologist, or school counselor on a screening basis in which a number of students may be tested in any one sitting. Achievement tests, various other NRTs that yield normative data, and infrequently used and very general CRTs are used. In short, survey level assessment relies heavily on the use of published materials and tests. The type of information derived at this level also is general enough that it provides a foundation for further diagnosis. With this information, tentative hypotheses regarding testee errors may be made.

Survey level assessment can be conducted by using NRTs that test any of the following areas (Blake, 1974):

Social Skills	Prevocational Skills
Self-Help Skills	Vocational Skills
Survey Battery(ies)	Spelling
Listening	Handwriting
Vocabulary	English Usage
Speech	Written Composition
Reading (survey)	Arithmetic (survey)
Reading (diagnostic)	Arithmetic (diagnostic)
Projective Tests	Diagnostic-Remedial Tests

Test names for each of these categories can be found in Buros (1978). Since these tests generally are NRTs, they are composed of a representative sample of behaviors that reflects a broader universe of information with varying degrees of validity and reliability.

Standardized or norm-referenced tests typically select representative samples of skills to be tested—ones that are somewhat different from those that will be taught eventually, and compare one student's performance to that of the population on which the test was standardized. Criterion-referenced tests are composed of larger and more representative numbers of items, assess a majority of the skills that eventually will be taught, and compare one student's performance only with that individual's past or future performance (Gronlund, 1973).

The standardized test that provides sufficient instructional information to classify it as a specific level evaluation instrument is rare; more often than not, it is categorized at the survey level. In addition, some general CRTs may be normed, categorized, and used as survey level instruments. Most frequently, however, CRTs have been developed for use on the specific level of evaluation. For examples of instruments in each of these categories, note Exhibit 9-1. Detailed and critical reviews of many of these tests may be found in Buros (1978).

Exhibit 9-1 Levels of Evaluation by Types of Tests Matrix

| | | LEVELS OF EVALUATION | |
	Survey	*Specific*	*Intensive*
Standardized or Norm-Referenced Tests	Key Math Wechsler Adult Intelligence Scales Stanford Achievement Test Wide Range Achievement Tests Comprehensive Tests of Basic Skills Metropolitan Achievement Test Gates-MacGinitie Reading Test	Woodcock Reading Mastery Scales Gates-McKillor Reading Diagnostic Tests Stanford Diagnostic Arithmetic Test	
Criterion-Referenced Tests	Oregon Math Inventory Oregon Reading Inventory Prescriptive Reading Inventory	Teacher-developed CRTs Curriculum pre/post tests Marketed CRTs not affiliated with marketed instructional programs	Curriculum Probes Marketed probes and CRTs not directly affiliated with marketed instructional programs

(TYPES OF TESTS)

What, then, is the major difference between survey level and specific level tests? The difference is defined as the type of information gained by each level of testing. Survey level tests do not usually yield information from which instruction may be developed; conversely, specific level testing does provide information that, in most cases, can be translated directly into the programming of instructional sequences. Information from survey level tests almost always is presented in terms of group comparisons.

For example, scores on the survey level Woodcock Reading Mastery Test may state that Beth is functioning on the 1.7-2.6 grade equivalent level in word attack skills. In contrast, data from a more specific teacher-developed CRT may demonstrate that Beth was able to identify orally the letter sounds [S], [T], [L], [N], [I], [R], [A], [F], [C], [D], [H], and [P] at a rate of 60 per minute with 100 percent accuracy but was unable to accurately blend two known sounds at a rate of 60 per minute without pausing between two sounds. In short, the types of information generated by both levels of evaluation vary dramatically. Procedural distinctions between use of the two levels are discussed later in this section.

Survey level information need not only be framed in terms of a test score, subtest scores, scattergrams, or profile analysis. Instead, a general sample of students' behavior on a given task can be obtained by observing them as they work on class assignments, NRTs, CRTs, or newly taught material (deriving information through both observation and test use is in the next section). Fact finding, then, represents an important first step of each level of evaluation.

Immediately thereafter, a close inspection of the content and a task analysis of the incorrect responses may be necessary. Based on error patterns that may be evident in the data, one or more hypotheses are generated. Finally, the hypotheses must be accepted or rejected, based upon further fact finding. Typically, further fact finding needed to confirm or negate a hypothesis means progressing from one to the next specific level of evaluation. Similarly, to validate the hypotheses on the specific level, the teacher may have to progress to an intensive level of evaluation.

Specific Level Evaluation

The purpose of specific level evaluation is to validate the hypotheses and/or confirm the conclusions reached at the survey level. Additional specific level test data also may suggest more numerous or more extensive hypotheses. These, in turn, can be validated by proceeding to the intensive level of evaluation. Teachers who rarely depend on NRTs and frequently use CRTs in their instructional evaluation very probably are entering the Trilevel Model directly at the specific level. In most cases, evaluation on only the specific level is sufficient for instructional purposes. In situations in which additional information is needed, evaluation proceeds to the intensive level.

Specific level diagnosis is geared more toward within-individual evaluation than is survey level diagnosis. In short, specific level evaluation should show most of what the student may or may not know about a specific content area. On the specific level, also, instruments that are composed of a very representative sample of test items derived from either a specific body of knowledge, a curriculum program, a unit of instruction, or a text chapter are used. Accordingly, the information on these tests frequently is relied upon for instruction, program development, and curriculum evaluation. These tests should be used only for the selection and classification of skills to be taught and, in some cases, for the assignment of LBP students to instructional groups according to ability levels. Classifying and labeling adolescents or assigning them to special education settings may occasionally be an appropriate use of specific level test data.

Intensive Level Evaluation

Intensive level evaluation is very similar to specific level evaluation. In fact, Howell et al. (1979) and Howell and Kaplan (1980) combine specific and intensive levels of evaluation under the heading specific level evaluation. The major discriminants between the two levels are (1) the degree of range and scope of the content, (2) the degree of representativeness of test items to the content, and (3) the ease with which intensive level tests can be constructed and given.

Intensive level tests, sometimes termed probes, typically are one-page documents. Eventually, all the test items are to be taught. Furthermore, the items are very specific in that the test constructor has analyzed the content of what is to be assessed as thoroughly and vigorously as possible. As a result, the representativeness of the test items is as thorough as is possible while still being practical.

If the skills to be taught are all addition facts for any number, 0 to 9, for example, then all possible combinations of addition math facts will be probed. Probe construction also allows the teacher to immediately determine the content that is known and the error patterns that may be produced (Exhibit 9-2).

Exhibit 9-3 is a Math Facts Probe that represents the following 11 single-digit (0-to-9) vertical addition math fact combinations:

A	B	C	D	E	F	G	H	I	J	K
0	□	□	□	□	□	□	□	□	□	□
+□	+0	+1	+2	+3	+4	+5	+6	+7	+8	+9

The probe is limited to only one area (addition math facts), while the range of content is clearly defined and limited (vertical addition math facts using only single digits 0 to 9). On this probe, heavy transverse lines have been drawn in after testing

Exhibit 9-2 Types of Math Facts Errors Observed in Elementary and Secondary School Pupils

---

ADDITION

Made errors in combinations
Made errors in counting
Lost added carried number
Forgot to add carried number
Wrote number to be carried
Performed irregular procedure
   in column
Carried wrong number
Grouped two or more numbers
Split numbers into parts
Used wrong fundamental operation
Depended on visualization
Disregarded column position
Repeated work after partly done
Omitted one or more digits

Made errors in reading numbers
Dropped back one or more places
Derived unknown combination from
   familiar one
Disregarded one column
Made error in writing answer
Skipped one or more decades
Carried when there was
   nothing to carry
Used scratch paper
Added in pairs, giving last
   even as answer
Added same digit in two columns
Wrote carried number in answer
Added same number twice
Lost place in column

Source: Adapted from G.T. Buswell & L. John, *Diagnostic studies in arithmetic*. Chicago: University of Chicago Press, 1926, p. 27.

---

to indicate each of these error categories. Students do not perceive these categories during testing and are directed to answer all problems in a left-to-right direction, starting with the problem at the upper left.

There are limitations in the types of data that can be derived from intensive level probes. These probes tell teachers a great deal about addition and subtraction math facts, percentages, or decimals but little about more general information such as part-whole relationships. A thorough specific level test of part-whole relationships, on the other hand, will show the students' skill level at converting decimals into percentages but will tell the teacher little about their ability to deal with rational numbers in a variety of ways.

Accordingly, a survey level test for mathematics—the Key Math Diagnostic Arithmetic Test, for instance—will tell the teacher about the students' general functioning level across most mathematics operations, processes, and products but may not provide specific or intensive level information regarding any one of these factors. In short, what is not tested should not be open to conjecture. It should, instead, be tested.

Exhibit 9-3 Addition Math Facts Probe[1]

CATEGORY GROUPS—ADDITION

Date: _____   Grade: _____   Time: _____   Name: _____

F	2 +4	7 +6	4 +2	2 +5	4 +1	1 +0	7 +8	4 +3	0 +8	7 +7	4 +9
H	9 +6	3 +2	3 +5	5 +1	4 +0	3 +8	0 +3	0 +7	5 +7	1 +9	9 +4
D	2 +2	1 +5	3 +1	9 +0	5 +8	6 +3	0 +3	0 +7	5 +9	4 +4	8 +6
G	4 +5	7 +1	2 +0	4 +8	5 +3	0 +4	9 +7	0 +9	3 +4	3 +6	8 +2
C	1 +1	8 +0	8 +8	3 +3	0 +5	1 +7	2 +9	1 +4	2 +6	7 +2	5 +5
B	6 +0	9 +8	8 +3	0 +6	4 +7	7 +9	6 +4	5 +6	6 +2	0 +5	9 +1
J	0 +8	2 +3	0 +1	8 +7	3 +9	7 +4	1 +6	1 +2	6 +5	6 +1	5 +0
E	7 +3	0 +9	3 +7	9 +9	8 +4	0 +6	9 +2	9 +5	8 +1	0 +0	6 +8
A	0 +2	6 +7	8 +9	5 +4	6 +6	0 +2	7 +5	2 +1	7 +0	2 +8	1 +3
	2 +7	6 +9	0 +4	4 +6	5 +2	8 +5	0 +1	3 +0	1 +8	9 +3	0 +10

I   K   F   H   D   G   C   B   J   E   A

1. Adjusted to show category groupings of single-digit vertical addition math facts. Each category grouping is a potential category of errors.

Source: Reprinted with permission from A. Hofmeister. *Diagnostic math facts test.* Exceptional child Center. Utah State University. 1972.

Three Levels by Four Stages

As noted in the discussion on survey level assessment and as shown in Figure 9-3, there are four steps in evaluating adolescents with learning and behavioral problems: fact finding or information gathering, data analysis, hypothesis formation, and hypothesis validation. These steps tend to clarify the differences between one level of evaluation and another, particularly since those distinctions often are vague. In fact, these distinctions consist only of the procedural steps needed to ascertain relevant instructional information.

The first step—fact finding—occurs during survey level evaluation. The last step—validating the hypothesis generated from this information—occurs at the specific level. In the interim, test users move from the survey to the specific levels by undertaking the second and third activities—analysis of the test items and formulation of hypotheses based on the analysis (Howell et al., 1979). Similarly, fact finding can occur on the specific level, with related hypotheses validated on the intensive level of evaluation; test users once again must utilize data analysis, hypothesis formation, and hypothesis validation activities.

Gathering Pupil Performance Information

Educators do not evaluate by tests alone. There are two major sources of obtaining information on pupil performance in the classroom. The first is through the use of either NRTs, CRTs, or a combination of the two; the second is through direct observation of the students interacting with their educational environment, as shown in Exhibit 9-4. A third, frequently used, option is to combine both test and observation data when making instructional decisions. In this section both the first and second options are reviewed; the third is discussed in the formative assessment procedural analysis later in this chapter.

Mention has been made of direct and indirect assessment. Direct assessment refers to evaluation based on the instructional materials or programs that will be used later in instruction. Indirect assessment refers to the evaluation of student performance using materials, tests, or instruments not directly developed from instructional programs (Howell et al., 1979). Direct measures usually yield voluminous and specific data, as teachers often use CRTs as direct assessment measures when monitoring specific progress. Indirect measures of performance, on the other hand, often yield more limited general information through the use of standardized achievement and diagnostic tests. These often measure related concepts that either have not been or will not be taught directly. In Exhibit 9-4, direct measures of performance are most likely to occur in options II and III; indirect measures in option I, and particularly in I.A.

Figure 9-3 Steps in Procedural Analysis

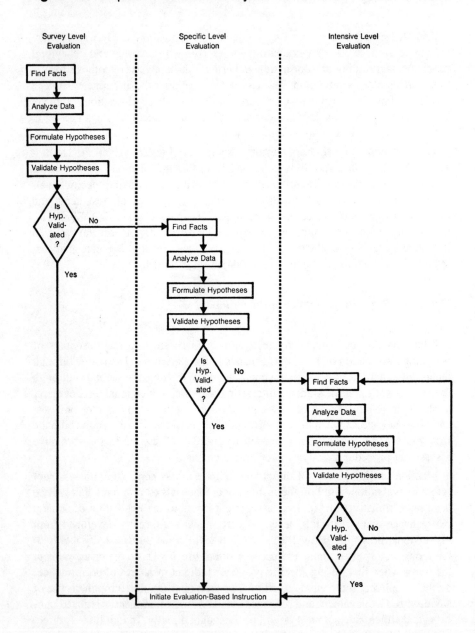

Exhibit 9-4 Sources of Student Performance Data

I. Test Data
   A. Norm-Referenced Test Data
   B. Criterion-Referenced Test Data

II. Direct Observation Data
   A. Direct Measurement of Lasting Products
   B. Direct Measurement of Performance
      1. Percentage Correct System
      2. Points Scored System
      3. Frequency System
      4. Rate System
   C. Observational Recording
      1. Continuous Recording
      2. Event Recording
      3. Duration Recording
      4. Interval Recording

III. Direct Observation of Test Situation Plus Test Data

NORM- AND CRITERION-REFERENCED EVALUATION

A frequent source of direct and indirect measurement data upon which instructional decisions are made is that derived from the administration of tests. How these tests compare with one another and how and under what conditions they may be used are analyzed briefly.

A Comparison of Test Types

The major differences between norm-referenced and criterion-referenced types of tests are outlined in Exhibit 9-5. Also included are some of the major strengths and weaknesses of each type as well as various limits on their use.

It is beyond the scope of this chapter to discuss test type differences in detail; however, helpful information may be found not only in Exhibit 9-5 but also in Alley and Foster (1978), Ebel (1975), Gronlund (1973), Howell et al. (1979), Howell and Kaplan (1980), and Popham (1976).

A Comparison of Test Use

As implied in Exhibit 9-5, NRTs differ from CRTs in terms of definition, emphasis, basis, type of items, and their assumptions and development. The

Exhibit 9-5 Comparison of the Two Types of Evaluation Instruments

Instrument Characteristics	Norm-Referenced	Criterion-Referenced
	Types of Tests	
CLASSIFICATION PURPOSES	Classifies student as high, middle, or low performer.	Classifies one student only in terms of skills known and skills not known, or in relation to a preestablished criterion.
TEST BASES	Is based on average test performance of specific populations of selected subjects. Variables controlled for are race, geographical area, socio-economic status, sex, etc.	Is based on specific task or objective sequences regardless of who exhibits the skills or how well they are being performed.
PERFORMANCE	Performance is relative and equated with a normal distribution.	Performance is an absolute "yes-no" or "can-cannot do" matter.
TYPES OF SCORES	a. grade equivalent scores b. percentile ranks c. standard scores d. stanine scores e. untransformed raw scores	a. learner has or has not reached criterion for acceptable performance in terms of percentage, rate, duration, precision, or quality criteria
APPROPRIATE USES	a. selection of students b. classification of students c. obtaining survey level instructional information	a. progress in skill or curricular sequence b. monitoring instructional and learning progress c. obtaining specific and intensive levels of instructional information
INAPPROPRIATE USES AND LIMITATIONS	a. not to be used for program or curriculum evaluation b. not used frequently in instruction	a. not for cross-curriculum comparisons b. not for classification and selection of students
DEFINITION/ INTERPRETATION	Individual's test performance is compared against others on the same test; discriminates performance between children.	Individual's test performance is compared against absolute standards; discriminates performance of one child across time.

Exhibit 9-5 continued

EMPHASIS	Emphasizes general individual differences by surveying generally accepted skills and knowledges. Used on survey level of evaluation.	Emphasizes specific individual differences by specific and intensive level assessment procedures. Objectives are usually related to curriculum content.
DEVELOPMENT ACTIVITIES	a. content area specified b. test items developed that tap skill or process areas c. norms established via formative evaluation d. reliability and validity measures determined e. cannot be easily developed by the teacher	a. curriculum or content area specified and analyzed b. test items written to reflect content and operations c. criteria established d. can be easily developed by teacher
TEST ITEM SAMPLING	Test items are a general and representative sampling of more global skill or process areas. It is assumed that the test items validly and reliably reflect the hypothetical construct.	Test items are a specific and general-to-absolute sampling of skills. Little or limited sampling is done. Test items should replicate behaviors called for in instruction.

manner in which each is used and the information that results also differentiate the two. For example, NRTs must be used as decreed by the test administration manual. CRT use, on the other hand, tends to be more flexible. Data derived from NRTs lend themselves to open, broad, and general interpretation, whereas CRT results are limited more to closed skill-oriented assessment of rather narrow scope. NRT raw scores, for instance, often must be transformed into normative, relative, or comparative numbers while CRTs' give general-to-specific indications of how well the students perform in some skill area in relation to some preestablished criterion for acceptable performance.

Because NRTs essentially are discriminatory by nature, their use increases the probability of the teacher's either purposely or inadvertently misusing the data (Ysseldyke & Regan, 1980). For this reason, a clamor has arisen calling for a moratorium on NRTs and for an increased emphasis on the primary or sole use of CRTs—a stance with which neither these authors nor the American Psychological Association (APA, 1966) necessarily agree.

The rationale behind the disagreement between advocates of criterion- and advocates of norm-referenced testing is that criterion data delineate only skill deficits in individual learners whereas normative data differentiate one student from another in terms of relative performance. In short, NRTs assess performances between and among youths, CRTs variations in each student's performance on a student-by-student basis. In this process NRT students generally are classified as high, middle, or low performers while the CRT rates each only in terms of what the person does and does not know.

In NRT use, performance is usually equated with their adolescent peers while CRT is more of a "yes-no" or "did the student reach the criterion?" matter. NRTs are relatively general in scope and context as compared to CRTs and are used most often for screening, survey, and global diagnosis. CRTs permit specific and intensive levels of diagnosis. Whereas educators should not teach to NRTs, they can use the CRT as an outline for instruction. NRTs also tend to be of the paper and pencil variety while there are many more possibilities for the student to respond using CRTs—an important consideration in working with LBP adolescents.

Because of the formality of NRT administration (as opposed to the informality of CRTs), the situation does not always allow for impromptu, in situ, or informal hypothesis testing. Furthermore, NRTs allow for only general error analyses while CRT data tend to be used in more specific hypothesis situations. The duration of NRTs tends to vary from one to the next but usually is strictly controlled by the instructions; CRT administration time, on the other hand, often is open ended. Finally, NRTs' results very often are used in conjunction with logistical, administrative, and placement decisions while CRT scores provide information more germane to individual instructional decisions.

In summary, the process of comparing NRTs to CRTs is somewhat akin to comparing cross-country with downhill skiing. Both activities need snow, use skiis, and are predicated on different outcomes desired from each sport. They are alike, yet so very different, that comparison activities can easily lose their meaning. In testing, as in skiing, being aware of the similarities, distractions, and conditions of appropriate and inappropriate use of each system helps educators decide which test should be used.

DIRECT OBSERVATION METHODS OF EVALUATION

The second option in instructional data collection is that of the direct observation of student behaviors during nontest situations. This general heading includes three data monitoring and formative assessment procedures: (1) direct measures of lasting products, (2) direct measures of performance, and (3) true observational recording (note Exhibit 9-4, supra). Each of these categories can be further analyzed into a series of discrete procedures.

The first and simplest of these—directly measuring lasting products—usually consists of nothing more than recording daily the number of work sheet pages done, pages read, lessons completed, and skills performed.

The second category—the direct measurement of performance—includes monitoring procedures such as percentage correct, points scored, and frequency, and/or rate. This last-named procedural category views student performance as adequate when it reaches or exceeds some predetermined accuracy, mastery, or maintenance criterion.

The third and least frequently used category is observational recording. This consists of procedures such as continuous, event or frequency, duration, and interval recording. Although applicable to the monitoring of academic behaviors, these procedures often are used in behavior management.

The Number of Lasting Products System

This first category of monitoring techniques is easily implemented in the classroom as it records only very generally how much work has been completed. The teacher need only keep a daily chart or graph of the number of items completed per student in any standard time period, such as:

1. the number of spelling words learned per half hour
2. the number of DISTAR lessons completed per hour
3. the number of math facts completed per 10 minutes

Cross-day comparisons must be made in terms of a standard time unit. If the performance time has changed (i.e., lengthened or shortened), the data become biased and must be adjusted proportionally to cancel out differences between the time units. Quality is not necessarily important since progress is determined by making day-to-day comparisons of the number of words, lessons, or pages completed within the stipulated time period. However, as shown in Figure 9-4, scoring conventions can be used to indicate whether or not the students have met the criterion.

When progress is monitored in terms of lasting products, both data recording and plotting activities are combined. To display these types of data, a simple graph is sufficient. By labeling the vertical axis in terms of the number of word units, lessons, pages, or tasks completed in the stipulated time period, and the horizontal axis in terms of the time unit, the teacher can rapidly record, plot, and display student performances as in Figure 9-4.

Figure 9-4 Lasting Products Data[1]

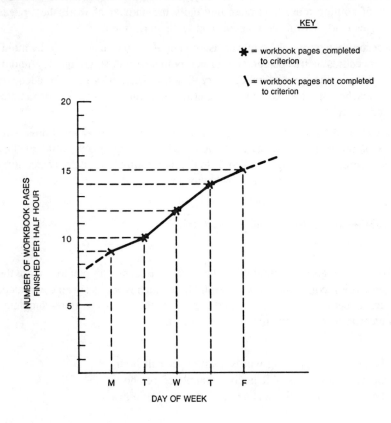

1. Plotted by date and number of items completed; pupil success (i.e., reaching or exceeding a criterion) also is noted.

The Direct Measures of Performance System

As indicated earlier, assessment can be either direct, in that it tests directly the matter to be taught, or indirect because it evaluates either already taught material in an indirect fashion or related material in a direct way. In this second category of measurement techniques—direct evaluation—the teacher is concerned not only with how much work is completed but how well and/or how fast it is done. Quality of performance therefore can be expressed by any or all of the direct measure methods: (1) the percentage correct system, (2) the points scored system, (3) the frequency system, and (4) the rate system. Each provides specific information regarding both the quality and quantity of student performance.

The Percentage Correct System

This first direct measurement system is the one most commonly used by teachers, probably because it is traditional, simple, and can be used rapidly. The percentage of correct responses is calculated by dividing the number of times a behavior is performed correctly by the number of times it is observed (whether it is incorrectly or correctly performed), and multiplying the result by 100.

$$\frac{\text{\# of Correct Trials}}{\text{Total \# of Trials}} \times 100 = \square \ \%$$

The recording of percent correct data is done simply by tallying the number of correct responses on scratch paper or on some established data form (three of which are shown in Figure 9-5). Typically, percentages are calculated on the form, as in example (c). In some cases the calculations may be dispensed with if percentage criterion levels are established beforehand and indicated on the form, as in example (a) (note the 80 percent and 90 percent criterion lines). At other times, simple data may be left in raw score form to be eyeballed, as in example (b).

The plotting and displaying of percent correct data require tallying responses as either correct or incorrect, comparing the number of correct ones with the total number of answers, and graphing each percentage as a data point on a standard graph form. Percentages of correct responses are plotted on the vertical axis; time is plotted on the horizontal axis.

The Points Scored System

This second direct measure of performance is used in programs in which student progress is defined in terms of both (1) how much teacher assistance has been and/or is being given during any one presentation, and (2) the decreasing degrees of teacher assistance across instructional time the adolescents require to perform a task (McCormack, 1976). This system is extremely sensitive in situations in which the students make few or small gains, or advance very slowly over time, or in which the teacher purposefully manipulates or fades assistance. The system is used often when teaching motor skills but is applicable to the instruction of many cognitive or knowing skills as well.

The recording of data on points scored is done in a very specific fashion. Given a task or content analysis, student performance on each step or substep is rated, and a total score summed for the points score. The analysis and scoring procedure are structured by the data form in Figure 9-6. A task analysis of the terminal behavior of face washing results in 17 discrete steps; the student's performance of each step is rated according to the range shown in the key at the bottom of the form. The

Figure 9-5 Three Data Recording Conventions in the Percentage Correct System*

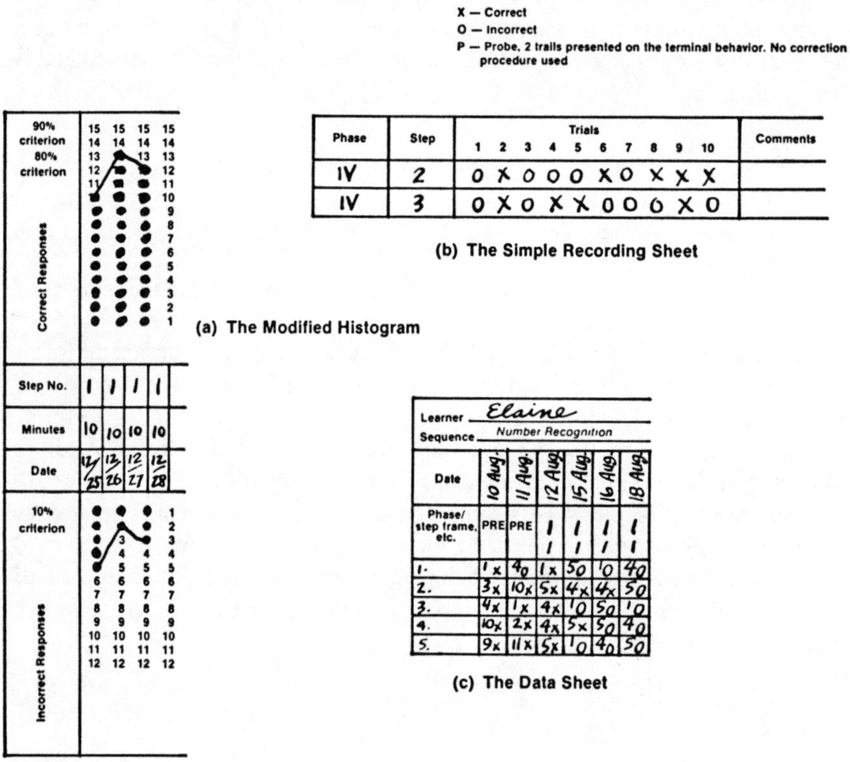

X — Correct
O — Incorrect
P — Probe, 2 trails presented on the terminal behavior. No correction procedure used

(a) The Modified Histogram

Phase	Step	Trials 1 2 3 4 5 6 7 8 9 10	Comments
IV	2	O X O O O X O X X X	
IV	3	O X O X X O O O X O	

(b) The Simple Recording Sheet

(c) The Data Sheet

*The modified histogram in (a) automatically records the number of correct and incorrect responses on a visually comparative basis. The simple recording sheet (b) shows only correct and incorrect responses out of a total of ten possible trials. The data sheet (c) records each response as incorrect (X) or correct (O) for a total number of correct responses (CR), which yields a percent CR or percentage correct measure.

Source: Reprinted with permission from Teaching Research, Monmouth, Ore., and Educational Associates, Manchester, Mass.

maximum that can be earned in this example is 6 (points per step) × 17 (steps), or 102 (points). Variant scoring conventions for the quality of performance of certain key steps is optional (for instance, items A and B are rated 4 = excellent to 1 = poor). As a general rule, the more independently and efficiently the students perform each step of an assigned task, the more points are awarded.

Figure 9-6 Points Scored Data Sheet for Teaching Face Washing

PROGRAM __Face Washing__   __1__ OF __1__ PAGES

DATE	2-1	2-4	2-8	2-11	2-15	2-18	2-23	2-25			
1. TURNS ON COLD WATER	5	5	6	6	6	6	6	6			
2. TURNS ON WARM WATER UNTIL WARM	3	4	5	6	6	6	6	6			
3. WETS WASHCLOTH	5	5	6	6	6	6	6	6			
4. PICKS UP SOAP	5	6	6	6	6	6	6	6			
5. RUBS SOAP ON WASHCLOTH	4	5	5	6	6	6	6	6			
6. PUTS SOAP DOWN	6	6	6	6	6	6	6	6			
7. WASHES CHEEKS	5	5	6	6	6	6	6	6			
8. WASHES CHIN AND NECK	4	5	4	6	6	6	6	6			
9. WASHES NOSE AND FOREHEAD	4	5	6	6	6	6	6	6			
10. RINSES WASHCLOTH THOROUGHLY	3	4	6	6	6	6	6	6			
11. RINSES ENTIRE FACE WITH WASHCLOTH	5	6	6	6	6	6	6	6			
12. PUTS WASHCLOTH BACK TO APPROPRIATE PLACE	5	5	6	6	6	6	6	6			
13. TURNS OFF WATER	5	5	6	6	6	6	6	6			
14. PICKS UP TOWEL	5	6	6	6	6	6	6	6			
15. DRIES FACE WITH TOWEL	5	6	6	6	6	6	6	6			
16. PUTS TOWEL BACK TO APPROPRIATE PLACE	5	5	5	6	5	6	6	6			
A. WASHING SCORE	2	2	3	3	3	4	4	4			
B. DRYING SCORE	3	3	3	4	4	4	4	4			
TOTAL	79	88	97	103	102	104	104	104			
STAFF	BJD	BJD	BJD	BJD	ND	ND	ND	BJD			

```
SCORING KEY:  6.  SELF-INITIATED AND TOTALLY INDEPENDENT
              5.  NEEDS VERBAL PROMPT ONLY ("WHAT DO YOU DO NOW?")
              4.  NEEDS STEP COMMAND ONLY ("PICK UP THE...")
              3.  PERFORMS STEP/TASK AFTER STEP COMMANDS PLUS MODELING
              2.  NEEDS STEP COMMAND AND PHYSICAL PROMPTS
              1.  NEEDS STEP COMMAN AND TOTAL PHYSICAL ASSISTANCE
              0.  CANNOT, DOES NOT, OR REFUSES TO DO STEP ITEM
SCORING FOR A & B: 4. EXCELLENT  3. GOOD  2. FAIR  1. POOR
Total Possible Points 104
```

Developing a hierarchy of "help ratings" is an arbitrary task. That is, the teacher can assign any number of points to any number of given levels of instructional assistance. McCormack (1976), for instance, suggests using a 6-point 0-to-5 rating system in lieu of the 7-point 0-to-6 scale in Figure 9-6:

(5) done by self
(4) needs verbal assistance
(3) needs demonstration
(2) needs partial physical assistance
(1) refuses to do step item (p. 3)

The points scored data sheet contains a space to score each step of the task analysis sequence. The actual steps may or may not be included—that is a matter of teacher preference. As the task is conducted, the teacher assigns points to each step based on the type of or amount of assistance preferred. The points are summed at the bottom of the form, then compared to the total possible points (usually the number of task steps times the highest possible rating).

Graphing the points scored data is simple. On a piece of standard graph paper, the sum of the accrued points is displayed in such a way that the total points scored are plotted on the vertical axis and subsequent program sessions on the horizontal axis. It should be remembered that these are points scored, not percentages.

Both the percent correct and points scored systems are used frequently in monitoring LBP students' progress. Their major drawback is that they do not contain a time reference for the recorded behavior. If the speed at which the students are to perform a skill is an important consideration, it is not appropriate to use either the percentage correct or points scored technique. In such cases, the teacher should turn to either the frequency or rate system since both measure the speed and accuracy of task completion.

The Frequency System

This third direct measure of student performance is used to record the number of times a behavior occurs in a preestablished time period—usually "*n*" number of seconds or minutes. The teacher first must determine the observation's length of time (five minutes, for example), then count the number of times the targeted behavior occurs during that span. In short, behavior "*A*" occurs "*X*" number of times in "*n*" minutes. When monitoring academic tasks, the teacher may want to collect frequency data on both correct and incorrect responses (Anderson et al., 1975). Since recording and display conventions for the frequency system are identical to those of the rate system, both are discussed.

The Rate System

This fourth direct measure of pupil performance is very similar to the frequency system. Rate is the average frequency of behavior adjusted mathematically to the number of times the behavior occurs per standard time period—one day, one hour, or one second. Increasingly, the common time unit is the minute. To determine response rate, the teacher first must count the number of correct, incorrect, or correct plus incorrect responses, then measure the time during which the behavior occurs. The total number of times a behavior occurs is divided by the total time spent observing the behavior:

$$\frac{\text{Total Number of Behaviors (correct or incorrect)}}{\text{Total Number of Observation Minutes}} = \frac{\text{``X'' Behaviors}}{\text{1 Minute}}$$

For example, Sandy completes 60 written single-digit answers on a math probe in one minute.

$$\frac{60 \text{ Digits}}{60 \text{ Seconds}} = 60 \text{ Digits/Minute}$$

If Sandy does better next week and correctly completes 90 digits in 60 seconds, the rate will increase accordingly:

$$\frac{90 \text{ Digits}}{60 \text{ Seconds}} = 90 \text{ Digits/Minute}$$

Recording either rate or frequency data is done easily by following these steps and by tallying both the adjusted number(s) of behaviors and the standardized time period(s) on scratch paper. The more frequent procedure is to skip the written data recording stage entirely. This is best done by counting behaviors while noting the time period, mathematically adjusting the time to one minute, and graphing the data immediately.

When considering the appropriateness of using the rate or frequency of response systems, two requirements must be met.

First, whatever behavior is recorded must be of a free operant nature—that is, one in which the students' response rate is limited only by their ability to reply to a stimulus presentation. A good example of a violation of this limitation is the inappropriate use of flashcards to test math fact rates. What would happen if the students were able to respond faster than the teacher could flash the cards? Would the recorded rate be indicative of the teenagers' math facts ability or the teacher's flashcard presentation ability? Certainly, the student rate scores would be deflated by the rate of flashcard presentation. Placing 150 cards neatly on a table in front of a student, who picks them up one at a time and identifies each orally, will limit the stimulus presentation problems and should increase the rate of responding. In short, rate data are not reliable if the teacher controls the speed at which the stimuli are presented.

The second requirement in recording rate or frequency data is that the responses be equivalent—that is, all questions should be of the same or of approximately equal difficulty. In another math situation, computing the rate of response on problems by tallying the total number of written digits provides more valid rate data than do problems scored by totaling the number of written answers. Single written digits are of relatively equal difficulty. Writing a four-digit answer not only is more difficult, it is more time consuming. For this reason the number of digits in multi-digit responses is added to obtain a total of single-digit answers. These then are used to determine the overall rate score.

Graphing rate or frequency data is recommended as such information is highly adaptable to graphic display (White & Haring, 1976). Once the data have been collected, they can be plotted or charted on various types of graph paper. The most common convention is the six-cycle semilogarithmic chart shown in Figure 9-7 and designed by the Kansas Behavior Research Company in the mid-1960s.

Behaviors that occur from .001 times/minutes (or once in an 18-hour "awake" day) to 1,000 times/minute can be plotted on the six-cycle log paper, an advantage in identifying behaviors with frequencies that vary greatly from day to day. Another advantage of the six-cycle log paper is the number of calendar days on which data points may be entered. Usually 140 days or 20 calendar weeks of data may be displayed on one sheet, allowing for the effective longitudinal analysis of the data.

When graphing frequency or rate data, the rate of occurrence is plotted on the vertical axis and the standardized time on the horizontal axis. Further information on recording, graphing, and interpreting rate and frequency data may be found in Haughton (1969), Howell et al. (1979), Lindsley, Haughton, and Starlin (1969), Waters and Galloway (1972), White and Alper (1970), and White and Haring (1976).

Observational Recording

This third category of monitoring techniques is used for measuring both academic and academic-related management behaviors. There may be occasions in the classroom when behaviors are observable but do not result in tangible products or are testable directly via NRTs and CRTs. In such situations it is necessary to assess behaviors through direct observation. Continuous, event or frequency, duration, and interval recording techniques all are procedures that require teachers to collect data while observing the conduct as it occurs.

Figure 9-7 Semilogarithmic Six-Cycle Graph Paper Used in Charting Data

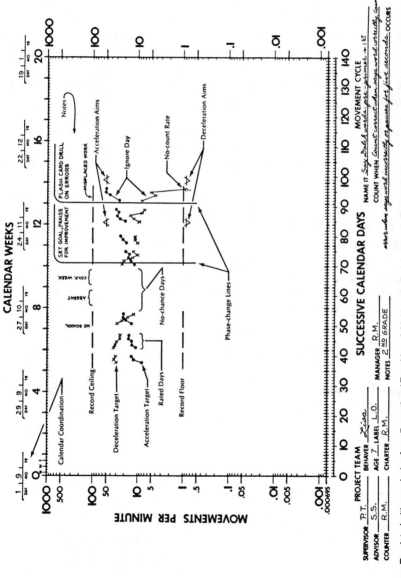

Continuous Recording

This first method of observational recording, sometimes termed specimen description or narrative recording, requires the teacher to describe, in continuous and objective terms, the students' actions as they occur. Specific target behaviors may not always be stipulated before observation begins because, in many cases, they have not yet been identified as problems. An advantage of the continuous recording system is that it can be used to ascertain patterns of stimulus and reinforcement variables that may be related to a target behavior. Continuous recording also allows the teacher to examine patterns of pupil interaction over extended periods of time and across settings.

The recording and displaying of continuous data usually are done in paragraph form. This should be easy to read; contain a time sequence for observation; be written in specific, observable, and nonjudgmental terms; and allow for the formulation of hypotheses or inferred motives that may help explain why the students acted in the way they did.

Exhibit 9-6 is an example of a format for a continuous recording procedure. When implementing this method, the following activities are suggested to teachers: (1) write the data in shorthand or telegraphese that will result in rapidly recorded yet understandable data, (2) record observations on one side of the page and related interpretations or hypotheses on the other side, (3) observe the students when they are relatively active, (4) record as much detail as is possible, and (5) continue the observation for a long enough time so that repetitive or recurring behavior patterns will begin to emerge.

Exhibit 9-6 Continuous Recording Procedure Format

Behaviors Observed	Goals/Motives Inferred
3/16/8__	
Jane lied about assignment.	Fear of being reprimanded.
3/17/8__	
Jane cheated on exam.	Fear of failure.
3/19/8__	
Jane stole pencil from Carol.	Did not like Carol and knew it would make her mad.
3/20/8__	
Jane lied about taking pencil when confronted.	Fear of being punished and/or embarrassed. Also would not want to give Carol satisfaction of catching her.

Event Recording

This second method of observational recording allows data to be taken on the occurrence of discrete and highly visible behaviors such as hand raising, correct oral responses, kicking, quarreling, etc. In this method, predetermined problem behaviors are targeted and each occurrence recorded during an observation period of specified length. As in the frequency and rate performance systems, the data most often describe the frequency or number of times a behavior occurs within consistently standard units of time, usually one-minute periods.

Advantages of the event recording system are numerous. It may be used with a wide variety of behaviors, and the data are easily computed and are best displayed graphically. A major disadvantage is the system's limited use with certain types of behaviors. It would be inappropriate, for instance, to use the event or frequency recording system with behaviors that continue for a long time, that do not have discrete beginning and ending points, that occur at very high rates, and that may last for highly variable lengths of time. In these cases, other observation recording procedures such as the duration or interval recording systems should be used.

The recording of event or frequency data is most effective when the observed behavior occurs between once per minute and 60 times per minute. Data recording may be done in either narrative or event counting forms. If narrative recording is used, the teacher should enter the observations in brief telegraphese fashion in the most appropriate of four columns, one each for time of behavior occurrence, antecedent or stimulus events, behavior, and consequent or reinforcing events (Exhibit 9-7).

The time that the observation begins and ends can be used to compute the total observation span. This in turn provides the time frame in which X number of behaviors occur and from which the frequency of the conduct can be computed. If an event counting format is used, the teacher should choose and consistently use a standard time unit when observing a specific problem behavior from day to day. If this is done, the written data recording stage can be skipped entirely and the material graphed immediately. A graph can be developed on which the number of counted behaviors is entered on the vertical axis and the observation session number/day/date on the horizontal axis. Since the time unit is kept standard, daily comparisons of current and previous data are made easily.

Exhibit 9-7 Narrative Recording Procedure Format

Time	Stimulus Events	Behavior	Reinforcing Events
1 min.	ǂǂǂ ǂǂǂ ǂǂǂ ///	Pencil Tapping	Math Problems

Duration Recording

The third system is termed duration recording. This is used when the length of a particular behavior is under examination. Many behaviors, such as sneezing, saying consonant sounds, or hitting a peer, occur very rapidly. Other behaviors such as being excessively off task, continually talking out in class, or muttering may occur for longer periods. If a frequency or event system were used to record behaviors of relatively long duration (such as a tantrum), the data would indicate how many times or how often it happened but not the length of its occurrence. In this case, measuring the length of the tantrum would yield data that present a truer picture of the behavior. Response latency—the amount of time between stimulus and response—also can be measured using this method.

Duration data are recorded most effectively by a stopwatch whenever the target behavior is occurring during an observation period of some predetermined length. This will establish how much time per observation period the students exhibit the behavior. The duration is calculated by summing the total number of minutes or seconds a behavior occurs in one observation and comparing this to the total length of the observation period. To compute the total observation time in which the behavior occurs, the following formula is used:

$$\frac{\text{Total Time Behavior Occurred}}{\text{Total Length of Observation Time}} \times 100 = \underline{\quad}\%$$

Behaviors often are described in terms of the percentage of time they occur within an observation period. For example, in such a period lasting 30 minutes, Randy spends 14 minutes making eye contact with the assigned reading material. By regarding "eye contact with academic materials" as being "on task," it is possible to compute the percentage of on-task time. If the total time of the observation is divided into what is spent making eye contact with the materials, and multiplied by 100, the results are in terms of percentage of occurrence:

$$\frac{14 \text{ Minutes}}{30 \text{ Minutes}} \times 100 = 46.67\%$$

In this example, Randy is on task only 46.67 percent of the instruction time.

Interval Recording

This fourth type of direct observational recording is very effective in measuring behavior as it allows the teacher to examine both the duration and frequency of the action simultaneously. By breaking the entire observation span into short, equal blocks of time, a series of intervals is established. The observer then records whether the behavior has occurred for at least part of each interval.

The length of the interval usually varies across observations of five seconds to one minute; however, it should remain constant within any one observation period. Interval length depends on both the rate of response and the average duration of the behavior. If the conduct occurs frequently or at a high rate, the interval should be small enough so that two complete responses do not occur in a single interval period. The interval length should approximate the average duration of the target behavior.

Interval recording may be applied to behaviors that are discrete, continuous, and frequent or sporadic. For this reason, it is a very good all-purpose method of recording behavior. An additional advantage is that the observer need not define a strictly discrete unit of behavior. As long as the conduct can be recorded as having occurred or not occurred, interval recording may be used.

The recording of interval data is more complex than that of the previous observational systems. When preparing to record interval data, the teacher first should: (1) define the behavior; (2) choose a code for each behavior if more than one is observed at a time (note the behavior code key in Table 9-1); (3) describe the observation situation briefly; (4) establish the time interval; and (5) determine the time interval between observations, if any, that will be used on the data sheet.

Unlike duration or frequency recording, interval recording requires a formal data sheet. This form structures the length of the time span period into intervals of equal length, usually five or ten seconds, for total observation periods of five, ten, or more minutes (Table 9-1). A blank interval recording form will suffice for most behaviors as long as only one is being studied.

In some cases, the observer may desire to monitor more than one behavior. This necessitates the inclusion of behavior codes in each interval space on the form, even if the action occurs more than once per interval. If the behavior occurs at least once during each interval, a slash mark is drawn across the code for that behavior. If it does not occur during the interval, the code is ignored. Slashed codes, therefore, represent at least one occurrence of that specific conduct.

Adding the total number of intervals during which the behavior occurs will indicate how long it took place during the observation period (its duration). If the summed number of occurrence intervals is divided by the entire number of observation intervals, a percentage of occurrence is derived. If the number of times the behavior occurs (equal to the number of occurrence intervals) is divided by the total length of observation, a rate or frequency of response is computed. With training, teachers can observe and record a number of behaviors across very short time intervals. For practical purposes, however, they should use time intervals of 5, 10, or 15 seconds each and pinpoint no more than one to four behaviors at a time.

Table 9-1 Interval Recording Form[1]

NAME _____   OBSERVER _____

SITUATION _____   DATE _____

	10 Seconds		10 Seconds		10 Seconds		10 Seconds		10 Seconds		10 Seconds	= 60 Sec.
Minute 1	CR OFT XEC	XCR ONT EC	CR OFT XEC	XCR ONT EC	CR OFT XEC	XCR ONT EC	CR OFT XEC	XCR ONT EC	CR OFT XEC	XCR ONT EC	CR OFT XEC	XCR ONT EC	
Minute 2	CR OFT XEC	XCR ONT EC	CR OFT XEC	XCR ONT EC	CR OFT XEC	XCR ONT EC	CR OFT XEC	XCR ONT EC	CR OFT XEC	XCR ONT EC	CR OFT XEC	XCR ONT EC	
Minute 3	CR OFT XEC	XCR ONT EC	CR OFT XEC	XCR ONT EC	CR OFT XEC	XCR ONT EC	CR OFT XEC	XCR ONT EC	CR OFT XEC	XCR ONT EC	CR OFT XEC	XCR ONT EC	
Minute 4	CR OFT XEC	XCR ONT EC	CR OFT XEC	XCR ONT EC	CR OFT XEC	XCR ONT EC	CR OFT XEC	XCR ONT EC	CR OFT XEC	XCR ONT EC	CR OFT XEC	XCR ONT EC	
Minute 5	CR OFT XEC	XCR ONT EC	CR OFT XEC	XCR ONT EC	CR OFT XEC	XCR ONT EC	CR OFT XEC	XCR ONT EC	CR OFT XEC	XCR ONT EC	CR OFT XEC	XCR ONT EC	
Minute 6	CR OFT XEC	XCR ONT EC	CR OFT XEC	XCR ONT EC	CR OFT XEC	XCR ONT EC	CR OFT XEC	XCR ONT EC	CR OFT XEC	XCR ONT EC	CR OFT XEC	XCR ONT EC	
Minute 7	CR OFT XEC	XCR ONT EC	CR OFT XEC	XCR ONT EC	CR OFT XEC	XCR ONT EC	CR OFT XEC	XCR ONT EC	CR OFT XEC	XCR ONT EC	CR OFT XEC	XCR ONT EC	
Minute 8	CR OFT XEC	XCR ONT EC	CR OFT XEC	XCR ONT EC	CR OFT XEC	XCR ONT EC	CR OFT XEC	XCR ONT EC	CR OFT XEC	XCR ONT EC	CR OFT XEC	XCR ONT EC	
Minute 9	CR OFT XEC	XCR ONT EC	CR OFT XEC	XCR ONT EC	CR OFT XEC	XCR ONT EC	CR OFT XEC	XCR ONT EC	CR OFT XEC	XCR ONT EC	CR OFT XEC	XCR ONT EC	
Minute 10	CR OFT XEC	XCR ONT EC	CR OFT XEC	XCR ONT EC	CR OFT XEC	XCR ONT EC	CR OFT XEC	XCR ONT EC	CR OFT XEC	XCR ONT EC	CR OFT XEC	XCR ONT EC	

BEHAVIOR KEY

	Inappropriate	Appropriate
	CR — Crying	XCR — Not Crying
	OFT — Off Task	ONT — On Task
	XEC — No Eye Contact	EC — Eye Contact

1. This format provides for monitoring six discrete behaviors involving three general categories across 60 10-second intervals for a total of 10 minutes of observation time. The teacher draws a slash mark across the appropriate code as behaviors occur.

To provide the duration data for the forms, some method of timing the intervals is required. The observer may use a wall clock or stopwatch. The former may not be effective, however, because the teacher must watch the clock while trying to observe the student. Audio cues such as beeper tapes have proved more effective. A beeper tape is a cassette tape that beeps every 5, 10, or 15 seconds, etc., with each beep indicating the start of a new interval. A different tape is required for each variance in time interval. These can be developed easily in the classroom, however, given a blank tape, a watch or clock, and a sound source (a kitchen timer, piano, clicker, etc.).

CHOOSING AN OBSERVATION SYSTEM

Which observation technique should be used, and under what conditions? A number of criteria can help determine the choice of methods: (1) the duration or discreteness of the student responses, (2) the visibility of the behavior, (3) the number of behaviors being recorded simultaneously, (4) the level of precision required in measurement, and (5) the time spans. Usually, one or more of these factors will decide which to use. The types of questions asked about student performance also can dictate the type of data collection method, as shown in Exhibit 9-8.

Exhibit 9-8 Questions on Data Collection Methods

Questions Asked	Type of Data Collection Method Used
(a) How long does the behavior occur?	(a) duration recording system
(b) How often does the behavior occur?	(b) frequency or event recording system
(c) Does the behavior continue for a long time?	(c) continuous or anecdotal recording system
(d) At what rate, or how fast, does the behavior occur?	(d) rate recording system
(e) How much teacher assistance, across time, must be provided to the students to allow them to perform a given task?	(e) points-scored recording system
(f) What percentage of correct/ incorrect or appropriate/ inappropriate responses occur in a given sitting?	(f) percentage correct/incorrect or appropriate/inappropriate recording system
(g) How many behaviors occur in a given preestablished time period, each of which results in a lasting product, i.e., the number of pages read, puzzles completed?	(g) recording of direct measurement of achieved tasks

A PROCEDURAL ANALYSIS

A number of formative assessment models were discussed earlier. Although they vary to a certain degree, all share one common attribute: data on student progress are systematically gathered, analyzed, and used in the instructional decision-making process.

As shown in Figure 9-1, supra, there are ten major steps in evaluating student progress in which the teacher will:

1. choose a content area
2. evaluate the student
3. develop or choose instructional program
4. develop formative assessment procedures and related data recording systems
5. initiate instruction
6. implement formative assessment and data recording procedures
7. analyze formative assessment data
8. make data-based instructional decisions
9. recycle assessment methods as needed
10. report evaluation information

Some of these activities have been alluded to or discussed briefly in this chapter; those and the others are outlined now in a step-by-step fashion.

Step 1: Choose a Content Area

In many cases, choosing a content area is an almost automatic process. Whenever a referral is made or an IEP team meets to develop a plan for a student, general subject areas usually are outlined. These may include skill areas across the affective, psychomotor, or cognitive domains, or in perceptual motor development, sensorimotor development, perception and memory, language, cognitive skills, social, and socioemotional skills (Bateman, 1971; Bloom et al., 1956; Krathwohl, Bloom, & Masia, 1964). Skills also may be categorized by the more traditional instructional areas of reading (decoding and comprehension), mathematics, geography, history, English, language arts, spelling, and vocational education.

Step 2: Evaluate the Student

Finding out facts about student performance is the next step. This is known as testing. The purpose of fact finding is to collect a general sample of student behavior in terms of both (1) performance on test items and (2) observation of behavior during the test situation. To do this, both stimulus (or test item) and response (or student answer) information is observed and collected whenever the adolescent makes an incorrect response. An overall test score also may be derived. Student evaluation, therefore, starts with three distinct activities: (1) conducting a survey level assessment, (2) identifying entry abilities and skill area deficits, and (3) conducting further survey and/or specific level assessments, as needed.

Step 3: Develop or Choose Instructional Program

Based on the content analysis of the academic behaviors that are to be taught and the assessment information derived from survey, specific, and/or intensive levels of evaluation, it now is time to develop or choose the student's instructional programs. Whether they are commercial or teacher-developed is important only in the context of budget, time, and classroom.

Whether writing or purchasing programs, teachers should keep two points in mind: (1) the instructional objectives should be defined objectively and broken down or task-analyzed; (2) the results of this analysis should be small, discrete, and easily acquired instructional steps.

Since programs are numerous, certain minimal criteria should be considered when making curricular decisions. When educators are reviewing a program for purchase or writing their own, Wilson (1982) suggests using a number of curricular, student, and teacher variables as criteria for determining the appropriateness of a given program.

Curricular variables include the following points: (1) the content of the program should be appropriate for the skill level and relevant for the educational needs of the student for whom it is being purchased/developed; (2) the specific skills taught in the classroom should be clearly delineated within the framework of the program; (3) the teaching methodology should be appropriate in terms of the student's ability level, chronological age, mental age, interests, and motivational factors; (4) the curriculum should be flexible enough to allow for teacher modification, should instructional needs arise.

Student variables include the LBP adolescent's instructional needs; current level of functioning; grouping possibilities; the type of presentation or programming options open to the teacher; response to specific teaching methods outlined in the program; and various physical, social, emotional, and psychological characteristics that may impede or accelerate learning.

Finally, a number of teacher variables are important, including the methods of instruction, what specific approaches the practitioner may be best at and most comfortable with, time limitations or constraints that may limit the program's use, any training that may be needed to use the program effectively, and the educational background the teacher may or may not have had in that particular content area.

Step 4: Develop Formative Assessment Procedures and Related Data Recording Systems

By this time the teacher has evaluated the student using survey level assessment instruments, hypothesized specific types of skill deficits, evaluated the hypotheses on the specific and—if need be—intensive level(s), and either confirmed or negated the hypotheses. Since it is almost time to start teaching those skills, attention should be directed first to the methods of continually monitoring and analyzing student progress. For example, approaches employing direct measures of performance most likely will look at the following:

1. the direction of change in behavior (increase, decrease, no change),
2. the rate of change in behavior,
3. the stability of change in behavior. (Smith & Snell, 1978, p. 28)

When choosing a method, the teachers should decide first whether the desired pupil target will be in terms of the direction, rate, stability, or amount of change in conduct. Next, and after reviewing the categories of observational and test procedures outlined in Exhibit 9-4, supra, that may be used to collect pupil performance data, the teachers should ask any or all of the questions in Exhibit 9-8. Following those steps, in that order, will help them in choosing which type of data collection system to use.

Collecting Data

The sole objective of data collection is that the teachers eventually will use the information. For this reason, the efficiency of any classroom data monitoring system is a function of: (1) the type of data collected, (2) the frequency with which the data are assembled, and (3) the analysis procedures used. Before discussing these points, several ground rules on data collection should be outlined. Teachers should:

1. collect only enough data to meet basic instructional needs
2. be aware of what type of information is needed for a given situation
3. understand that raw data, or the material to be analyzed, must be summarized somewhere; how this is done involves the way the data are collected, the amount, and the range of tasks covered
4. realize that some environmental or instructional variable may be affecting the target behavior and in such cases should take data while they are occurring; on the other hand, if the behavior is a free operant, data should be taken at random periods throughout the student's day, using many short observation periods instead of a few long ones

Prerequisite to adopting a data collection system is the generation of a list of hypotheses and questions that teachers must verify and/or answer. Questions regarding behavior of these LBP adolescents are derived directly from assessment information about instructional and environmental variables. The primary purpose of any data collection system, then, is to answer the following questions: "Is what I'm doing working?" If no, "What do I need to change to make learning take place?" If yes, "What can I change to make learning more effective?"

Once questions on student performance have been formulated, the next step is to determine what information is needed to answer the questions; that is, what general categories of behaviors and environmental/instructional variables are to be measured, maintained, or manipulated? Should any of the instructional conditions be modified? The behavior itself? Or the reinforcer or consequence conditions? While modifying instructional, behavioral, or reinforcer variables, which one is the most appropriate data recording method to use that would effectively monitor progress?

In summary, seven important activities are to be conducted before or concurrent with instruction, all of them crucial in implementing evaluation and data monitoring procedures in the classroom. Teachers should:

1. define the target behavior(s) in specific and observable terms
2. determine what type of data will be collected
3. determine the appropriate method of observation based on the behavior(s) observed and type(s) of data desired
4. design observation instruments such as data recording and plotting forms
5. obtain any materials that may improve the effectiveness of the observation, such as counters, stopwatches, kitchen timers, etc.
6. implement the method, obtaining frequent and periodic data
7. display the data in summarized and/or graphic form

Establishing a Data Communications System

Once a data collection system is chosen and put into effect, it soon will accumulate so much information that a method for managing the material will be necessary. For this reason, some manner of formalized classroom communications system is recommended. Since special education teachers now are legally responsible (P.L. 94-142) for knowing and communicating specifics about which skills a student may or may not know, and for doing so effectively among multidisciplinary staff members, parents, paraprofessionals, and numerous other parties, the need for methods for information gathering and communication is extremely important.

Communication in the classroom occurs on a verbal or written basis. The former is less desirable because "though person-to-person interaction is usually the preferred means of communication . . . it has drawbacks (e.g., time consuming, depends on memory) and is often virtually impossible in a setting with a continuous flow of specialists, aides, volunteers'' (McCormack & Chalmers, 1978, p. 79). Hence, a written form of continuing performance evaluation usually is more desirable and effective.

Since many of the professionals and paraprofessionals providing services to the students do so on a transient or year-to-year basis, the responsibility for coordinating and maintaining communication efforts rests with the teachers. A written communication system in the classroom enables them to coordinate the efforts of the instructional personnel more easily. They also can monitor the specifics of student performances and communicate such information to parents and next year's teacher(s) more effectively. If the maximum benefits of specific instruction and/or multidisciplinary settings are to be achieved, some type of written communications system should be developed and implemented on a continuing basis.

Criteria for an Effective System

Of what should such an information gathering and communicating system consist? McCormack and Chalmers (1978) suggest the following:

1. a focus on quantifiable behaviors
2. a description of training procedures in clear, operational terms that others can follow successfully
3. the identification of a procedure for assigning who does what, with whom, when, where, and how
4. the provision of a centralized written record for reporting learner behavior on each task
5. procedures to analyze data on common ordinates (e.g., percentage, rate) for all students on all tasks
6. the organization of a central data file across learners and tasks

Since a number of these criteria, particularly the first four, already are part of the student's IEP, special attention should be given to the last two.

Components of an Effective System

To meet these six criteria, a communications system should consist of a periodic planning sheet, the instructional programs, related instructional materials, a program and data file, one or more methods of data recording, and teacher decisions (Figure 9-8).

The Periodic Planning Sheet. The periodic planning sheet stipulates who does what with whom, when, where, and how. Usually more specific than a schedule for weekly lesson plans, the sheet should include space in which to write perform-

Figure 9-8 The Classroom Communications System

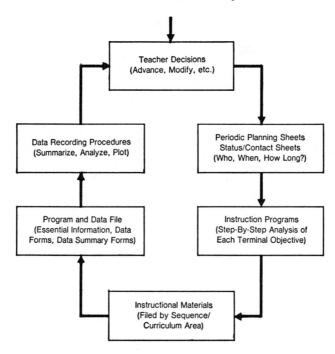

Source: Reprinted with permission from *Early Cognitive Instruction for the Moderately and Severely Handicapped: Program Guide* by J.E. McCormack and J.A. Chalmers, Research Press Company, © 1978.

ance information adjacent to the task statement (Figure 9-9). During morning planning sessions, the teacher should write in the task statement (i.e., what is to be taught), the criteria for acceptable performance (i.e., how well the student is to perform what is taught), and the name of the staff member responsible for the instruction of that specific skill. Session dates and instructional times can be added later by the staff member involved. These forms are called by various other names—weekly planning sheets, status sheets, contact sheets, and individual assignment sheets, among others.

Instructional Programs. These programs are any commercially marketed or teacher-developed instructional sequences, units, lessons, skills continua, etc. These should be filed by the name of the educational objective and should provide essential information such as what materials are needed, how to prepare and present them, what the student must do, how many trials or times the instructional sequence should be presented, criteria for acceptable performance, and any other pertinent points.

Figure 9-9 The Periodic Planning Sheet

STUDENT'S NAME: _____   CLASSROOM: _____

Page _____ of _____ pages

Date of Session	Total Time	Staff	Task Statement	Criteria for Acceptable Performance	Results and Comments

Instructional Materials. These are the ones called for by the programs. They may be either teacher-made, commercially produced, or marketed with teacher adaptations. Materials can be filed and/or stored by either curriculum area or by program name. Storing materials in clearly labeled shoeboxes, Manila envelopes, coffee cans, cardboard ice cream containers, etc., will keep materials sets neatly organized. These should be kept in each classroom so as to be readily accessible to teachers, staff, and paraprofessionals.

Program and Data File. Once the instructional program and any type of information or data sheet(s) associated with it are prepared, these should be put into some type of centralized file, one file per student. A file is any system of categorizing the program/data sheets. This may be done simply by placing them in one file folder, three-ring binder, or clipboard per student. If the materials or programs are too cumbersome to be included in the file, they should be stored nearby. Each student's file should be accessible enough so that the information may be retrieved at a moment's notice. Generally, these are used on a daily basis for any data recording that may take place. Including a copy of the student's IEP in the file will allow for quick reference, update, and the addition to or modification of any related content.

Methods of Data Recording. These may be any of the techniques discussed earlier in this chapter. They should. be both predetermined and established: predetermined in the sense that the teacher, anticipating what type of data may be needed, will have chosen the specific system and developed related data sheets before instruction begins; established in the sense that the teacher, knowing which recording system will be (or is) installed, will have become fully familiar with how to use it before instruction begins.

Teacher Decisions. These are based on the preceding five communication components. For instance, based on specific level instructional data gathered on a periodic basis, the teacher may decide a student should advance, maintain position, or step back on a given program, or to modify the program itself.

With this or a similar system, the teacher can determine quickly how well a student is performing with other teachers, therapists, or tutors, which instructional objectives are being taught, and how fast they are being learned. This information provides the teacher with the knowledge necessary to answer questions about both the teenagers and the instructional procedures being used. Usually, these procedures for periodically monitoring performance across time are conducted informally in the minds of most teachers. However, by externalizing or putting into written form each component of the system, teachers can greatly increase the efficiency and probability of success of any activity.

In viewing the communications system in terms of its importance in the overall formative evaluation of the performance of LBP adolescents, it is easily recognized that each step of the procedure depends upon data-based decisions. The communications system incorporates all aspects of formative evaluation insofar as effective instructional decisions and programs cannot be made or performed without a data base from which to proceed. In essence, the communications system serves as the centralized information storage and retrieval mechanism in the classroom.

Step 5: Initiate Instruction

Now it is time to start teaching. The instruction should be based on the entry level of the students and the content and range of academic behaviors outlined in the table of specifications.

Step 6: Implement Formative Assessment and Data Recording Procedures

Depending on the data recording method used, this step may occur either after or during the implementation of instruction (Step 5). For instance, the practitioner may teach for two, three, four, or five days, then use probes or time trials to determine what has been learned. Or, the teacher may complete only one instructional session, then turn to probes or time trials. In either case, evaluation procedures are suspended for the time actual instruction occurs but may be implemented upon the termination of the teaching. In rare situations, evaluation may occur on a trial-by-trial basis concurrently with instruction.

Whether evaluation efforts occur during, immediately after, or periodically during instruction depends entirely on the task, the teaching procedures, the students' acquisition rate, the amount of data the educator desires, and a variety of other factors. In any case, evaluation should be conducted on a frequent, consistent, and continuing basis.

Step 7: Analyze Formative Assessment Data

It is time now to look at the collected data with a critical eye. As mentioned, data are amassed exclusively with the idea that the teacher somehow, sometime, will respond to the information by analyzing and employing it as a foundation for routine decision-making procedures in the classroom.

Monitoring students' performances need not cause the teacher to change an instructional program or the way it is being presented—they may be doing well, making few errors, and exhibiting satisfactory progress. In such a case, the data are used only to monitor student progress periodically. Not only are they doing well but their teacher is certain they are. Occasionally, though, little or no instructional progress may be made. When this occurs, the data are used in a different fashion. With the techniques described in this chapter, they should serve as an impetus for the teacher to change or modify the students' program.

Step 8: Make Data-Based Instructional Decisions

The teacher makes instructional decisions that are a direct result of a five-step analysis sequence.

First, the initial definition of the problem must be defined clearly. Saying that Sandy cannot read is a general, descriptive statement but does not clearly define the problem. Saying that Sandy has problems in quickly blending certain specific letter sounds gives the teacher a better starting point for the decision-making process. Usually this information is generated by the specific level evaluation.

Second, the teacher must determine what, if any, further information will help in arriving at a final solution. In Sandy's case, knowing what specific letter sounds are causing problems, how quickly the student must blend them, and how well or accurately this must be done will greatly aid the decision-making process. Thus, proceeding to a more specific level of evaluation may be necessary.

Third, a strategy must be formulated to meet the problem. This is termed a modification (if a program already exists) or a program (if no instruction is being provided).

Fourth, the teacher must implement the modification or initiate the program in an active and dynamic sense in classroom presentations.

Fifth, the decision maker evaluates the effectiveness of the modification by continually monitoring student progress across time. If no changes in performance indicators are evident after a few days, the decision-making process should be recycled through the third, fourth, and fifth steps. That is, the practitioner must reformulate, reimplement, and reevaluate a new modification and continue to do so until student progress is reflected in the data. It is evident that if there are no specific data or a management system to store and analyze it, the teacher cannot use such a process effectively. At best, program and instructional modifications then would be based on hunches and intuition and implemented somewhat like a shot in the dark.

What does the teacher modify? Usually the environmental and instructional variables that can be easily and consistently adapted in such a way that student performance will improve. These commonly fall into one of the following three categories: antecedent, behavior, and consequential conditions.

Antecedent conditions are the stimulus situations in which the target behavior usually occurs. These include the instructional setting, the time of day, and the materials being used. The most important antecedent conditions usually are those that occur just prior to the targeted behavior. These may include:

1. Organismic Variables (learner characteristics)
   a. learner input functions
   b. learner input modality
2. Stimulus Variables (materials dimensions)
   a. stimulus input characteristics
   b. presentation format
3. Presentation Variables (presentation/procedural variables)
   a. stimulus presentation characteristics
   b. stimulus pacing characteristics
   c. group size during presentation
   d. distribution of practice

Behavior conditions include considerations such as the frequency with which the LBP adolescents independently perform the target behavior and how much of that conduct can occur without teacher assistance (Smith & Snell, 1978). They also include variables such as the type of response required of the students, the characteristics of the responses that are closely related to the stimulus, how the responses are organized during emission, and how well certain behaviors may be retrieved from memory. These include:

1. Organismic Characteristics
   a. learner output functions

2. Response (Output) Characteristics
   a. response abstractness
   b. response complexity
   c. number of responses
   d. interresponse similarity
   e. response rate
3. Response Organization
   a. temporal continuity
   b. task component continuity
4. Storage Interval (memory over time)
5. Retrieval Performance (over time)

Third, reinforcement or consequential conditions may be modified by the teacher to improve students' performance. These include the types of actions taken and comments made immediately after the targeted behavior occurs. Other conditions include:

1. Effect of the Reinforcer
2. Type of Reinforcer
3. Amount of Reinforcer
4. Reinforcement Ratio
5. Delay of Reinforcement

If analysis results in identifying what appears to be the variable or combination of variables that consistently hinders or improves student progress—usually termed the causal variable—the teacher can then systematically adapt the factors to determine whether it actually is the causal variable. If it is, and if it is modified accordingly, the data soon will reflect this change.

For example, if data indicate that the teenager performs poorly because there is little incentive or reward for doing well, the teacher may modify the instruction by increasing either the level, amount, or type of reinforcement, contingent upon good performance. After a few days of this new variable condition, the teacher should check whether student performance has improved. If it has, the new reinforcing condition can be maintained. If performance levels remain unchanged, inadequate, or drop, the teacher has not yet identified the variable or combination of variables hindering progress. If that is the case, further analysis is necessary.

How often should data be collected and analyzed and related decisions made? The general rule of thumb is to do so at "appropriate" intervals. As would be expected, that term is difficult to define—what is appropriate for one student and teacher may not necessarily be so for others. "Periodically" is another term hard to define. For most researchers, the two terms mean both collecting and analyzing data on a daily basis.

Of course, the realities of teaching may determine how much time can be spent on such activities. Such realities also may dictate that occasionally days will be missed. On the other hand, too many missed days seriously reduce the quality of the information gathered. For this reason, every attempt should be made to gather data as frequently as is needed. In some cases, such as when a great deal of data are to be plotted and analyzed, it may be more efficient to conduct analysis and make instructional decisions two (Wednesday and Friday) or three (Monday, Wednesday, and Friday) days per week. Data not analyzed for a week or more accumulate rapidly. Handling large amounts of data can prove to be an aversive task and may identify problems that occurred a week or more ago.

Obtaining and analyzing data on almost a daily basis, then, not only is the most effective but the most efficient method in terms of use of teacher time. In so doing, data can be continually interpreted in light of the students' instructional programming, both within tasks and across the goals and objectives outlined in the IEPs.

Step 9: Recycle Assessment Methods as Needed

One of the more important steps of the formative evaluation process, this provides for the continuity of data collection, recording, managing, and analysis procedures that result in sound instructional decisions. Following the first eight steps, it now is time to recycle the assessment and data monitoring systems as needed.

In this step, a variety of options are open to teachers. For example, if all needed skills in a subject area have been learned, it may be time to recycle to Step 1 and choose another topic. Before doing this, however, the educators may want to verify their teaching in a posttest situation by recycling back to Step 2 and evaluating students on the survey level assessment instruments initially used as pretests. Teachers also may want to recycle back to Step 4 and evaluate the students using specific and/or intensive level posttest assessment procedures. In any case, the whole process starts all over again.

Step 10: Report Evaluation Information

Although not strictly necessary for the effective formative evaluation of student progress, it occasionally is desirable and sometimes required that a summary report be developed outlining what the adolescents know, what they do not know, and what they should be taught. Since much of the information traditionally found in a summary report is in each student's IEP, close attention should be paid to that document's content and format. These concerns are addressed at some length in Chapter 8.

Should a summary report be necessary, the outline in Exhibit 9-9 should be used to draw together much of the information discussed in this chapter. Although no set

Exhibit 9-9 Format for Year-End Summary Evaluation

1. General Area
2. Survey Level Tests Used
3. Description of:
   3a. Test(s):
   3b. Score(s):
   3c. Summary:
4. Survey Level Error Analysis and/or Hypothesis of Facts
5. Specific Level Tests Used
6. Description of:
   6a. Test(s):
   6b. Score(s):
   6c. Summary:
7. Specific Level Error Analysis and/or Hypothesis of Facts
8. Specification of Instructional Objectives in Order of Difficulty, Based on Table of Specifications
9. General Testing/Teaching Recommendations

---

or standard format is used, the one proposed here not only includes all of the pertinent information that may be collected but also orders the content in a logical survey-to-intensive levels order. Educators can freely adapt this outline, however, to meet any report requirements stipulated by a school or district.

SUMMARY

This lengthy chapter addresses a variety of pragmatic concerns related to the role of formative instructional evaluation of adolescents with LBPs. The first section—Evaluation and Exceptional Learners—asks a number of cogent questions while presenting logistical, pragmatic, and instructional reasons for evaluation. A number of basic assumptions underlying formative instructional evaluation are presented.

The second section—Formative Evaluation—reviews a number of simplified models, discusses the role of formative assessment in the classroom, presents a generic instructionally based model of formative evaluation, compares test types and uses related to norm-referenced and criterion-referenced evaluation, and outlines a number of direct observation methods of evaluation.

In the third section—A Procedural Analysis—a number of previously discussed concepts and methods are included in a ten-step process for teachers interested in developing their evaluation techniques to include skills other than simply testing students. The analysis also proposes methods of organizing, storing, retrieving, using, and reporting data-based information in the classroom.

Certain evaluation and instructional implications are suggested in this chapter and its evaluation model. The first is that the use of both continuing and specific evaluation may be most instructionally effective for most exceptional learners.

Second, educators and teacher trainees should obtain or improve upon their working knowledge of basic testing and assessment concepts. This includes becoming familiar with: (1) a variety of NRTs and CRTs; (2) the characteristics, appropriate use, and inappropriate use of NRTs and CRTs; (3) the content and operations of what is to be tested and taught; and (4) NRT and CRT/probe construction. It also includes becoming facile at formulating and evaluating hypotheses generated from limited test data; becoming adept at identifying instructional problems, analyzing information, specifying goals and objectives, generating alternatives to established tests, and evaluating the alternatives; and, finally, becoming more concerned with the utility-related, as opposed to the issue-related, use of NRT and CRT evaluation instruments.

Third, it is the authors' contention that the use of a set of formalized procedures nested in a general model of evaluation that emphasizes the utility of specific levels of information across both NRT and CRT test conditions will yield a fruitful and valuable methodology for evaluating the instructional performance of adolescents with LBPs.

Chapter 10

Applied Research Techniques for LBP Adolescents

David A. Sabatino and Patrick J. Schloss

INTRODUCTION

A decade or two ago a major argument consumed the thoughts of many educators: was education an art form and its practitioners artists or were teachers scientists who were concerned with understanding human behavior, curricula, and the interaction between the two? The issue was that as artists, educators' subjective response to learners was stylistic and was not concerned with a systematic search for objective data to enter into the instructional decision-making process. On the other hand, if educators were scientists, then the instructional process should be viewed objectively, beginning with a statement of the problem, goals to be achieved and the systematic recording of data from students. Not only should the data be recorded, they also should be analyzed and interpreted, using procedures to ensure that they would be usable, if indeed not capable of being generalized to different groups of youths or to other learning environments.

The 1970s brought an end to the academic rhetoric. Huge federal expenditures during the 1960s generated an urgent national requirement—accountability. No longer was it important whether educators were stylistic or scientifically inclined. Local education agencies and state and federal offices and departments of education required an evaluation of the instructional process if federal monies were spent. Increasing pressure was brought to bear on special educators to provide evidence that efforts with exceptional children were beneficial (Lessinger, 1971). It was a professional expectation that all teachers: (1) delineate program outcomes objectively and precisely, (2) present evidence of the achievement capability of those results, (3) offer validity statements on cost and time efficiency in light of learning effectiveness, and (4) establish that the efforts reflected a best practice procedure. Once again, the rhetoric was brilliant. However, the average educational practitioner, even after completing a preservice training program within the preceding five years, was simply overwhelmed.

315

Secondary special educators functioning in the classroom, resource room, or technical assistance capacity (instructional adviser), faced with the day-to-day reality of teaching learning and behaviorally disordered youths, did not have the time or interest in learning another obtuse theoretical mode. Having heard the arguments against research in the past, they were critical of researchers, the research literature, and the value of data approaches. Ohrtman (1972) aptly describes the "in and out researcher . . . who gets two groups of kids, does A to one group and B to another, compares them, and one group does better at the .01 level—then off to the next project" (p. 377).

Vergason (1973), in response to the evaluation requirements of that period, noted that the results were meaningless until a standardized communication system was available. The feeling among practitioners was that the time and effort required did not generate information of value. Data on the instructional process did not provide answers as to why a program failed, only that it did so. In short, data on instruction did not provide a solution to learning deficits that the educators knew existed. It only amplified a known fact, not offering a solution or even focal point for initiating either a different educational delivery system or an alternate instructional and behavioral management approach.

Jones (1973) states that before a school system considers adapting an accountability (evaluation) system, it must answer four questions:

1. What are the common and specific goals to which the teacher and school are striving?
2. What student, community, or societal need inventories are available to indicate change strategies that should be undertaken?
3. What specific and measurable performance objectives have been written that would enable parents, students, and teachers to understand the minimum expectations of the unstructured programs?
4. What analysis of the existing delivery system is available to indicate that the current educational input approach is manageable as compared to the alternatives?

Public Law 94-142 (1975) requires that each student's individualized education program (IEP) be monitored yearly. The call for accountability continues but with little additional prescribed direction for users. Teachers, now having received inservice and preservice professional preparation on evaluation processes as well as alternatives to the traditional group comparison research paradigm, have not received meaningful feedback on evaluation data supplied to their local administrators. To compound the problem, the existence of a bottleneck for promoting meaningful research frequently is denied by local special education directors (Weatherly & Lipsky, 1977).

To bridge this informational gap, the specific focus of this chapter is to:

1. review traditional applied research methodology
2. present a simplified classroom evaluation system
3. discuss single-subject research design and time series technique
4. present a brief review of research describing adolescents with learning and behavioral problems (LBPs) in which usable results have been ascertained
5. provide examples of applied research and evaluation utility in the classroom

In so doing, this chapter is dedicated to secondary special educators, whose need for usable data has reached a level of urgency. If preschool programs seek to prevent academic deficiencies and elementary programs purport to remediate academic and social skill deficits, then secondary efforts should provide a setting in which skills can be directed to life's goals. The success of this endeavor would enhance the development of a most valuable resource, the young men and women with learning and behavioral handicapping conditions. Without effective and efficient program development and validation capabilities, educators' goals for these adolescents may be jeopardized.

TRADITIONAL RESEARCH APPLICATION

Specific principles using statistical procedures require that data be entered into a mathematical analysis reflecting a sound design with reasonable control of the variables that may influence the results. There exists in educational circles an erroneous belief that statistics and research are synonymous. Research is viewed as good (or as bad) as the statistical manipulation of numbers. This belief undermines the importance of the question being researched, the design used to ascertain the data, and their interpretation. In 1923, McCall noted, "There are excellent books and courses of instruction dealing with the statistical manipulation of experimental data, but there is little help to be found on the methods of securing adequate and proper data to which to apply statistical procedures" (p. 41). This statement remains true today.

The field of special education is in a position somewhat similar to medicine in the mid-1800s. Prior to Pasteur's isolation of bacteria, disease was attributed to a variety of presumed conditions. Similarly, it is recognized that there are developmental rules for learning, but they cannot be defined. Further, the manner in which the nervous system processes information is known (L'Bate, 1969; Mark, 1962; Sabatino, 1968), but its effectiveness cannot be maximized. As Pasteur charged the medical community to learn to wash its hands, so the profession of special education is charged with systematically observing and recording learner responses to instructional approaches and to the methods of educational delivery.

There exists an attitude of pessimism and indifference toward the utility of research. In some circles, the major assumption is that research precludes or diminishes the effectiveness of service delivery. This attitude is augmented by the view that most research in special education is so tainted by design flaw that it is not usable.

The following section examines the reasons for this negative view of research and reviews factors that must be considered in developing paradigms that are understandable and meaningful to educational practitioners.

Teacher Attitude toward Research

Good and Scates (1954) document a persistent pessimistic attitude toward research by many educators dating back to 1935. Gallagher (1975) and Krathwohl (1977) describe teachers' continued negative attitude on research. Yet DeVault (1965) clearly indicates that teachers are the keys to the implementation of applied research in their schools. Why is this?

Marks (1972) notes that few teachers receive either the preservice or inservice preparation necessary to understand or appreciate laboratory research. Isakson and Ellsworth (1979), measuring education students' attitudes toward research, find that, having completed a course well taught on research application, they demonstrate a much more positive attitude ($p < .05$ level of confidence) than those not having had such a course. Johnson's (1966) data support the hypothesis that there is a strong positive correlation between department heads and staff in interest and willingness to conduct research. Therefore, it would appear that one fruitful area to increase educational research is to provide supervisors and administrators with inservice training on this subject. Another way would be early introduction to research, and required competence in applied research at the undergraduate level of teacher preparation.

Kerlinger (1977) identifies two common misconceptions associated with research:

1. Pragmatic-Practical Misconception: Research cannot solve education's problems or improve its practices. Traditional research can only identify a solution on the concept "if one practice is better than another for a group," an outcome that at best is implied, not inherent. It is inconceivable that scientific research will provide a decision improving education in general. The quality of instruction may be improved by being based on solid data rather than its overdependence on subjective teacher or administrator opinion.
2. Demand for Relevance: Research may supply understanding and explanation but not relevance to applied situations. As a point in fact: teacher A, using the same program as teacher B, with a matched group of children, gets

better results year after year. Research may provide understanding. Teacher A is a joy to be around, a charming, stimulating person; teacher B has an affectless personality. Relevance, in this case, is to fire teacher B, and that is not possible with tenure laws. The relevance of the research is dependent upon the use to which the data are placed. The purpose of educational research is to understand the instructional process. That does not mean research data will change that process, but it may supply the reason for someone to make that highly relevant decision. In other words, what if the school district had a policy saying no persons with affectless personalities were to be employed because it was speculated that they were less effective in the classroom although data on a population of teachers, ranked on effect, refuted that speculation?

Changes in attitude will result only when professional practitioners and teachers see their role in the applied research process. Research these days is considered a practice of academic educators. Professional burnout and staff management planning are topics of great concern so it is important to know who survives in the field and who doesn't. If a new 22-year-old teacher enters a self-contained high school classroom for behaviorally disordered boys, can that person be expected to still be interested in working with such students in 30 years? If so, what personal and professional characteristics should such a teacher have?

The issue is that research on teachers should excite the profession. The fact that it does not stems from (1) a fear of knowing, since educators never have, and (2) the fact that most preservice undergraduate teachers rarely receive a course in educational research application.

The goal of research is simply to uncover answers to questions. However, as Clifford (1973) reports, research in education has had little discernible effect on educational practice. One persistent problem is that a distinction is needed between applied and basic research. Shaver (1979) addresses the question by noting that both are needed if productivity of educational research is to be realized. He concludes, "Developing of the scientific potential of educational research will depend principally upon the building of appropriate training programs for prospective researchers" (p. 8). Could professional preparation be the culprit?

Technique vs. Technician

Slavin (1978) in a powerful argument writes, "What is needed in education is more, not less, research directed at the improvement of instruction and of the schooling experience for children . . . such research needs to be made programmatic, systematic, useful, and cumulative" (p. 17). Could it be that most teachers and few schools have bothered to believe in, support, reward, or require research? Is it that the profession lacks the technique or the technician? The technique can be taught, the technician employed. There is little excuse for not placing greater emphasis on research in the classroom. That, too, must come from the top down, and public school administration has not been emphasizing research.

Administrators have not found research data to assist them in responding to the questions they face in the decision-making process. It is not that data are not available nor that meaningful interpretations have not been made from them. It is the fact that confidence in, and respect for, much of the data available has fallen to a low level of trust as a result of the poor design of many of the studies conducted, and the inability of researchers to replicate them (Erickson, 1979).

Before a simplified classroom evaluation technique is discussed, it is worthwhile reviewing one basic aspect necessary to the next three sections—validity. Researchers use two terms: (1) internal validity and (2) external validity. Internal validity addresses issues of the design, its application, recording of data, and whether the user of the materials can believe in them. For example, did an experimental treatment in fact generate the difference in data among treatments and among groups? External validity encompasses the data generalizable to other populations.

Internal Validity

Campbell and Stanley (1963) list eight variables affecting validity that can confound experimental design, destroying the effect of a treatment:

1. *History,* specific events occur between the first (pre) and second (post) measurement.
2. *Maturation,* control for processes within the respondents operating as a function of the passage of time and not the influence of the treatment.
3. *Testing,* the effects of taking an initial (pre) test upon the scores of a second (post) test.
4. *Instrumentation,* the data are seldom more valid than the test instument or observation is reliable.
5. *Statistical regression,* operates when groups have been selected on the basis of their extreme scores (particularly important for special education populations).
6. *Biases* may result from the differential selection of students in comparison (particularly control) groups.
7. *Experimental mortality,* or differential loss of respondents from the comparison groups.
8. *Selection-maturation interaction,* etc., which in certain of the multiple-group quasi-experimental designs, is confounded with, i.e., might be mistaken for, the effect of the experimental variable. (Campbell & Stanley, 1963, p. 5)

External Validity

Bracht and Glass (1968) further break out external validity into (1) population validity and (2) ecological validity.

Population validity.
Generalizing from the sample of subjects studied to the total population of subjects about whom the researcher is interested.
Ecological validity.
1. *Independent Variable*: Specificity in describing the variable manipulated is necessary for the generalization and replication of the experimental results.
2. *Multiple-Treatment Interference*: Factors which may interact and mask experimental effects when two or more treatments are administered consecutively to the same persons within the same or different studies.
3. *Hawthorne Effect*: A subject's behavior may be influenced partly by his perception of the experiment and how he should respond to the experimental stimuli.
4. *Novelty and Disruptive Effects*: The experimental results may be due partly to the enthusiasm or disruption generated by the newness of the treatment.
5. *Experimental Effect*: The behavior of the subjects may be unintentionally influenced by certain characteristics or behaviors of the experimenter.
6. *Pretest Sensitization*: When a pretest has been administered, the experimental results may *partly* be a result of the sensitization to the content of the treatment.
7. *Post-Test Sensitization:* Treatment effects may be latent or incomplete and appear only when a post-experimental test is administered.
8. *Interaction of Treatment Effects*: The results may be unique because of "extraneous" events occurring at the time of the experiment.
9. *Dependent Variable*: Generalization of results depends on the reliability with a specific population of an instrument designed to measure these variables.
10. *Time of Measurement and Treatment Effects*: Measurement of the dependent variable at two different times may produce different results. (Bracht & Glass, 1968, pp. 438-439)

There are two applied alternatives to traditional group comparison research—a simplified classroom evaluation model and a single-subject one.

A SIMPLIFIED CLASSROOM EVALUATION MODEL

Evaluation is the procedure by which instructional decision making is held accountable. Stufflebeam (1972) assumes that the fundamental goal of evaluation is to determine the value of a particular educational program or instructional activity. Originally, Stufflebeam (1969) saw evaluation as a systematic process of "delineating, obtaining, and providing useful information for judging decision alternatives" (p. 129). The model he developed represents a frame of reference for presenting alternatives to decision makers and can provide classroom teachers with information about the program. However, that evaluation model is too complex for daily use in the classroom.

Other evaluators have discussed plans for curriculum and course evaluation (Cronbach, 1963; Krathwohl, 1965; Lindvall, Nardozza, & Felton, 1964; Michael & Metfessel, 1967; Popham, 1969) while still others have presented theoretical evaluation models (Aikin, 1969; Hammond, 1969; Provus, 1970). These plans generally represent similar processes for conducting educational evaluations, but they do not offer a simplified procedure for the already overburdened classroom teacher to use.

What the practicing special educator must have is a simple, manageable evaluation plan that will provide information and feedback for determining whether instructional strategies are working and, if not, why not. The model presented here (Figure 10-1) is an attempt to provide a practical approach to conducting an evaluation that follows a logical plan. Teachers should be able to apply it to everyday classroom situations.

This evaluation process contains three major stages: the presituational, the situational, and the postsituational.

During the first stage (presituational) the goals and objectives of the program are defined.

During the situational stage, data are collected that allow judgments (valuations) to be made (for example, statements about particular behavioral objectives that demonstrate attainment of desired goals). This step is essential if the evaluation is to provide any information regarding objectives, goals, and their attainment. The information may be collected by questionnaires, interviews, observations, etc. The data obtained during this stage must be prepared descriptively so that their meaning and utility will be apparent. This involves representing graphically or otherwise the results of the valuations and defines the next step of the model. If the goals are not being met, the teacher can relate this information back to the first stage and either formulate new objectives or agree upon new ones. However, if the goals are being met, the teacher then proceeds to the postsituational stage.

The postsituational stage involves determining which parts of the program are effective for obtaining the objectives and goals. The major function is to establish

Figure 10-1 A Simplified Evaluation Process

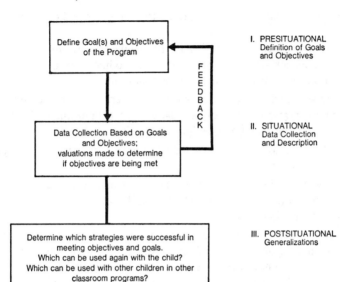

Source: Reprinted with permission from "Program and Teacher Evaluation" by R.F. Algozzine, S.K. Alper, and D.A. Sabatino in *Learning Disabilities Handbook: A Technical Guide to Program Development*, D.A. Sabatino (Ed.), Northern Illinois University Press, © 1976.

the relationship between the program goals and the successful achievement of objectives that lead to those results.

To summarize, the presituational stage involves defining the goals and objectives of the program to be evaluated. In the situational stage, information is collected, described, and related to the desired objectives and goals. In the postsituational stage, the obtained information is compared to what is intended.

A Practical Evaluation Design

The following example illustrates how a special educator can implement a proposed design to evaluate a unit on word-recognition skills for a learning disabled adolescent. This is not to recommend that a phonics approach be used to teach word-recognition skills in all situations; it is used here merely as an example. The steps in each stage are not all-inclusive but represent possible choices in a sequenced flow of instructional activities. It remains for the teacher to determine which strategies will be most effective for the individual youths.

Presituational Stage

The purpose of this stage is to state clearly the goals and objectives:

- Gather assessment information on the student from other personnel (for example, check school records, test results, other teachers' reports, etc., to gather any information that might pertain to the overall goal).
- Administer teacher-made informal tests to determine the adolescent's level of functioning (response to previous instruction). (For example, the student can recognize letter combinations but not words.)
- Specify behaviors in need of remediation (recognizing initial consonant blends, for example).
- Specify instructional strategies (methods and materials) to be used in achieving the behavioral objectives (task analysis, behavior modification principles, types of remedial materials).
- Develop a hierarchy of sequential behavioral objectives based on the above information regarding the student's strengths and weaknesses. At this point the teacher will have defined goal(s) in an instructional area and specified a sequence of behavioral objectives that should lead the youth toward mastery of the major aims of the program.

Situational Stage

The purpose of this stage is to collect and describe data based on the goals and objectives defined in the first phase:

- Administer teacher-made, criterion-referenced tests to determine whether the LBP student has mastered the behavioral objectives being taught.
- Gather information from the youth, parents, other teachers, etc., such as attitudinal information on study habits at home, and so on.
- Consult with others if necessary, e.g., resource teacher, supervisor, school psychologist. Self-determination of the classroom climate (teacher-curriculum interaction) may be helpful at this point.
- Feed back this information to the original objectives in order to determine the student's performance in interacting with the curriculum according to the standards specified.

At this point, the teacher may want to ask questions such as "Are the objectives being met? Are the behavioral objectives, teaching materials, and instructional strategies appropriate for the youth?" This information can be used to determine whether continuation, modification, or termination of the original objectives is warranted.

It might be determined, for example, that the work in the regular classroom is too difficult and that the student does not know the reading vocabulary in most of the required courses. The task is to determine whether that vocabulary can be learned in some or all of the teenager's classes or if work in the resource room must be substituted for regular classwork.

Postsituational Stage

The purpose of this stage is to make comparisons, predictions, and generalizations based on the data obtained in the situational stage as they relate to achieving the desired goals. The teacher should:

- Administer criterion-referenced tests to determine where the student is functioning now in relation to the hierarchy of behavioral objectives. How do strengths and weaknesses change as remediation is applied and what new goals and behavioral objectives seem appropriate?
- Determine which instructional strategies were successful and which were not. Which ones, totally or in part, can be used again as work is initiated on new goals and objectives?
- Determine which techniques might be successful for use with other youths with similar problems.

The answers to these questions provide the teacher with evaluative information about the program. They help explain which aspects of the teaching plan were effective and require systematic recordkeeping of the students' progress. Next is a second alternative to traditional group comparison research—the single-case approach.

Single-Subject Design

The special education classroom is especially appropriate for single-subject research. This research is a viable alternative to group study for a number of reasons. First, statistical significance obtained through inferential statistics does not necessarily support the clinical significance of treatment. For example, a reduction in reliably measured aggressive outbursts from 100 per day for a group of 20 individuals to 60 a day may be statistically significant although a majority of individuals still would be candidates for a correctional facility. The effectiveness of applied research, on the other hand, is judged by the difference between the strength of the behavior before and after treatment of any one individual. Reducing aggressive outbursts for an individual from eight per day to two would not be considered a successful intervention if the teacher had expected their complete elimination.

Individual responses to treatment are highlighted in the single-case approach while differential responses are averaged across a number of youths in the group approach. A revolutionary reading effort may substantially increase reading scores for only six of ten LBP students producing a group difference of sufficient magnitude to validate the program's effectiveness. A single-case approach allows the practitioner to specify the conditions under which the program is and is not effective, thereby enhancing the teacher's ability to match the reading program to the needs of individual youths. In general, the single-case approach allows the teacher to generalize information from student to student rather than from group to group or from group to youth (Bergin, 1966).

Failure to control for variability within groups has been a major obstacle in special education research (Cronbach & Snow, 1977). Many potentially effective educational practices have not demonstrated statistical success because of differences in the characteristics of adolescents who were in the experimental and control groups. While some students excel through the educational procedure, others show little progress. These within-group differences obscure the potential value of the procedure for some youths.

The single-case approach minimizes the interference of between-subject differences. Single-subject designs evaluate the individual's variability of behavior across program conditions without relying on the presence or absence of variability between one subject and another. For example, a self-instructional program may be demonstrated to be effective in increasing math performance for Individual A by comparing data collected under normal program conditions, then under self-instruction conditions, and again normal program conditions. In the process, no comparison is made between Individual A's behavior and that of another student.

The major disadvantage of single-case research methodology lies in the limited confidence users may have in generalizing findings from one individual to another (Kiesler, 1971). This objection is addressed in the "technique building" approach described by Bergin and Strupp (1972) in which single-case studies are used to develop specific treatment packages to be used with well-defined treatment groups. A large group design then may be used to evaluate the treatment approaches, thereby increasing the teacher's confidence in the generalization of findings. A second approach to generalization is through systematic replications of single-case research.

Countering the criticism of generalizability, the application of single-case experimental methodology to special education classrooms is encouraged by six major features:

1. It relies on the practitioner's assessment of the learning characteristics of the handicapped youth.
2. It facilitates the matching of innovative educational practices with identified learning characteristics of the adolescent.

3. It supports the systematic application of educational approaches.
4. It is sufficiently flexible to allow the modification of educational strategies as indicated by the student's performance.
5. It does not rely on the comparison of separate individuals but on the progress of one student under different program conditions.
6. It allows the practitioner to validly and reliably assess the effectiveness of a given educational practice.

For the practitioner to employ the single-case approach effectively, an accurate assessment must be made of the subject's current level of functioning as well as the environmental factors impinging upon the student's behavior.

BEHAVIORAL ASSESSMENT

Applied research generally is concerned with demonstrating that a specific approach is effective in influencing the target behavior(s) of an individual. The initial step involves a behavioral assessment, which serves two purposes: (1) it identifies specific and relevant conduct and environmental target areas that may be subject to change and (2) it facilitates the identification of a specific behavior change procedure (Goldfield & Pomerang, 1968).

In general, behavioral assessment identifies and defines the target behavior and generates teacher "hunches" about functional relations between the activity and specific events. Events that are hypothesized to be functionally related to the target behavior become the independent (treatment) variable while measures of the strength of the target conduct become the dependent variable. A single-case experimental design is applied to demonstrate that a functional relation does, in fact, exist.

For example, following a behavioral assessment, a teacher may hypothesize that Judy's talking-out behavior is functionally related to peer attention. Frequency of talk-outs is the dependent variable and peer attention the independent variable. A single-case experimental design can test peer attention's influence on talking-out. A relevant conclusion may be that the removal of peer attention following Judy's talk-outs reduced all such behaviors while reinstating peer attention increased them. Therefore, talk-outs are functionally related to peer attention. A valid functional analysis requires that the target behavior be functionally defined and that environmental target areas be isolated.

Definition of the Target Behavior

The target behavior should be defined clearly, objectively, and completely (Hawkins & Dobes, 1975). The use of descriptors such as inattentive, lacking motivation, depressed, hyperactive, etc., invariably produces unreliable assessment data. Statements such as "fails to look at the teacher during class demonstrations," "fails to complete assigned homework," "cries frequently while in class," and "is often out of the seat during math class without teacher premission" are likely to produce reliable assessment data.

Examples of clear, objective, and complete response definitions include:

- Praise: ". . . verbal praise, encouragement, positive evaluative comments, and statements of approval of the child's general behavior or work, e.g., 'That's very good' and 'You're working well.' " (Stokes, Fowler, & Baer, 1978)
- Spelling behavior: ". . . the number of words the children spelled correctly on daily six-word spelling tests." (Axelrod & Palushka, 1973)
- On-task behavior: ". . . engaged in behavior relevant to the assigned academic activity—for instance, reading in the assigned book, writing on a work sheet, or looking at the teacher when she was presenting material . . ." (Siegel & Steinman, 1973)

Having carefully defined the target behavior(s), the practitioner must identify conditions that may be associated with variability.

Identifying Environmental Target Areas

Environmental target areas include events that may influence occurrence or nonoccurrence of the behavior. Specific environmental targets can include: antecedent events that may cue the desired or undesired behavior, consequent events that may increase or decrease the likelihood that the conduct will recur, and mediational responses or cognitions that influence the activity.

A study that targets antecedent conditions is described by Lovitt and Curtis (1968). They demonstrate that a student's correct answer rate on math problems increases while the error rate decreases as the result of verbalizing the problems before making a written response. Schumaker, Havell, and Sherman (1977) present a study that focuses on consequent conditions. They implement a procedure whereby improved school performance is followed by praise from parents and by special privileges. They report the program elevated the percentage of rules followed in class and the percentage of classwork points earned from a baseline of approximately 50 to an average treatment percentage exceeding 90.

Bornstein and Querillon (1976) demonstrate the effectiveness of a two-hour self-instructional package in altering inferred mediational events. The instructional procedure involves encouraging the students to think to themselves: (1) questions about the teacher's expectations, (2) answers to the questions in the form of cognitive rehearsals, (3) self-instructions that guide them through the task, and (4) self-praise. They report the mediational procedure reduced excessive classroom activity with three overactive 14-year-olds.

Measures of Behavior Strength

Single-case experimental research requires the continuous monitoring of the target behavior (dependent variable) throughout baseline and treatment conditions. This feature is particularly useful to teachers in special education classrooms. Such continuous monitoring facilitates the evaluation of intervention plans. An ineffective educational approach can be identified and modified quickly and subsequent data can test the efficacy of the altered approach.

The validity of single-case findings is intimately associated with that of the dependent data. As with inferential statistics, the most elegant and sophisticated research design cannot produce important findings from contrived data. Sulzer-Azaroff & Mayer (1977) offer three major criteria for precise behavioral measurement: (1) observations must be objective in that personal interpretations and feelings do not influence the data; (2) observations must be valid, measuring the behavior they intend to influence directly, and (3) observations must be reliable.

The reliability of data is judged by the extent to which a measurement procedure will lead to similar results when used by independent observers. In most cases, direct naturalistic observations using a well-defined target behavior meet these criteria (Jones, Reid, & Patterson, 1975). The direct measurement of behavior can be conducted through a number of techniques.

Event Recording

This probably is the most useful and least time consuming of all measures of behavior strength. The frequency with which a target behavior occurs in LBP adolescents is determined by counting each episode of the action through a specified period of time. Frequency measures are appropriate when (1) the response has a distinct start and stop such as words spoken, steps taken, or balls thrown, and (2) when the response lasts a relatively constant time (Kazdin, 1980). Event recording should be avoided when measuring behaviors that are not discrete or of constant duration. For example, a treatment may effectively reduce the duration of crying episodes from two hours to ten minutes but not alter the number of such behaviors. Therefore, a frequency measure would not be sensitive to the change in conduct.

Frequency data from day to day often are not directly comparable because of varying times available for observation. A student may be in a class for four hours one day and six hours the next. There may be two aggressive outbursts on the first day and three on the second. It cannot be concluded that the behavior is stronger on the second day because the amount of time observed confounds the data.

The frequency of response can be transformed to a rate of response that gives comparable data across observation periods. The rate of response is computed by dividing the number of occurrences (frequency) by the amount of time observed. In the previous example, there were two aggressive outbursts in four hours on the first day, yielding a rate of .5 per hour,

$$\text{Rate} = \frac{\text{Frequency}}{\text{Time}} = \frac{2}{4} = .5$$

while there were three in six hours on the second day, producing the same rate per hour (i.e., 3/6 = .5).

A number of devices have been used to reduce the amount of staff time involved in event recording. For example, Mahoney (1974) reports using an abacus watchband and Lindsley (1968) a golf stroke counter. These devices are especially useful in classrooms because they require only one hand to make a tally, can be carried by the teacher, and can be operated without disrupting student activities. Regardless of the instrument used, a recording sheet that stores data from day to day is essential. Exhibit 10-1 illustrates a commonly used data sheet for observations of varying length.

Measurement of Personal Product

This is a recording procedure similar to frequency recording. It is particularly useful in special education classes in which academic behavior often results in some quantifiable product. Single-case studies that demonstrate effective academic remediation procedures often focus on the outcome of academic exercises as the dependent measure. For example, Trap, Milner-Davis, Shirley, and Cooper (1978) report developing an elaborate scoring procedure to determine the correctness of cursive letters. The percentage of correctly trained letter strokes

---

Exhibit 10-1 Recording Sheet for Rate Data

Date	Start	Stop	Total	Frequency	Rate[1]
		Time			
3/3	8:00	11:00	180 mins.	36	.2
3/4	8:10	10:10	120 mins.	14	.1
3/5	8:30	10:30	120 mins.	18	.4

[1]Rate per hour of observed behavior.

becomes the dependent measure for a study that evaluates the influence of feedback, rewriting, and reinforcement on cursive letter formation.

When using the permanent product as a dependent variable, the examiner must demonstrate that the demands are relatively stable through the study so that the individual's performance level is not obscured by tasks that vary in difficulty from session to session. When an individual is expected to perform a different number of tasks from day to day, permanent product data should be expressed as the percentage of correct responses over the number of opportunities to respond.

Interval Recording

This commonly is used to determine the strength of behaviors that do not have discrete start or stop times and that vary in length (e.g., singing, hand waving, talking, attending, sitting, etc.). Interval data are collected by dividing a long period of time into shorter periods. For example, a 20-minute class may be divided into 40 half-minute intervals. The behavior is scored as occurred or not occurred in each of the intervals. The actual number of occurrences in the interval does not affect the scoring. Often, interval data are time sampled (i.e., taken in random periods of time through the day that are expected to approximate the strength of the behavior throughout the day).

Kazdin (1980) describes an interval procedure by which a number of students in a classroom can be observed over the same period of time. The first youth is observed in the first interval, the second in the second interval, and so on, until all are observed. The recorder then returns to the initial student until the entire class has been observed for a number of intervals. Another variation of this procedure involves observing the youth through an interval, then taking a short time to record the response before beginning the second interval. For example, observation intervals may be 15 seconds in length and scoring intervals 5 seconds.

Figure 10-2 represents a scoring sheet commonly used with interval recording. The numbers over each square denote the time of the interval. A + or a – is used to indicate the occurrence or nonoccurrence of the behavior. The interval data are transformed to the percentage of intervals in which the behavior occurs by dividing the number of occurrences by the number of intervals.

Marholin and Steinman (1977) assess on-task behavior of adolescents with academic and behavioral problems using a time-sampling procedure. The researchers divide 5-minute observation periods into twenty 10-second intervals, with 5 seconds for recording (i.e., 10-second observation followed by 5-second recording, repeat). An observation interval is scored as on-task if the student engages in an assigned task for at least 9 seconds of the 10-second interval. The researchers demonstrate that in generalizing behavioral gains outside the teacher's presence, reinforcing a teenager for completed work is superior to reinforcing specific on-task conduct.

Figure 10-2 Scoring Sheet for Interval Recording

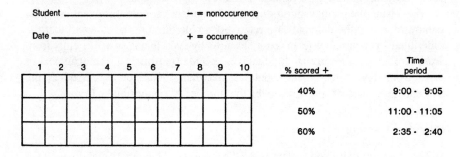

Duration Recording

This is useful when the intervention approach is expected to increase or decrease the amount of time an individual engages in an activity. An investigator may seek to increase the amount of time a student spends on homework or decrease the time in the halls between classes. In these cases, the dependent measure is duration. Whitman, Mercurio, and Caponigri (1970) utilize duration data in a study designed to evaluate the effectiveness of a social interaction training procedure, measuring the number of minutes spent in such activity by program participants. Subjects showed a progressive increase in social interaction during the reinforcement period.

Response Latency

This is a variation of duration data used when the dependent measure is the amount of time from some event to a specific response. Phillips (1968) uses latency data to assess the effectiveness of a strategy designed to reduce tardiness of predelinquent youths. Results indicated a significant reduction in tardiness among youths studied.

Interobserver Reliability

An overriding methodological issue in single-subject research is the extent to which an observational procedure produces a reliable assessment of the target behavior. Interobserver reliability in single-subject research is determined by assessing the degree to which independent observers agree on the occurrence/nonoccurrence, duration, or strength of the conduct. In general, reliability indicates the consistency with which the behavior is observed and scored (Kazdin, 1980). High reliability is essential so that variability in data can be attributed confidently to the treatment procedure rather than observer error.

Poor interobserver reliability often is the result of an inadequate response definition or observational procedure. For example, it is unlikely that independent observers can agree on the occurrence of hyperactive behavior using a frequency measure (e.g., number of hyperactive episodes). On the other hand, if the response definition is changed to number of times out of seat, two observers probably can agree fairly consistently on the occurrence of that conduct.

Interobserver reliability for frequency measures is determined by two individuals' checking the student for the same period of time. The lower frequency of occurrences then is divided by the higher frequency to produce the reliability coefficient (i.e., percentage of agreement between two observers).

For example, a teacher and aide both record the number of swear words uttered by a youth in a two-hour period. The teacher records ten, the aide eight. The resulting reliability coefficient is computed by dividing the smaller number of observations (eight) by the larger (ten), producing 80 percent agreement:

$$\frac{\text{smaller frequency}}{\text{larger frequency}} = \frac{8}{10} = .80$$

Reliability in duration recording is computed by dividing the shorter time reported by the longer duration clocked by two independent observers:

$$\frac{\text{shorter duration}}{\text{longer duration}} = \frac{25}{30} = .83$$

The reliability coefficient in interval recording is determined by dividing the number of intervals in which both observers score an occurrence by the number of their agreements and disagreements. Intervals in which both observers do not score an occurrence are excluded from the computation:

$$\frac{\text{\# agreements}}{\substack{\text{\# agreements \& disagreements} \\ \text{excluding nonoccurrences}}} = \frac{5}{7} = .71$$

Interobserver reliability should be evaluated before initiating baseline, during baseline, and every three to five days throughout the study. Baseline refers to the period of data collection when intervention is not occurring. Reliability should be tested at a level of .80 or better before the initiation of baseline. Consistently high reliability (e.g., .98) requires fewer checks. As was mentioned, low reliability prior to baseline may indicate the inadequacy of the response definition or of the observation procedure. Before continuing with data collection, the examiner should redefine the target behavior and/or modify the observation procedure until reliability exceeds .80.

Research demonstrates that observers obtain higher rates of agreement when they are aware that a reliability check is being made as compared to when they are not aware (Kent, O'Leary, Dietz, & Diament, 1979). These findings suggest that, for a more conservative estimate of reliability, the primary observer should not be aware of times when checks are made.

Unfortunately, practical limitations often make this difficult, if not impossible. Taplin and Reid (1973) suggest that researchers increase the frequency of reliability checks throughout the study, in lieu of blind ones. In general, if the datakeeping system, response definition, and method of collecting reliability data are structured by the classroom teacher/researcher to reduce or eliminate subjective judgment and bias, the reliability of the obtained data will be defensible and, more importantly, usable for decision-making purposes in the classroom.

Collecting Baseline Data

The common characteristic of all single-subject research is the continuous measurement of the target conduct (dependent measure) through a baseline phase (A) and treatment phase (B). The baseline provides a measure of behavior strength under natural conditions, against which subsequent treatment effects may be compared. For comparisons to be valid, the baseline must be representative of the true behavior strength under normal program conditions. A valid representation of behavior strength is achieved by collecting reliable baseline data through four or more days in which there is neither an ascending trend, when a reductive intervention is planned, nor descending trend, when an accelerative intervention is planned. There also should be some degree of stability in the data.

An ascending trend indicates that the dependent measure is increasing in strength, a descending trend the reverse. In either case, if the examiner shifts to the B phase while a baseline trend is present in the desired direction of treatment, comparisons between phases are of questionable validity. For example, Figure 10-3 shows descending baseline data and subsequent treatment data. The effect of treatment on the dependent variable is not clear because there is no abrupt shift in the strength of the target behavior when treatment is introduced. Similarly, when an ascending baseline precedes a treatment designed to strengthen a target behavior, the influence of treatment on the conduct is not clear. A possible solution to this problem involves continuing baseline conditions until a plateau is reached or until the behavior attains acceptable levels through natural program conditions.

A similar pattern involves an ascending baseline preceding a deceleration program, or the inverse, a descending baseline preceding an acceleration program. In such cases, the trend in baseline data indicates a deterioration in the behavior that treatment is designed to improve. This pattern presents less of a concern to applied researchers than the previous one because treatment effects can be ascertained from a redirection of the dependent variable.

Figure 10-3 Improper Descending Baseline Trend

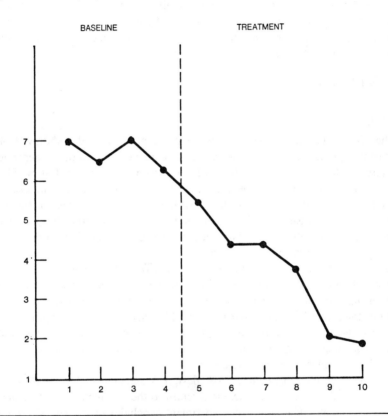

The final pattern of concern is the unstable baseline. Gross variations in baseline data collected over short periods of time reduce the teacher's ability to ascertain the strength of the target behavior if treatment were not applied. An unstable baseline can be corrected by delaying the introduction of the B phase until some degree of stability is obtained or until sufficient baseline information is accumulated to demonstrate that the data are neither ascending nor descending under natural conditions.

Reactivity (i.e., the influence of the observer on behavior strength) is the final consideration in designing valid baseline observations. White (1977) demonstrates that the mere presence of observers may influence the occurrence or nonoccurrence of the target behavior. While other researchers present contradictory findings (Mercatoris & Craighead, 1974; Nelson, Kapist, & Dorsey, 1978), there is general agreement in the literature that investigators should guard against reactivity as a contaminating influence on behavioral data (Kazdin, 1980).

Reactivity can be minimized by (1) taking extended baseline data, thereby reducing the novel effect of datakeeping and allowing the student to acclimate to the observation procedure, (2) using individuals frequently present in the setting as data takers, and (3) taking data covertly (e.g., behind a one-way mirror, with a counter hidden in the teacher's pocket or desk, etc.).

Reversal Designs[1]

A-B-A Design

The A-B-A design involves the systematic application and withdrawal of a treatment approach to demonstrate the reinforcement's control of the dependent measure. A stable low rate of behavior in the first baseline phase, followed by a high rate in the treatment phase, followed by a low rate in the second baseline phase allows the examiner to conclude that the treatment produced an increased rate of conduct over baseline. Confident statements of causation can be made when the behavior improves during treatment and reverses to its original baseline level following the withdrawal of treatment.

Figure 10-4 is an example of an A-B-A design. This design was modified by the chapter authors to relate to an adolescent type behavior to demonstrate a functional relationship between teacher attention and the use of profanity by an adolescent. A study of their data in Figure 10-4 reveals a high and somewhat variable rate of profanity under baseline conditions. Profanity is reduced dramatically under the B phase (teacher attention). The conduct begins to return to its original baseline rate when the examiner withdraws treatment.

The major limitation of the A-B-A design is apparent in Figure 10-4. The experimental design does not include a return to the treatment procedure that it sought to validate. Therefore, the experiment concludes under natural program conditions that are demonstrated to be inferior to the treatment condition. The A-B-A-B design, presented in the following section, resolves this criticism.

A-B-A-B Design

The A-B-A-B design differs from the A-B-A in that a treatment phase is reinstated following the second baseline phase. The A-B-A-B design is superior to the A-B-A for both ethical and methodological reasons. The return to treatment allows two comparisons to be made between it and baseline conditions. The first A-B compares baseline to the initial treatment phase; the second A-B compares the subsequent treatment to the baseline phase. Thus, the behavior change can be expected to coincide with the introduction of treatment on two occasions.

Fox, Copeland, Harris, Rieth, and Hall (1973) utilize an A-B-A-B design to demonstrate the effectiveness of a token economy system in reducing the number of interruptive behaviors of an adolescent in a junior high school special education

Figure 10-4 A-B-A Design: Teacher Attention and Profanity

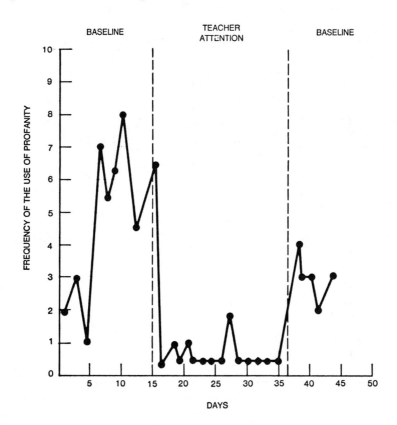

classroom. Their data, in Figure 10-5, show a high rate of interruptive behavior in the first baseline phase. The initial treatment phase dramatically reduces the number of interruptions from an average of 10 to 4. The subsequent return to baseline results in an increase in the target behavior to a mean of 5.8. This is reduced to a mean of .6 in the final treatment phase. It is important to note that the behavior does not return to the original baseline level in the second baseline phase. This reduces educators' confidence in the influence of treatment on the target behavior. Changes in conduct may be attributed to maturation, teacher effectiveness, or other variables not isolated by the experimental design. The authors of this chapter are painfully aware, however, that applied research data do not always parallel textbook models because of the inherent difficulty of controlling the numerous variables encountered in natural settings. The confidence teachers may have in this or other applied research data must be left to their discretion.

Figure 10-5 A-B-A-B Design for Token Economy in Reducing Interruptive
Behaviors

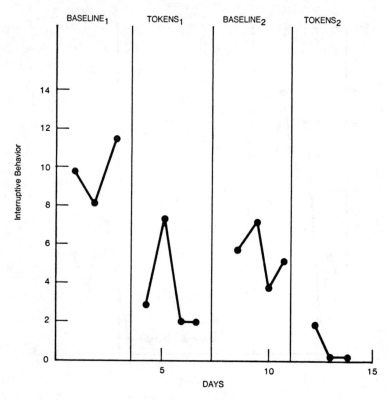

Source: Adapted with permission from "A Computerized System for Selecting Responsive Teaching Studies, Catalogued Along Twenty-Eight Important Dimensions" by R.G. Fox, R.E. Copeland, S.W. Harris, H.J. Rieth, and R.V. Hall in *Behavior Analysis: Areas of Research and Application*, E. Ramp and G. Semb (Eds.), Prentice-Hall, Inc., © 1973, p. 151.

B-A-B Design

The B-A-B design is useful in evaluating the effectiveness of an educational procedure initiated before the start of a formal study. The first phase (B) usually includes the continuing educational procedure, the second phase (A) the discontinuation of the procedure, and the final phase (B) its reinstatement.

For example, the authors were asked to determine whether a study carrel being used with a mildly retarded adolescent in a vocational training program was effective in improving her speed of production. Production rate data were taken for one week with the carrel in place. The carrel then was removed for a ten-day baseline period. Finally, the carrel was reinstated. Data in both treatment phases were stable at an average of .3 units per minute. The baseline phase produced unstable production rate data averaging .1 unit per minute. The conclusion was that the removal of the carrel was functionally related to an erratic and low speed production for this adolescent.

Concerns in Using Reversal Designs

Each of the preceding designs relies on the withdrawal of treatment and subsequent deterioration of the target behavior to demonstrate experimental control. This characteristic of the A-B-A, A-B-A-B, and B-A-B design limits their usefulness. It is difficult and sometimes unethical to withdraw a viable teaching strategy simply to demonstrate its validity.

For example, the authors were asked to design a program to reduce the frequency and strength of aggressive episodes displayed by a highly disruptive 14-year-old boy. The teacher reported four to seven hitting episodes per day through a five-day baseline period. (It should be noted that "natural conditions" associated with baseline imply that the teacher followed the general approach of isolating and reprimanding the youth.) The experimental approach of verbal praise coupled with a tangible reinforcement (Popsicle) was introduced and the number of aggressive episodes reduced to one a week. Returning to baseline to demonstrate the control of treatment over aggressive episodes could not be considered because the potential (and predicted) increase in disruptive behaviors would threaten the safety of other students in the classroom. A reversal phase would have been needed to control for extraneous variables.

In some cases, A-B-A, A-B-A-B, and B-A-B designs are contraindicated because the withdrawal of treatment is not expected to produce a return to baseline rate. For example, a self-control program may propose to train unseen mediational statements that may motivate homework completion. Withdrawal of the training procedure would not be expected to result in the deterioration of homework performance since the mediational responses are expected to be independent of external intervention. Failure of the behavior to return to baseline rates following training would reduce confidence in the validity of the treatment approach. Fortunately, other designs can be used that do not require the withdrawal of the intervention to make confident causal statements. These are presented in the following four sections.

Multiple Baseline Designs

These offer an alternative to the reversal designs when ethical and practical constraints dictate against the removal of a successful treatment approach (Barlow

& Hersen, 1973; Kazdin, 1980). Three general types of multiple baseline designs may be used: (1) across behaviors, (2) across settings, and (3) across individuals. In each variation, the systematic approach to treatment remains the same while the target of the intervention differs.

Multiple Baseline across Behaviors

Multiple baseline across behaviors involves collecting baseline data across three or more actions by an individual. Once stability exists in each baseline, the intervention procedure is initiated with the first behavior. After that becomes stable, intervention is introduced to the second behavior. When the second is stable, the intervention procedure is applied to the final one. While this discussion includes only three behaviors, a stronger statement of the treatment effect can be made by sequentially introducing treatment for four or more.

An example of the multiple baseline across behaviors design is reported by Furman, Geller, Simon, and Kelley (1979) in their validation of a job interview training program for psychiatric patients. As can be seen by their data in Figure 10-6, the examiners collect baseline data on three behaviors: positive information, questions to interviewer, and expressions of enthusiasm. Once improvement and stability are achieved in the positive information baseline, a behavior rehearsal procedure is introduced to teach the client to offer positive information about any employment and educational history. After the rate of positive information improved and stabilized, behavior rehearsals focused on increasing appropriate questions asked of the interviewer. Following improvement and stabilization in the higher rate of appropriate questions, the behavior rehearsals focus on the third target—expressions of enthusiasm. It is apparent from these data that the behavior rehearsal procedure is effective in improving the three target actions.

Multiple Baseline across Settings

This design involves collecting baseline data on the same conduct in three distinct settings. Once a stable rate of the behavior is represented in each baseline, the intervention procedure is applied in the first setting. As the behavior stabilizes in the first setting, the intervention is applied in the second, and so on. Control of the dependent measure by the intervention procedure is established by substantial changes in the strength of the target behavior that occur only as the experimental procedure is initiated. Figure 10-7 represents a multiple baseline design used by the authors to evaluate the effectiveness of a positive practice procedure in reducing irrational verbalization of an emotionally disturbed adolescent in a vocational training setting. Baseline data were collected in the workshop, music classroom, and physical education room. Each time the intervention procedure

Figure 10-6 Multiple Baseline across Behaviors Design

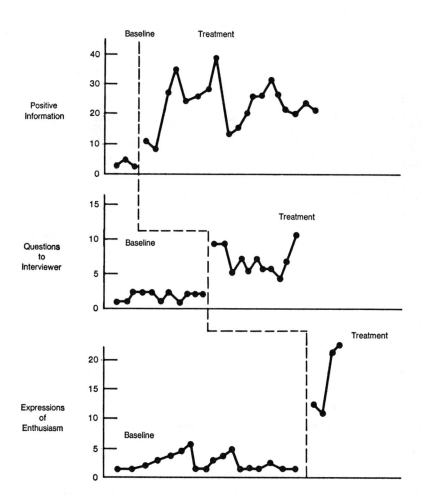

Source: Reprinted with permission from "The Use of a Behavioral Rehearsal Procedure for Teaching Job Interviewing Skills to Psychiatric Patients" by W. Furman, M. Geller, S.J. Simon, and J.A. Kelley, *Behavior Therapy, 10,* pp. 157-167, © 1979.

was implemented in a different setting there was a dramatic change in the frequency of irrational verbalizations. The association of the intervention with a reduction in the target behavior across each setting demonstrates that the positive practice procedure was effective in reducing the conduct.

Figure 10-7 Design To Validate a Positive Practice Procedure

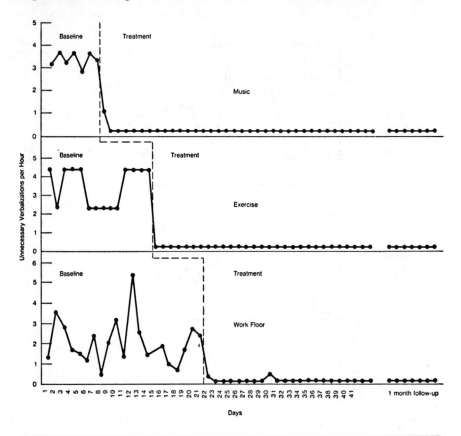

Multiple Baseline across Individuals

This design involves collecting baseline data across the same behavior of three or more individuals. Once stability exists in the three baselines, the intervention procedure is applied with the first person. As that individual's conduct becomes stable, the intervention is applied with the second person and, once stabilized, with the third. Control of the dependent variable by the intervention is established as the strength of the target behavior for each individual changes concurrently with the introduction of treatment.

Schumaker, Havell, and Sherman (1977) report a study demonstrating the use of a multiple baseline design across individuals. They evaluate the effectiveness of a daily report card system in modifying the school conduct of problem junior high students. The report card system was applied systematically to each of three students; a substantial increase in the percentage of class rules followed. The systematic introduction of the report card system and concurrent change in rate of the target behavior for each of three subjects demonstrate the validity of the intervention approach.

Concerns in Using Multiple Baseline Design

Multiple baseline designs involve the systematic application of treatment to several behaviors, individuals, or settings. There is no need to interrupt treatment (amid predictions of the return of inappropriate or undesirable behavior) to demonstrate experimental control. To the contrary, in many cases the multiple baseline design provides a systematic framework in which to conduct positive programming.

For example, the authors were asked to design a training program to develop socially skillful behaviors with severely withdrawn adolescents. Following a careful behavior analysis, it was determined that (1) the behaviors may not have been in the individuals' repertoire, (2) the classroom conditions did not motivate the use of socially skillful behavior, and (3) it was unlikely that the students would acquire and demonstrate a large number of skills in a short time.

The resulting program involved teaching and motivating one behavior (saying hello to people entering the room) until a specified criterion was reached, then teaching and motivating a second behavior (saying goodbye to people leaving the room) and so on until four behaviors were learned and used in the natural environment. The design of multiple baselines across behaviors not only validated the training procedure but also provided a positive and systematic approach to teaching social skills. New concepts were introduced only as previous skills were mastered. The expectations for the adolescents on any given day were clearly specified by the design. Finally, at no time did the number of demands placed on the adolescents exceed their ability to respond successfully.

There is one major limitation to the multiple baseline design. The effect of the treatment is demonstrated strongly only if the target behavior changes as the intervention is applied. If the behavior begins to improve before treatment, a clear statement supporting its effectiveness cannot be made. The likelihood that this confounding influence can arise is addressed by several studies. For example, Kazdin (1973a) demonstrates that a treatment applied to one type of conduct may improve other behaviors. The improvement in one individual's behavior may result in the improvement of another's (Kazdin, 1979), and the application of an intervention procedure in one setting may generalize to another (Kazdin, 1973b). While the unexpected improvement in untreated behaviors may be a welcome problem, it significantly reduces users' confidence in the validity of the treatment procedure. When a spontaneous generalization of treatment effects across people, settings, or behaviors can be anticipated, an alternate design should be employed.

Changing Criterion Design

The final single-case experimental option in this chapter is the changing criterion design. This does not rely on a reversal or multiple baseline to demonstrate experimental control. Rather, validity is established when the individual's behavior continually exceeds a specified criterion for reinforcement. The person's behavior is expected to change commensurate with a series of more stringent criteria for reinforcement.

Baseline data are collected on the target behavior. Once stability is achieved, a criterion for reinforcement, slightly higher than the baseline level, is established. When the behavior is equal to or greater than the first criterion for a number of sessions, the level is elevated. As the behavior consistently exceeds the second criterion, a third, more stringent one is imposed, and so on until the conduct reaches a level specified by the program objective. Experimental control is established by the target behavior's continually increasing (or decreasing) in strength to meet the criterion for reinforcement.

Hartman and Hall (1976) report the use of a changing criterion design in increasing the number of math problems completed by a behaviorally disordered youth. A baseline phase is established in which the teacher gives the student a work sheet containing nine math problems. Following baseline, a criterion for reinforcement is set at two problems, the next highest whole problem over the mean of the baseline. The consequence of meeting or exceeding the criterion includes extra time playing basketball. Failure to meet the criterion results in extra math time. Following three successful sessions at the first level, the criterion is elevated to three, then to four, and so on until all nine problems are completed. The functional relationship between reinforcement and math assignment completion is established as the individual's behavior changes to conform to the requirements for reinforcement.

Concerns in Using a Changing Criterion Design

The changing criterion design is not compatible with behavior change procedures expected to produce a dramatic increase or decrease in conduct over a short time. A reinforcement procedure that is expected to rapidly increase the strength of a response will not produce a number of sessions in which behavior strength adjusts to a more stringent criterion. One or two increases in behavior that exceed the criterion for reinforcement do not clearly demonstrate the effect of treatment on the conduct. Numerous confounding variables are not controlled for when there is not a demonstrable association between the behavior strength and criterion for reinforcement.

On the other hand, the changing criterion design provides a logical, systematic, and positive framework for training that is expected to produce a gradual increase in the skill level of an individual. The teacher can begin the study with very modest student expectations, thereby ensuring success. Once the initial criterion is met, a slightly more demanding one is established. The progression from the initial to the final criterion can be sufficiently gradual to ensure that the youth will adapt to more stringent task demands without excessive frustration or failure.

This section has described three major single-subject design options: reversal, multiple baseline, and changing criterion. The practitioner can use these research tools to validate a wide range of intervention/instructional procedures in the special education classroom. By carefully selecting a specific design based on (1) the response characteristics of the adolescent, (2) the nature of the intervention procedure, (3) the number of participants with similar characteristics, (4) the anticipated outcome of the intervention, and (5) the practical limitations of the classroom setting, the teacher can identify a research option that does not interfere with the continuing educational activities of the class.

APPLIED RESEARCH WITH MILDLY HANDICAPPED

This section briefly reviews a sample of the research conducted with learning and behaviorally disordered adolescent youths. Three research issues are studied: (1) the characteristics of the learning and behavioral disordered adolescent; (2) the effects of various instructional approaches with these youths, and (3) the influence of various instructional environments (program delivery systems), i.e., learning centers, career information centers, resource rooms, etc.

The brevity of the section reflects its two intents: (1) to examine the research method and (2) to discuss the impact of that research for educators. By no means should it be assumed that this section reflects an in-depth review of the literature; other books and periodicals accomplish that objective quite nicely. In addition, the literature is cited extensively, in almost every chapter of this book.

Research on Learning Characteristics

One mark of adolescence as a unique period is that a balance of independence and dependence within selected social and personal relationships could be hypothesized if these young people are to evidence positive adjustment. The struggle between independence and dependence, in the context of the social agency known as the schools, has caused educators to raise serious questions concerning the influence of academic progress on social-personal adjustment. Rapid physical growth, newfound concerns for a place in an enlarged world, the establishment of sex role relationships, and intense pressures from without to accept the adult world and establish an earned place in it, all interact to create tremendous internal needs that may meet acute frustration if academic failure is experienced. Add to those dimensions the combination of school and societal failure, overlaid by a handi-capping condition. Yet the secondary schools steadfastly remain academically oriented, functionally denying the existence of "problem youths."

Deshler (1978), reviewing school records in search of characteristics of learning disabled adolescents, observes, "By adolescence there is a high probability that learning disabled students will experience the indirect effects of a learning handi-cap as manifest by poor self-perception, lowered self-concept, or reduced motiva-tion" (p. 68). In short, research can be as simple as going to school records and abstracting the data in them in a systematic manner.

What, then, is the influence of learning disability on self-concept? One tech-nique for answering that question is to administer self-concept tests to groups of secondary learning disabled students. That is the procedure Brookover, Erickson, and Joiner (1967) use in reporting a high positive correlation between academic achievement and self-concept. It is important that a correlation not be viewed as a cause-and-effect relationship but merely as an occurrence of two events. There-fore, the question of which comes first, the chicken or the egg, the academic deficit or poor self-concept, remains open for future longitudinal research.

There simply are no longitudinal data available on learning disabled students. Hogenson (1974) advances the following hypotheses:

1. Continued failure in reading is a deeply frustrating experience.
2. Continued frustration over prolonged periods of time will result in aggres-sive behavior.
3. Confined delinquent boys who have failed in reading will have behavioral histories showing more antisocial aggression than able readers.

To conduct such a study, Hogenson randomly selected two populations of boys from institutions for delinquent youths. The researcher then administered a number of reading tests, examined records, and gathered data from the school backgrounds on each youth. The results yielded correlations of .33 and .40 for the two groups between reading and aggression. Hogenson interprets that finding as a significant correlation (although a low moderate one). The implications are that (1) greater emphasis should be placed on increasing remedial reading programs in the primary schools, (2) remedial reading programs should be designed to meet individual learning needs, (3) reading instruction should be delayed until the student is developmentally and cognitively able to understand failure, and (4) remediation should be continued as long as necessary.

This is an example of overdrawing conclusions on the basis of the data available. The relationship between the conclusions and the data is purely coincidental. Sparkling accounts exist of pedagogical methods and appropriate principles for secondary learning disabled students, but there are insufficient data to support such positions since most of the standardized group and individual diagnostic tests have been designed for the elementary grades.

The tangled cause-and-effect relationship between learning problems and juvenile delinquency often results in argumentation as to whether these two disorders are correlated. Some researchers prefer to circumvent this issue and go directly to the problem of providing assistance to juvenile offenders with learning problems. Bachara and Zaba (1978) studied the effects of remediation in the form of special education placement, tutoring, and perceptual motor training on 79 juvenile delinquents ranging from 14 to 16, of normal intelligence, and at least two years behind in reading as measured by the Wide Range Achievement Test. They report that the rate of recidivism for subjects in the remediation group is significantly lower ($p \leq .01$, df $= 1$) than the group not receiving educational assistance.

In a follow-up of poor readers in elementary school, Muehl and Forrell (1973) isolated a group of 43 students (mean placement at the time of initial assessment was the fifth grade) who showed a delay of three years in reading. The study of learner characteristics showed that (1) the group continued to be poor readers in secondary schools, (2) there was no relationship between electroencephalograms (EEG) classifications at diagnosis and high school reading scores, and (3) verbal intelligence and chronological age at the time of the initial diagnosis in elementary school were significantly related to reading in high school.

Research on Type of Instruction

Research on type of instruction is limited. A number of articles in the literature report what to teach but few have data to support the effectiveness of the teaching methods.

One excellent piece of work is reported by Bursuk (1971) in which he hypothesizes that: (1) adolescent retarded readers taught by a combined aural-visual approach will achieve greater gains in reading comprehension than those taught by a predominantly visual approach and (2) there will be a significant relationship between sensory modality preference and emphasis of instruction with reference to comprehension. (The aural-visual approach is more effective in improving comprehension for auditory learners and those without a sensory preference than for visual learners; the reverse is true with the mainly visual approach.)

Bursuk administered several tests to a population of 132 adolescents. The test data were used to classify the subjects as to modality preference. After classification, groups of 30 were established and further separated into experimental and control groups differing as to remedial technique used; there were 90 adolescents used in this research study.

After a semester of instruction differing in emphasis on visual or aural comprehension, a reading achievement posttest was administered. The two hypotheses were supported. Bursuk concluded that the mode of instruction should be consistent with students' preferred learning style. If that is not possible, an integrative, multimodal approach is preferred.

Many publications describe successful reading intervention techniques used with secondary learning disabled students. Cole (1967) utilizes a rehabilitation program in which reading skills are developed by considering the students' environment and future aspirations. Neeley (1972) uses driving manuals to develop skills in nonreaders. Behavior modification is used by Nolen, Kunzelmann, and Haring (1967) to help secondary learning disabled students to complete reading tasks with increased demands. Page, Prentice, and Thomas (1967) facilitate cross-age tutorial programs singly and in coordination with other techniques to improve reading ability. Interrelating listening, speaking, reading, and writing activities increased reading comprehension in an investigation by Scott (1971).

Bendell, Tollefson, and Fine (1980) investigated the interaction of locus of control orientation with two conditions of learning on the performance of learning disabled adolescents. A sample of 50 learning disabled adolescents was divided into two divergent samples on the basis of the locus of control variables assessed via the Intellectual Achievement Responsibility Questionnaire. The youths were administered a list of spelling words under two conditions of learning—highly structured reinforcement and lowly structured reinforcement.

The results of a repeated measures analysis of covariance indicate that adolescents who view their performance as related to their own behavior and efforts (internal locus of control) perform significantly better in the low structure reinforcement condition while those with an external locus of control perform better in spelling under highly structured reinforcement conditions.

Deshler (1975) administered five school-related tasks requiring the student to monitor either self-generated or externally generated errors. Two groups of students (36 in each) were selected; one group was known to exhibit learning disabilities, the other was normal. The same tasks were administered to both and were scored to determine whether the groups could be differentiated on a variety of error measures. The results indicated that:

1. on the creative writing task, significant differences were found between the variances and means on the measures of errors, errors detected, percent errors detected, nonerrors detected, and percent errors corrected for both groups
2. on the editing task, significant differences were found between the means and variances on the measures of errors detected, percent errors detected, nonerrors detected, and percent errors corrected (for both groups, no significant difference was found on errors corrected)
3. on the yes-no spelling task, a significant difference was found in detectability of errors

4. on the vocabulary task, a significant difference was found on their detecting of errors in vocabulary usage (however, the learning disabled group did better on this task than on spelling).

Analysis of the results suggests that these tasks are effective discriminators and that the monitoring is a necessary diagnostic method for learning disabled students at the high school level. However, these results should be treated as preliminary in nature and suggestive for future research efforts and refinements.

Research on the Instructional Environment

There is a possibility that some secondary students are more effectively, if not more efficiently, served in one type of setting than another.

Landis, Jones, and Kennedy (1973) report the results of a one-year secondary reading program for learning disabled students in which the textbook-oriented instruction was replaced by a multisensory approach. Behavioral objectives were written by the teachers, and materials were developed to meet those goals. Neither assessment instruments nor test data were reported.

Program descriptions of secondary programs abound in the literature. Behan (1968) describes a junior high school resource room but does not measure its effectiveness. Brutten (1966) tells of a vocational education program but again, no data. Cole (1967) and Colella (1973) discuss an integrated vocational rehabilitation program and a career development center, respectively. Again, no data.

A cross-tutorial program was instituted by Lane, Pollack, and Sher (1972). Secondary learning disabled students tutored third and fourth grade pupils twice a week for seven months. Behavior modification techniques were used at weekly rap sessions to help improve behavior and strengthen the self-images of the secondary students. They achieved an average gain of 19 months, as measured by the Metropolitan Achievement Test. Their classroom behavior was graded satisfactory by counselors while the students rated themselves as less angry, more confident, and responsible. Again, no effective method measurement—no data.

Dillner (1971) studied the effectiveness of a cross-age tutoring design in teaching remedial reading. Standardized reading and self-concept tests were given to experimental and control groups in pretesting and posttesting in order to assess growth. The tutoring took place once a week with the tutors having a training session the day before to plan the lesson. A short seminar followed each session in an effort to evaluate and improve the tutoring techniques.

Although the tutors gained in many areas, the only significant differences between the two groups were in reading skills (in poetry comprehension) and in self-concept (autonomy). No significant difference existed in the relationship between reading and self-concept or between reading and attitude toward school. But when each group was looked at separately for this factor, the experimental group exhibited a relationship between growth in reading as well as in attitude toward school.

Implications in that dissertation are that the classroom teacher has the main responsibility for the success of the program but that cross-age tutoring has much applicability for the average classroom.

Another approach is to provide the youths rather than the teacher with the skills necessary for the students to personally rearrange critical aspects of their environment in order to help promote desirable behavior. In a study by Marshall and Heward (1979), eight institutionalized male juvenile delinquents participated in a 13-session course on principles and techniques of self-management. The course was conducted in a specially designed classroom in which each student responded on an overhead projector built into his desk.

The results showed students had increased their verbal knowledge of behavioral principles, correctly implemented self-management techniques presented in the course, and showed improvement on selected target behaviors during intervention. In addition, seven of the eight felt their self-management projects were successful in significantly modifying their chosen target behaviors.

SUMMARY

This chapter has provided educators of secondary mildly handicapped students with both an understanding of current research practices and the means whereby they can be implemented by practitioners in the classroom. The intent has been to bridge the information gap between those conducting research with an often unserved or underserved population and those held accountable for providing adequate educational services to adolescents with learning and/or behavioral problems.

NOTE

1. The reader is directed to Hersen, M., & Barlow, D.H. *Single case experimental designs: Strategies for studying behavior change*. New York: Pergamon Press, 1978, for a comprehensive explanation of the experimental designs presented in this section.

Part IV

Alternative Models to Traditional Secondary Programming

The last part of this text addresses program alternatives. It is a logical extension of the curricula section (Part III), broadening the earlier discussion to include instructional delivery, beginning with mainstreaming as a conceptual and operational process. Chapter 11 reviews mainstreaming as a structure within which a curriculum flow can be effective. Chapter 12, on parallel alternative curricula, offers a step-by-step procedure for installing a mainstreaming approach.

Chapter 13 looks at that all-important alternative to traditional academic dependence—career-vocational education as a concept and how to process it. Finally, Chapter 14 examines alternative schools and programs offered as a second chance for those who have failed continually in a rigid system. That chapter moves this section from an internal view of the regular classroom, where mainstreaming is practiced, through vocational-technical programming in the social-personal development of job preparedness known as career education, to external (to school) alternative types of programs. Thus, educators can move from the regular classroom, using specialized instruction, to any setting, using an integrated career education approach, to school-community related programming in a variety of settings.

It should be kept in mind that this section forms the container for the information in the earlier sections—especially Part III. In perusing this final section, educators should reread earlier chapters, fitting information together to provide a clear concept of adolescents with learning and behavior problems, an approach for setting an appropriate task, a process for reporting that process (IEP), ending in discussions on alternatives to regular, vocational, and special education curricula and programs for LBP secondary youths.

Chapter 11

Mainstreaming LBP Adolescents

Harold Wm. Heller

INTRODUCTION

Perhaps no other single word in the history of special education has more dominated its terminology than "mainstreaming." This has come to mean many things to many different people, in both regular and special education. The problem with any term is the degree to which it communicates adequately what it is attempting to say.

The word mainstreaming in the vernacular of the special educator has been developed to indicate a program that seeks to integrate and/or retain handicapped individuals to the maximum extent possible in a regular school placement. It implies that the place where most education occurs is the so-called mainstream. The mainstream then becomes regular educational programs because the majority of all schooling in the United States is provided in regular classrooms.

THE CONCEPT

The concept of mainstreaming definitely is not new. In 1953, the Illinois Commission for Handicapped Children conducted its Tenth Annual Governor's Conference on Exceptional Children in Chicago and titled it "The Handicapped Child in the Mainstream." This conference focused on finding ways to ensure that handicapped learners would not be segregated and isolated in their daily activities while assuring them at the same time the special services needed so they could develop into useful and well-adjusted adult citizens.

Since 1953, educators have pressed efforts for meaningful integration of handicapped learners into the regular classroom and/or school situation. This is predicated on the belief that the regular education program should accommodate the needs of the handicapped in both academic and social ways, integrating "the whole adolescent." This concept of integration goes beyond the mere inclusion of handicapped adolescents with normal peers to require that such placements facilitate the total acceptance of these individuals into the classroom both socially and academically. The problems inherent in the realization of the latter are almost the same in the 1980s as they apparently were in 1953.

The revival of the term mainstreaming in the 1960s was not a return to the 50s but rather a realization that many of the ideals established in specialized educational services were not being realized.

The mainstreaming concept received major impetus from a 1968 article by Dunn titled, "Special Education for the Mildly Retarded—Is Much of It Justifiable?" Dunn brought to the surface placement practices for special education classrooms that at best were highly questionable. His basic contention was that special classes were becoming dumping grounds for socioculturally deprived children and youths. He felt that many of these persons were not mentally retarded but rather environmentally deprived, which caused them to function psychometrically in a manner analogous to individuals characterized by low IQ scores.

Dunn's article precipitated considerable discussion in the field of special education and resulted in numerous other articles that looked at placement processes as well as the possible retention of students in regular classroom settings. While the article often was misinterpreted and misunderstood, nevertheless it probably more than any single incident caused special educators to look at themselves, their programs, and the degree to which they were effectively serving handicapped students.

Although journalistic rhetoric caught the attention of special educators, more persuasive techniques were needed to convince many teachers and administrators of handicapped students' right to be educated in the mainstream. Initially it was necessary to resort to litigation to ensure this right. The following sections present (a) definitions of mainstreaming, (b) an overview of the legal basis for the mainstreaming of handicapped students, (c) moral and ethical basis, and (d) placement considerations.

DEFINITIONS

There are a number of definitions of the term mainstream in the literature. Individuals' points of view or positions often determine the definition they choose. For purposes of perspective, several are presented here, albeit they are by no means all-inclusive of the variety of definitions that exist.

A simplistic definition is that formulated by Birch (cited in Jordan, 1974) that refers to mainstreaming as the practice of placing exceptional children in regular classes and providing special educational services for them to function in those settings. A somewhat more comprehensive definition is that developed by Kauffman, Gottlieb, Agard, and Kukic (1975):

Mainstreaming refers to the temporal, instructional and social integration of eligible exceptional children with normal peers based on on-
going, individually determined, educational planning and programming
process and requires clarification of responsibility among regular and
special education administrative, instructive, and supportive personnel.
(pp. 40-41)

In 1976, the Council for Exceptional Children adopted the following definition
of mainstreaming:

Mainstreaming is a belief which involves an educational placement
procedure and process for exceptional children, based on the conviction
that each such child should be educated in the least restrictive environment in which his educational and related needs can be satisfactorily
provided. This concept recognizes that exceptional children have a wide
range of special education needs, varying greatly in intensity and duration; that there is a recognized continuum of educational settings which
may, at a given time, be appropriate for an individual child's needs; that
to the maximum extent appropriate, exceptional children should be
educated with nonexceptional children; and that special classes, separate
schooling, or other removal of an exceptional child from education with
nonexceptional children should occur only when the intensity of the
child's special education and related needs is such that it cannot be
satisfied in an environment including nonexceptional children, even
with the provision of supplementary aids and services. (Official Actions
of the Delegate Assembly of the 54th Annual Council for Exceptional
Children International Convention in Chicago, Illinois. *Exceptional
Children,* Vol. 43, p. 43, 1976.)

Wiederholt, Hammill, and Brown (1978) define mainstreaming as a "noncate-
gorical resource program . . . designed to meet the . . . needs of children with
mild or moderate learning and/or behavior problems" (p. 7). Castor (1975)
attempts to define mainstreaming by indicating what it is and what it is not.
According to Castor, mainstreaming is:

• Providing the most appropriate education for each child in the least
restrictive setting.
• Looking at the educational needs of children instead of clinical or
diagnostic labels such as mentally handicapped, learning disabled,
physically handicapped, hearing impaired or gifted.

- Looking for and creating alternatives that will help general educators serve children with learning or adjustment problems in a regular setting. Some approaches being used to help achieve this are consulting teachers, methods and materials specialists, itinerate teachers and resource room teachers.
- Uniting the skills of general education and special education so that all children may have equal educational opportunity. (p. 174)

According to Castor, mainstreaming is not:

- Wholesale return of all exceptional children in special classes to regular classes.
- Permitting children with special needs to remain in regular classrooms without support services that they need.
- Ignoring the need of some children for a more specialized program that can be provided in a general education program.
- Less costly than serving children in special self-contained classrooms. (p. 174)

Turnbull and Schulz (1979) declare that "mainstreaming is the educational arrangement of placing handicapped students in regular classes with their handicapped peers to the maximum extent appropriate" (p. 52). They, like Castor, attempt to clarify what mainstreaming is by saying what it is not. In so doing, they cite the following:

- Mainstreaming is not the wholesale elimination of special education self-contained classes. It does not mean that all handicapped students will be placed in regular classes. Further, it does not automatically imply that those handicapped students who are placed in regular classes will be in that setting for the entire day.
- Total mainstreaming is not an arrangement that can be accomplished overnight in a school system. Instant change often leads to threatening and unstable classroom environments.
- Mainstreaming is not just the physical presence of a handicapped student in the regular class.
- Mainstreaming does not mean that the placement of handicapped students in regular classes creates jeopardy for the academic progress of nonhandicapped students.
- Mainstreaming does not mean that the total responsibility for the education of handicapped students placed in regular classes will fall to the regular class teacher.

- Mainstreaming does not mean putting educators "out on a limb" and expecting them to accomplish tasks for which they are not prepared. (pp. 52-53)

These definitions are indicative of the problems in using the term. Views and opinions of what mainstreaming is are mixed and unclarified. Common to all of them, however, is the concept that placement in a regular classroom is a desired goal but may not be possible for all handicapped children. Further, they contend that no effort to mainstream should preclude the opportunity for the handicapped to obtain the services that will provide them with maximum benefit from the educational setting.

LEGAL BASIS

The basic constitutional premise that handicapped children and youths are entitled to the equal protection of the law and, therefore, may not be treated differently without due process of law, has been used successfully in recent years to guarantee their right to a free appropriate public education and to prevent their exclusion from its programs. Focusing on this constitutional assumption, a federal court in *Pennsylvania Association for Retarded Children (P.A.R.C.) v. Commonwealth of Pennsylvania,* 343 F. Supp. 279 (E.D. Pa. 1972), declared that Pennsylvania did indeed owe its retarded children and youths an appropriate program of education and training. According to Gilhool (1976), "If schooling is provided to children generally and, indeed, to most handicapped children, it must be provided to all handicapped children; hence, zero-reject education" (p. 12). Zero-reject means that there is very little reason why any and all children should not receive a free and appropriate public education.

Zero-reject and integration imperatives have their modern source in *Brown v. Board of Education,* which stated in 1954,

These days, it is doubtful that any child may reasonably be expected to succeed in life if he is denied the opportunity of an education. Such an opportunity, where the state has undertaken to provide it, is a right which must be made available to all on equal terms. (347 U.S. 483, 493)

As an aftermath of the Pennsylvania case, many right-to-education suits were initiated across the nation. Federal legislation ultimately was developed to ensure that the intent of these decisions was in fact realized. Thus, it was that Public Law 93-112, the Rehabilitation Act of 1973, included Section 504, which protected the handicapped from being excluded from participation in, the benefits of, or discrimination under any program or activity receiving federal assistance. Small wonder it is that P.L. 94-142, The Education for All Handicapped Children Act, was passed in 1975 and defined special education as "specially designed instruction, at no cost to parents or guardians, to meet the unique needs of a handicapped child, including classroom instruction, instruction in physical education, home instruction, and instruction in hospitals and institutions" (§ 4(a)(16)).

This definition focuses on instruction and a free and appropriate education in the least restrictive environment. The act also requires that individualized education programs (IEPs) be developed for handicapped students. There are those who argue that the least restrictive environment aspect of P.L. 94-142 is synonymous with mainstreaming. However, the terms are not interchangeable and, in the case of least restrictive environment, the focus is on the instructional setting for the student, whereas in mainstreaming the focus is on regular class placement with supportive services.

The individualized education specified in P.L. 94-142 has long been sought for handicapped students. Perhaps no other characteristic so precipitated the development of self-contained classrooms than the principle of the individualization of instruction. In the past, as today, regular education classrooms remain large in student-teacher ratio and are not able to cope with individualized instruction. Individualization, therefore, is necessary to meet the unique needs of the handicapped students who require specially designed instruction. According to Abeson and Weintraub (1977), P.L. 94-142 has four primary purposes:

1. To guarantee the availability of special education programming to handicapped children and youth who require it.
2. To assure fairness and appropriateness in decision-making about the provision of special education to handicapped children and youth.
3. To establish clear management in auditing requirements in procedures regarding special education at all levels of government.
4. To financially assist the efforts of state and local government through the use of federal funds. (p. 4)

The legal basis for placement of adolescents with learning and behavioral problems in a mainstream setting has now been made possible through the enactment of P.L. 94-142. However, merely because laws exist does not necessarily result in their intent becoming widespread and fully implemented. The intent of P.L. 94-142 must be the rule rather than the exception if handicapped students are to benefit from its existence.

MORAL AND ETHICAL BASIS

Sarason (1978) is most accurate when he states, "At its roots, mainstreaming is a moral issue" (p. 38). The basic issues and questions raised regarding the dilemma of segregation emerge again when arguments for mainstreaming are formulated. What right does a minority have in encroaching upon the rights of the majority? How does society define the rights of the majority as they relate to the basic rights and expectations of the minority in a given setting? As professionals view the educational setting, is it different from or the same as that of society in general?

Those who view education as a microcosm of society generally feel that without exposure to the minority, the majority never will be able to see life as it really is. Similarly, the fact that the handicapped must deal with nonhandicapped persons on a day-by-day basis in society also is life as it really is. The nonhandicapped need to learn what it is like to cope, compensate, and adapt.

Special educators as a group tend to characterize themselves as individuals interested in doing "good" things for people who generally have had very few good things happen to them. Therefore, this makes special educators feel good.

However, the issue is whether or not regular educators who must deal with the handicapped in the mainstream are as intent on being "good" as are special educators. This surfaces the issue of what is "good" and what is "not good." For example, some regular educators argue that they chose to teach normal students because they did not feel comfortable with individuals who had handicaps. This is not to suggest that the reason for their choice of regular as opposed to special education causes them to be "not good." Rather, it suggests teachers, like other individuals, have basic choices to make that they hope will be respected. The dilemma becomes one of whether or not an individual's right to choose to teach in a regular class setting includes an equal right to deny a handicapped student an opportunity to participate in it. What are the rights of teachers as opposed to the rights of the decision maker to force upon them groupings of students they neither wish, nor feel competent, to teach?

Ethically, a teacher teaches students regardless of who they are, whence they come, or whether they are black, handicapped, sweet, or mean. No teachers knowingly have been prepared to select out only the "choice" students and teach them, thereby having nothing to do with those who, in their estimation, might not be choice. Teacher training programs deal with the all-encompassing concept of the average, which includes all types of students.

But there are no ethical codes to apply to the behavior of teachers who do not wish to teach LBP adolescents with the same enthusiasm as they do youths who do not have similar problems. There are no ethical codes to impact on teachers who choose to reject students who are different. As a result, there have been few, if any, malpractice suits brought against teachers for failure to provide an appropriate education in their classrooms for LBP students. Given present constructs of ethical practice, there is every reason to believe that such cases will continue to surface infrequently.

The tragedy is that, in some cases, teachers who view their teaching as "good" are in fact probably performing in an unethical manner when it relates to the provision of adequate information for LBP adolescents. This is because they lack the skills to provide an appropriate education for such students.

In spite of these difficulties, and questions that must be raised concerning moral issues, there is general agreement among both regular and special educators alike that handicapped adolescents should be provided an education in as proximate a context as possible with their normal peer group. It is indeed unfortunate that it required congressional action to ensure for the handicapped the right to a free and appropriate education in the least restrictive environment. But Sarason (1978) provides a true appraisal of reality when he states:

> Rhetoric aside, mainstreaming challenges the very nature of our society and it would be foolhardy to face the future as if that challenge will not be met by efforts to blunt it. Society and its dominant institutions do not change quickly. (p. 37)

Schools tend to reflect the priorities of society. As those priorities change to give greater emphasis to handicapped individuals, schools' acceptance of LBP adolescents into regular education can be expected to grow. This transformation already is occurring as cities act to bevel curbs and widen doorways, to provide parking spaces for the disabled, and to seek input from persons with handicaps on decision-making boards and councils.

Laws often must delineate what the real moral issues are before society itself incorporates them as a matter of practice. The laws established on behalf of the handicapped have evolved from a combination of advocates. These have included persons with handicaps themselves, special educators and others in education concerned about improper placement practices and undue segregation of the handicapped from society as a whole, parents, and other supporters who have tried to place in proper perspective the rights of all persons.

PLACEMENT CONSIDERATIONS

The determination that an LBP adolescent is to be retained in, or returned to, a mainstream setting is a serious problem. The decision makers must consider not only the whole student but also the whole situation into which the adolescent will be placed. The following points were articulated by the National Education Association in 1977 as being essential for effective implementation of P.L. 94-142:

a. A favorable learning experience must be created both for handicapped and nonhandicapped students.

b. Regular and special education teachers and administrators must share equally in planning and implementation for the disabled.

c. All staff should be adequately prepared for their roles through inservice training and retraining.
d. All students should be adequately prepared for the program.
e. The appropriateness of educational methods, materials, and supportive services must be determined in cooperation with classroom teachers.
f. The classroom teacher(s) should have an appeal procedure regarding the implementation of the program, especially in terms of student placement.
g. Modifications should be made in class size, using a weighted formula, scheduling, and curriculum design to accommodate the demands of the program.
h. There must be a systematic evaluation and reporting of program developments using a plan which recognizes individual differences.
i. Adequate funding must be provided and then used exclusively for this program.
j. The classroom teacher(s) must have a major role in determining individual educational programs and should become members of school assessment teams.
k. Adequate released time must be made available for teachers so that they can carry out the increased demands upon them.
l. Staff reduction will not result from implementation of the program.
m. Additional benefits negotiated for handicapped students through local collective bargaining agreements must be honored.
n. Communication among all involved parties is essential to the success of the program. (p. 52)

The problem is that the list of essentials identified by the NEA has not been realized in practice. P.L. 94-142 has moved forward undaunted by the public schools' lack of readiness to effect its intent. As a result, one of the basic considerations rests with the students' IEPs as developed by the placement committee. That group must recognize its responsibility and the implications of its decision for the LBP adolescents who will not be functioning in a self-contained setting but in a highly departmentalized one with little planned individualization of instruction—a characteristic of most junior and senior high schools. The placement committee needs to know something about adolescence and adolescents before it embarks on IEP development. Adolescence, complicated with the additional problems of either learning or behavior problems, requires a decision that is unique and cognizant of psychophysical changes occurring in the youngsters.

Steps need to be taken, therefore, that ensure that the mainstream will be supportive, regardless of whether or not strict adherence to the IEP is realized. The most helpful steps to be taken relate to: (a) a reduction in class size, (b) teacher receptivity, (c) general education student receptivity, and (d) the structural (governance) aspects of the school and/or classrooms.

Class Size

There is a tremendous aura of contradiction between what is the intent of P.L. 94-142 and actual conditions in the public schools. The most obvious contradiction relates to the concept of individualization. A serious question can be raised about a practice that requires an individual student to be provided with an IEP when there is every likelihood that placement will be in a class of 25 or more. To expect individualization in such a situation is analogous to the eternal optimism expressed by educators that schools will become a higher priority in Washington than the military. Yet without smaller class sizes, the chances for mainstreaming to be effective are seriously reduced and, perhaps, truly constitute an effort in futility.

The research on class size is rather clear when that size is related to achievement. The work by Glass, Cahen, Smith, and Filby (1979) under the auspices of the Far West Laboratory for Educational Research and Development is indicative of the advantages of reduced class size. Glass et al. reviewed nearly 80 studies on the relationship between class size and pupil achievement. Their studies dated as far back as 1900 and involved more than 900,000 pupils. They describe the results of this review as follows:

> Imagine that a typical pupil in a typical class of 40 scores at the 50th percentile (i.e., the median) of an achievement test. The same pupil, taught in a group of 20, would have scored at the 55th percentile; in a group of 15, at the 58th percentile; in a group of 10, at the 65th percentile; and in a group of 5, at the 74th percentile. A pupil in a group of 40, then, would score 24 percentile ranks higher if taught in a group of 5 pupils.

> Our conclusion is that average pupil achievement increases as class size decreases. The typical achievement of pupils in instructional groups of 15 and fewer is several percentile ranks above that of pupils in classes of 25 and 30.

> We found, too, that for every pupil by which class size is reduced below 20, the class's average achievement improves substantially more for each pupil by which class size is reduced between 30 and 20. (p. 43)

The problem of class size in junior and senior high schools is well known and need not be elaborated upon further here. The evidence presented by Glass et al. is sufficiently conclusive in stating the problem clearly and in emphasizing class size as a consideration for placement in the mainstream. As noted previously, class size requirements should be addressed in the IEP and no student should be placed in a setting where individualization is clearly, at best, a remote possibility.

There are no gimmicks that can alter the benefits of a small teacher-pupil ratio. While paraprofessionals may help reduce the ill effects of a poor ratio, they are not the answer. In fact, the use of paraprofessionals to serve the mildly handicapped in regular classrooms has not met with a high degree of acceptance by administrators for reasons that may be obvious, such as lowered professional esteem by lay persons of educators. The major reason is cost. The same reason, incidentally, is given when the issue of reducing class size is presented to school administrators. If mainstreaming is to be realized, cost must be faced. After all, if the only hurdle to solving the class size dilemma is cost, then it simply becomes a matter of priority. Since P.L. 94-142 mandates placements in the least restrictive setting, it seems appropriate that regular education should seek to reduce class sizes. The ultimate result will be worthwhile to both the handicapped and the nonhandicapped.

Teacher Receptivity

Teachers in regular classrooms not only must be effective as educators but also must be positive in their view of the potential inherent in LBP students. Likewise, they must be cognizant of the difference between a learning problem and a behavior problem and be able to divorce these from the stereotyped concepts that teachers (and others) often have of adolescents. Many teachers are apprehensive about teaching in the junior and senior high schools. The result of the views of adolescence held by many teachers is that junior high and middle school positions frequently are the least sought and the last filled, even in times of teacher shortages. For students with behavior problems, this stereotype has major implications because they may not receive help for a problem that is unrelated to their being adolescents. In short, because all adolescents are viewed by some as problems, it often takes a great degree of nonconformity (beyond the perceived adolescent pattern) to be viewed as atypical.

Therefore, teacher receptivity must include both a desire to help adolescents and, more importantly, a desire to help LBP youths. This desire may have to be developed because many teachers choose not to teach the handicapped for both personal and professional reasons. This capability can be developed through inservice training, staff development, and selective employment over time.

Inservice education therefore should focus on expanding both the knowledge and skill base for every teacher who might balk at having an LBP student in the classroom because the practitioner feels deficient in either the knowledge or skills necessary to deal effectively with such an adolescent as a learner. Again, there are (it seems) an infinite variety of models for developing a viable inservice program. Since the advent of P.L. 94-142, inservice training for regular classroom teachers has been the rule, not the exception. However, the problem is that what is being transmitted is often information about due process and the development of IEPs. Little of a substantive nature is provided to teachers as to how to manage students who are acting out or how to assist those who may be having difficulties in perception. If the how-to were provided, the probability of the teacher's being confident enough to teach these students would be greatly enhanced. Add to such teachers a clear understanding of LBP learners as individuals and very likely they will feel almost as comfortable teaching those students as nonproblem ones.

Educators' receptivity goes far beyond the acceptance involved in the teacher-learner relationship. Receptivity also means that teachers will be supportive of the various programming alternatives, whether their role is as crisis resource educators or as teacher consultants. No matter how good teachers are (skill) or how accepting (attitude), they are likely to need varying degrees of support to accommodate the LBP students.

Inability to effectively interact with and benefit from assistance from external sources can result in even greater difficulties from a long-term viewpoint.

A final word: where compulsory assignments are made and teachers' objections are relegated to second or third priority, the placement of LBP adolescents is totally without justification. Every effort must be made to ensure that the psychological climate in the classroom for LBP students is as positive as it can possibly be. The likelihood of such a climate's existing without the personal support of the teacher is not high. Therefore, the school system and all parties involved in a placement decision must make every effort to determine whether the teachers with whom the students will be placed are receptive to having LBP adolescents assigned to their instructional care. Mainstreaming, as has been implied throughout this chapter, is highly contingent upon a strong, positive interpersonal climate in the classroom—and that must include both students and teacher.

Student Receptivity

Students, like teachers, have feelings, attitudes, biases, and prejudices. Like adults, many have developed strong points of view regarding individuals with handicaps. They often apply such verbal descriptives as "dummy," "retard," "crazy," etc., based on their assessment of a fellow student's performance or behavior. While the sources of these points of view vary considerably, nonetheless they do exist and have a dramatic impact on LBP students' acceptance of themselves as well as great implications for the development of their ultimate self-concept.

Because LBP adolescents spend much of their time with normal peers, it is imperative that the latter be receptive and supportively tolerant of them and their problems. The peers must interact and communicate with the handicapped students in a manner that does not accent their weaknesses nor suggest that they are being accepted on any basis other than for their own personal worth. If nonhandicapped students' acceptance of a LBP one is negative, the psychological climate of the classroom becomes extremely repressive. This is perhaps the single most crucial aspect of the instructional environment and requires that utmost concern be given to it in determining or implementing placement decisions. Yet in far too many decisions, it is given little, if any, emphasis.

Just as an assessment of the teacher's receptivity to the learning and/or behavior problems is needed, so too must an evaluation be made of nonhandicapped students' reactions. Once an assessment has been conducted, a systematic plan to build awareness, knowledge, understanding, tolerance, and acceptance needs to be implemented. Such plans preferably should be directed through teachers to ensure that they can be continuously reinforced and monitored. The teachers can use the process of communicating a better understanding of the disabled to nonhandicapped students as a system to also reinforce their own knowledge and information base regarding these LBPs. In fact, the inservice instruction provided to teachers would be appropriate, with minor adaptations and modifications, to disseminate to nonhandicapped students.

For LBP adolescents, the value of peer receptivity cannot be understated. All students, as indicated, need to be accepted, involved, and feel wanted. It is important that students who have not been exposed to or acquainted with handicapped individuals have an opportunity to acquire accurate information and knowledge regarding those with LBPs. Essentially, this information may be provided through the teacher's instruction, through independent readings, and/or through adolescents who have had occasion to interact with those with handicaps.

The major principle to understand is that the nonhandicapped peer's acceptance of an LBP student must be an objective one and not one of a superficial nature. Acceptance must not occur simply because the teacher says it is "the right thing to do." There must be a genuine feeling of acceptance if the LBP students are truly to appreciate and benefit from interpersonal relationships with peer groups. LBP students ask for no special favors and just want to be accepted for what they are and what they can be when they are part of the total group. Unless the LBP adolescents can truly become a part of the total group, the advantage of mainstreaming for them is very nebulous indeed.

Programmatically, normal peer acceptance of LBP students may be achieved if teachers:

1. Utilize normal students to the maximum in the development of informational concepts relative to understanding the handicapped.
2. Infuse into classes, where appropriate, elements relating to differences.
3. Use peer models who may be identified in the school as having positive attitudes toward persons with handicaps.

4. Use handicapped students, whenever and wherever possible, to communicate their personal feelings and concerns about being a part of the total school and its activities.

In summary, the following are some possible advantages of effective mainstreaming placement for LBP adolescents:

1. They have the opportunity to participate with their peer group, socially and academically.
2. They are provided an opportunity for self-analysis of their own strengths and weaknesses in competition with normal peers.
3. They may escape the labeling process.
4. Their interaction with normal youngsters will increase the motivation to learn.
5. They can become more self-sufficient, self-assured, and self-confident as a result of placement in a normalized setting.
6. Their opportunity to be maximally involved in the neighborhood will be increased as a result of interacting with peers in the regular classroom.
7. They can be expected, if placed in the mainstream, to be better able to adjust and cope with society upon termination of their formal schooling.
8. They provide, if placed in the mainstream, a comparison point for the understanding of individual differences by their normal peer groups.
9. Their parents are more receptive to such a placement because they understand better the nature of the regular curriculum and therefore the teaching the LBP students are receiving.

Just as there are advantages to placement of LBP adolescents in the mainstream, there also are disadvantages:

1. Regular classroom teachers may not accept the additional responsibility imposed by LBP students.
2. Large class sizes may reduce the opportunity for the LBP students to receive the advantage of individualized instruction.
3. Curricular content (and adaptive methodologies for such content) often is not appropriate to meet the learning needs of the handicapped.
4. Support services for technical assistance and supplementation of the classroom teacher's effort often are in short supply.
5. Normal students may assign labels to the students that are damaging to their self-concept and inhibit the development of a positive ego.
6. Parents may develop unrealistic aspirations for their students because of their concept of regular education.

7. The school may overtly resist removing the LBP students from the regular class if that is indeed perceived to be the most optimum placement.

Another important variable in successful mainstreaming of LBP adolescents is the structural aspects of schools and classrooms. These are presented next.

STRUCTURAL ASPECTS

Schools, like communities, often have their own unique personalities. After all, schools, like communities, are composed of different types of people who have different goals, desires, likes, and dislikes. When lumped together, these unique types of characteristics compose a climate that permeates the total school situation. The school also can take on a structural climate that is determined largely by the authority figures responsible for its operation. The structure that a given school may operate under and impose upon its students is quite obvious upon stepping into a school building.

For example, some schools are highly discipline oriented, others are highly nonstructured and facilitate maximum student progressiveness, and still others combine those two extremes. The process of mainstreaming may be realized differently in each of these settings and the prospects for its success likewise are contingent upon the structural (governance) aspects of the school and/or classroom. Essentially, these structural aspects represent one of three types: (1) laissez faire (permissive), (2) democratic, and (3) autocratic.

The Laissez Faire (Permissive) School and Class

The laissez-faire structure is open and progressive in nature. The dominant aspect is that all students play major roles in determining the structure as well as being responsible for ensuring that the structure has meaning for them. The authority figures in such a school and/or classroom situation serve primarily as catalysts who guide the students in their functioning within the bounds of the permissiveness inherent in organization. The degree of directiveness is miniscule. Maynard (1978) classifies this school or classroom as a "school climate model" that essentially results in student ownership. Such a school, according to Maynard, emphasizes the following:

- Educational quality and individual self-worth;
- trust;
- open and honest communication;
- shared leadership;

- heightened involvement of staff and students;
- acquisition of skills to accomplish the above. (p. 359)

The laissez-faire school also may be characterized as one that has very few disruptions among students. There are many reasons for this, but foremost among them is the fact that it is a learning environment where students and teachers have a stake in the school itself and in its curriculum. As a result, when students seek to disrupt the school, they are reacting to a situation they helped develop. In short, they place themselves in a conflict, not with the school but with themselves.

Much of the research on the concept of the open school and other similar alternative constructs seems to indicate that where students have an involvement in decision making, there is a positive effect on discipline problems, reducing their occurrence. Thus, for many students with behavioral problems this type of structure also has a beneficial effect.

A further supportive element is the wide array of programs from which the students can select those they perceive as most interesting and most important. While not every course is amenable to self-selection, nevertheless, every effort is made to provide a variety of options. For students with behavior problems, this eclecticism is most beneficial because it affords them an opportunity to develop their own curricula and thereby implement the structure within which they personally must accomplish certain educational goals. It is interesting that students usually select courses very analogous to those they would have been assigned had there been a mandatory type of scheduling.

Finally, the laissez-faire school should not be viewed as an institution where "anything goes." Controls are built into such a school or classroom setting; however, the major control point is focused within, not outside, the students. The laissez-faire school does take a particular type of teacher to function within it and an administrator willing to support it with the great flexibility it needs and provides. For persons who need a high degree of structure and organization, the laissez-faire school is not the place. For those who function best without a great deal of overt direction and/or external interference, the opportunity for maximizing individual freedom of choice and action is most gratifying and rewarding. The fluency of such a situation should be maximally supportive of the mainstream construct with regard to placement of adolescents with learning and behavior problems.

The Democratic School and Class

The democratic school or classroom provides freedom in a context of some specific parameters of organization. Options may be provided to the students, but these must be implemented within the constraints of prescribed rules and regulations that are established both to ensure a sense of order and to protect the rights of the majority from being infringed upon or violated by the so-called minority students in a given class or structure.

For example, adolescents with learning handicaps in a democratic setting generally will receive teacher help to the extent that they do not take time or resources from those who do not have such problems. The practitioner in this setting teaches to the majority in the class. Therefore, if the majority is able to read on a ninth grade level, then that is where the level of instruction will be focused. For those who cannot read at that level, the material must be provided on an individual basis or some special kind of grouping if they are to receive the same content at a level they can understand. Unlike the laissez-faire classroom or school where the students can seek a level at which they are most comfortable, in the democratic setting the level provided is the one at which most adolescents can function. As a result, most decisions involving a democratic setting are on a group basis, albeit each student may tend to have a reasonable expectation of providing input.

Many educators feel strongly that the type of program and curriculum offered in a democratic setting is the most appropriate because it acclimates students to the so-called real world. In the real world, the majority rules. This observation, say those who support the democratic type of classroom, needs to be made clear. This provides a degree of realism that is important, and it matters not whether the students are handicapped; they will have to interact in a world founded on democratic principles. Handicapped adolescents in a classroom or school are in the same minority role they will occupy in the community at large. Therefore, they must learn to synthesize the rights and privileges of their minority in relation to those exercised by the majority.

Placement of the handicapped in a democratic setting by no means limits them from having certain options or making certain choices. However, those choices and options generally reflect those of the majority of the students in a classroom or school. Thus, it is important that the classroom teacher be provided an opportunity, to the maximum extent possible, to individualize instruction to ensure that the needs of the minority learners are accommodated. If the teacher provides a truly democratic setting, the LBP adolescents will be given as much recognition and opportunity to realize their potential as will students in the majority.

For LBP adolescents, the democratic classroom has both advantages and disadvantages. The advantages are that the parameters of expected performance are fairly clear and the curriculum is that of the majority. It is not a watered-down or reduced curriculum made appropriate because the students purportedly cannot learn or meet the required standards. Therefore, handicapped students are getting what every youth is getting.

The disadvantages are that such a classroom or school emphasizes the majority and therefore denies equal opportunity for the handicapped to acquire the same content at the same degree of understanding. Options available to the LBP students often are constrained by the choices of the majority. The teacher, as a result, must ensure that the integrity of the choice or option selected by the handicapped has a reasonable expectation of being realized.

Most of today's classrooms may be classified as democratic in nature. Their curriculum is that of the majority learners. For example, ninth graders are expected to be learning specific content in a given class so the teacher teaches to that material.

Many schools seek to minimize the likelihood that minority learners will be penalized by their placement with the nonhandicapped through grouping or tracking based on ability levels. Using such an approach, the ninth graders with the lowest ability in math will be grouped with others having similar problems, and those with the greatest abilities will be grouped together. While grouping may be compensatory in nature, it does violate the principle by which the democratic classroom and/or school is founded. That principle is that each student should function in context with every other student regardless of ability and that the curriculum will be focused at the ability level of the majority. Whether a school uses grouping or the democratic classroom in its purest sense, there are advantages and disadvantages for learners with handicaps.

In a pure democratic classroom, handicapped adolescents are kept in context with the types of individuals with whom they will have to interact throughout the remainder of their lives. The heterogeneous nature of the classroom is the way the real world actually is. The handicapped can be assured of receiving in some form the same basic content as that of the nonhandicapped.

However, there are disadvantages that perhaps constitute the major obstacle to implementation of the mainstream construct. As noted, most practitioners teach to a majority, with obvious disadvantages for handicapped learners. The possibilities of differentiating content into the appropriate levels for the two types of students are extremely minute. Since the teacher focuses on meeting the needs of the majority, the minority cannot receive the same type of attention.

Thus, the factor of class size becomes highly important in a situation predicated on the democratic construct because the only way adolescents with learning or behavior problems can receive an equivalent amount of subject content is to have the teacher provide sufficient time.

The concept of the democratic ideal is noble and is the one to which most educators and others subscribe without serious question. However, in the context of an instructional setting or school organization, the emphasis on the needs of the majority does create serious problems for individuals with LBPs. Just as the rights of the minorities in society at large must be protected, so too must those of minority learners in the regular classroom or school. This requires individualization, access to instruction, opportunity for input, and ability accommodation.

The democratic classroom has the potential to meet each of these requirements only if maximum attention is given to the needs of the handicapped. Equality of instruction, however, does not just happen; it requires careful and conscientious planning even in the so-called democratic school and classroom.

The Autocratic School and Class

Contrary to what many educators would like to believe, some schools and classrooms operate on a very autocratic basis. In such situations, the absolute dictates of the teacher and/or authority figure constitute what is good for all children to learn. The opportunities for adolescents' freedom of expression and selection of curricular offerings are minimal at best. This applies regardless of whether the students are handicapped or nonhandicapped.

Some individuals state that adolescents with behavioral disorders need such an autocratic environment because it eliminates the necessity for them to make choices and provides a high degree of the structure they so greatly need. There is no evidence to prove or disprove this theory, but many of those who are knowledgeable regarding the education of youths with behavior problems would argue against it. For example, Hewett (1974) in discussing structure states:

> Here we are at the core of a basic issue in special education. Am I really talking about a teacher who is behavior-oriented fully—who is bigger, more powerful, and authoritarian than the child and given to using manipulation and control for their own sake? I am not. Somewhere in the often foolish debate among the behaviorists, the humanists, the psycho-educationists, and the psychodynamicists, the point has been lost that trust and belief in human goodness are far more the issues than professional identity or theoretical affiliation. (p. 120)

The school or classroom operated by a first sergeant is not conducive to the development of controls in the individual. Individuals in such a setting perform in a manner analogous to the game of table tennis, bouncing back and forth from one limit to another without ever really understanding why they exist in the first place. Many traditionalists feel that the key to effective learning is maximal structure accented with strict discipline. This Three Rs with a hickory stick approach has been winning greater and greater advocacy in this country. As the public looks at achievement scores on competency tests, there is increasing alarm that the schools are failing.

There are those who would argue that education has become too permissive and is controlled by students and their parents, rather than by educators. They contend that quality will reappear with the return to a traditional school pattern that emphasizes structure and discipline. Whether or not such a return is truly realized as the educational pendulum swings remains to be seen. Further, programs for disruptive youths comprise about a third of existing alternative programs in the United States (Arnove & Strout, 1980). This suggests that the conventional school, whether democratic or autocratic, affords LBP students the kind of environment conducive to improving their conduct from the standpoint of learning and of behavior.

When the autocratic school is analyzed from the viewpoint of whether or not mainstreaming of LBP adolescents would be successful in such a setting, a different conclusion might be reached. Given the likelihood that a directive would be carried out with precision and efficiency, it is very plausible to assume that the autocratic school would best facilitate the implementation of the mainstreaming approach. Directives can be given to principles and teachers and will be carried out without question and/or second-guessing. Students can be placed or maintained in such settings quite easily. Therefore, from an administrative viewpoint, the autocratic school has distinct advantages for the implementation of main-streaming.

The point that must be made is not what is efficient administratively. From the onset of the movement to mainstream the handicapped, the intent has been to provide an environment that maximizes the opportunity for such persons to truly function as individuals and to interact with the nonhandicapped. The emphasis then must be on the interpersonal relationships between the handicapped students and their teachers, as well as peers who may or may not be disabled.

Administrative expediency has little correlation with classroom climate. It is the latter that is basic to the realization of the underlying concept of mainstreaming. Without an appropriate and adequate supporting climate, both instructionally and psychologically, handicapped students can gain little from mainstream placement. Thus, the autocratic classroom whose primary advantage is administrative has as its major disadvantage the fact that it often is impersonal in application. As a structure for placement of adolescent children with learning and behavioral problems, the autocratic school or classroom has little to offer. Yet there is every reason to believe that such structures probably have been used to meet the dictates of P.L. 94-142 more than any other model. Educators are hoping that the evolving pattern of looking at students on an individual basis in an instructional setting that emphasizes the value and uniqueness of each one will lead to more, not fewer, alternative school patterns.

The preceding points dealt with elements to consider when making mainstream placements of adolescents with learning and behavioral problems. A multitude of other kinds of considerations might be reviewed, but basically those cited are considered by the author to be most significant. Of those discussed, the necessity for teacher and student receptivity is of maximum importance. For the handicapped to benefit from any mainstream placement they must have acceptance by the teacher and student peers.

Young (1976) summarizes the steps taken by Philadelphia to accomplish mainstreaming. These are worthy of note here because they underscore the necessity for careful and conscientious consideration in mainstream implementation and the ultimate placements that follow it. The following is a synthesis of the principles and processes used to accomplish mainstreaming for the educable mentally retarded in the Philadelphia public school system:

1. Broad-based educational activities directed toward the interpretation of the concept of mainstreaming and the rationale for its adoption as a strategy to provide appropriate education for pupils should be initiated.
2. Technical assistance and consultive help from professional sources such as universities and state education agencies should be obtained.
3. Staff development for all teachers in a building expected to instruct exceptional pupils in their classrooms should be planned and started.
4. Cooperative relationships with collective bargaining units, where they exist, should be developed.
5. Models for implementing mainstreaming at the local level should be built in accordance with the unique service needs of a particular school.
6. Parents should be maximally involved and given ample opportunity to have provided an interpretation as well as the rationale for mainstreaming.
7. Students should be encouraged to participate in the development of models for local schools.
8. Effective models should be replicated throughout the school system based on interest and action rather than on imposition of a total systemwide plan for mainstreaming.
9. Efforts must be made to build community understanding of the goals, concept, and implementation of mainstreaming.
10. Adequate physical support must be provided to ensure successful implementation.

This program is indicative of the kind of concern that must be present when considering placement decisions. The uniqueness of each school is emphasized in relation to the type of model a given school will select for implementation. Implementation of the mainstreaming concept and ensuing placement considerations are closely intertwined. Even if careful steps are taken to implement mainstreaming, there will be no assurance of its success without serious consideration of placement decisions.

Whether or not the mainstream becomes an advantageous or disadvantageous placement is determined by the extent to which those involved work together to make it happen. The following section describes the necessary interaction of key figures in a successful mainstream scenario.

ROLE INTERACTIONS

The educational scenario for LBP adolescents in a mainstream setting has a cast of three types of actors, all of whom must interact and interrelate effectively if the student is to realize maximum benefits: parents, teachers, and administrators. Each of these has a major role to play. If any one of these roles is not fulfilled to the maximum, the students very likely will suffer the consequences. Therefore, it is essential that these roles and the nature of their interaction be reviewed to fully understand their impact on mainstreaming LBP adolescents.

The Parents' Role

There is little argument that those most responsible for what students are and become are the parents. No other individuals spend as much time with the adolescents, either directly or indirectly, than do the parents. However, the extent of the interaction and time expenditure decreases as students proceed through the educational years. Such a decrease is noticeable by only a cursory review of the attendance at parent-teacher association meetings in the elementary school as opposed to reduced participation in sessions at the high school level.

This is not to imply that the parents think any less of their youngsters once they become adolescents. However, parents' interest or participation on an active basis in their youngsters' educational program does decline. This continues in spite of the fact that P.L. 94-142 guarantees parents maximum opportunities to participate in the planning of their adolescents' schooling. In addition to due process safeguards, P.L. 94-142 entitles parents to receive:

1. prior notice of any special educational diagnosis being or planned to be performed
2. prior notice before any change in the students' program can be made
3. full access to school records related to their adolescents' classroom situation
4. designation of a "surrogate parent" on behalf of students who are wards of the state or who are not residing with parents or do not have them available

The impetus of P.L. 94-142 has brought to a more meaningful level than ever before the role parents should and must play in the formulation of their adolescent's educational program. This role, which involves them in the planning process, changes considerably the previous perceptions of the teacher-parent interaction. The old concept of in loco parentis for the teacher no longer has the strength it once had. Parents now have the right (and more and more are exercising it) to become involved in and knowledgeable about what teachers are or are not doing for their teenagers.

The parents' role has to be more than as a mere advocate for their youngsters. They have an obligation to become familiar with the purposes of education and especially what the concept of mainstreaming means. Many parents believe that placement of their adolescents into the mainstream means the students will have to be able to measure up to the regular classroom's expectation and to whatever goals and objectives have been established for the nonhandicapped.

Given such a feeling, it is understandable why some parents may be apprehensive, especially if the students are being moved into the mainstream from a special education setting. There are parents who still remember what mainstreaming did not do for their teenagers when they were in it previously. Therefore, they do not want their youngsters to undergo a similar experience if the ultimate result is going to be a failure. Parents also must understand that placement of their youngsters in regular classes does not mean that LBP students will achieve at the same level or meet the same objectives as the nonhandicapped. The aspirations for the adolescents still must be kept in focus with regard to their abilities.

Once parents have achieved an understanding of the role of the school and better understand what mainstreaming means, they are in a position to play a responsible role in their youngsters' education. Acting responsibly requires parents to accomplish the following:

1. maintain close contact with the adolescents' teachers
2. maintain close contact with the school administrators
3. seek to monitor the adolescents' progress in school and relate it to their progress outside the formal school structure
4. become knowledgeable regarding the students' curriculum and its implications for the adolescents' ultimate success as adults upon completion of school
5. become knowledgeable about the total school, including extracurricular programs, whether or not the youngsters are participating in them or receiving services from support programs such as guidance and vocational education
6. maintain contacts with other parents of LBP adolescents in similar programs
7. always ask when in doubt

To reiterate, the parents' role is an important one and thanks to P.L. 94-142 is an integral part of any decision-making process that involves their youngsters. The role is not made any easier by virtue of the act nor is the pressure any less on the parents. But teachers and school administrators no longer can avoid involving parents in the decision-making process and, as a result, must seek to establish clearer and more effective interaction. The ultimate beneficiary of this interaction will be the adolescents.

The Teacher's Role

Much attention has been devoted to teachers and their role in implementing mainstreaming of the LBP adolescents. This discussion turns to the teacher's role as it relates to the parents and to the school administration. In the interactive triad of school-teacher-parent, it is imperative that the teacher work to maintain clear channels of communication with both the parents and the administrator. It also is the teacher's responsibility to continuously inform the administrator as to how well mainstreaming actually is working for the LBP adolescents.

To be most effective in their work with parents, teachers should:

1. schedule frequent parent-teacher conferences and orient parents to providing a positive rather than a negative view of the students' progress
2. pay home visits as often as possible to the parents and the adolescents
3. help parents to understand the concept of mainstreaming and how they may become active in its implementation
4. work to involve parents in conferences and other contacts with the home
5. involve the parents whenever decisions are made that may affect the teenagers' retention in the mainstream
6. communicate with the parents in a manner (whether written or oral) that is understandable, factual, nonemotional, jargon-less, and free of personal viewpoints
7. be prepared to deal with questions from parents of nonhandicapped students
8. acquaint the parents with the total school

Dealing with parents of LBP adolescents never has been easy for classroom teachers. Historically, teachers have been ill prepared to deal with parents, who in turn have been reluctant to become involved with the program once their child reaches adolescence. This caused junior high and senior high teachers to be even more unfamiliar with teenagers' parents.

With the advent of mainstreaming and the due process safeguards of P.L. 94-142, the situation has changed. More and more, teachers now must be able to communicate to parents why the mainstreamed LBP adolescents are or are not performing up to their expectations. Dealing with any parents is likely to be difficult for most teachers. The prospect of handling those of LBP students for a teacher whose primary training has been with nonhandicapped adolescents makes the situation even more difficult and somewhat fear-inducing. What is needed, therefore, is for the teacher to obtain background and practice in dealing with parents. The use of techniques such as those of social workers and counselors can be valuable; however, to be most effective, the teacher will need to rely on the two most important ingredients of any effective interaction—trust and honesty.

Administrator's Role

The principal is accountable to the community for what does or does not occur in a school and the superintendent for the total school system. This accountability is a. tremendous burden, but it is an essential part of the role that any good administrator must handle competently and effectively. Mainstreaming, for many administrators, emerged without the preparation and the resources to implement it adequately. Unquestionably, there still are administrators who actively oppose further implementation of the concept except as it may produce an economic advantage. It is to be hoped that there are but a few of these administrators because there is no question that mainstreaming will not be successful without the full support of those in charge of it. Just as teachers must be positive toward mainstreaming and the desirability of placing LBP adolescents in regular junior or senior high classrooms, so too must the school principal and other administrators be supportive of such a decision. As a result, the administrator must be highly positive and supportive.

Reynolds and Birch (1977) have developed a set of contrasts between prevailing and preferred practices in educational planning and parental involvement. These contrasts are presented here to clarify the role of the administrator in relation to interaction with parents and the facilitation of mainstreaming:

Prevailing Practices

1. Planning for individual pupils is informal and nondocumented in terms of specific objectives and processes.
2. Educational plans are made strictly by professionals.
3. Responsibilities for implementing educational plans are relatively unspecified.
4. Disagreements about educational plans or placements are essentially decided locally by professionals—with no "formal" hearings.
5. Children are examined by psychologists and other specialists by referral from teachers and principals.
6. School records are not reviewable by parents of children.
7. Most parent conferences are arranged by special education teachers and supervisors, social workers, or psychologists.

Preferred Practices

1. Individualized educational programs are drawn up recurrently and specifically for each child, listing specific objectives and procedures.
2. Educational plans are negotiated by professionals with students and parents.

3. Responsibilities for delivery on individualized educational programs are clearly specified.
4. All parties to educational plans per child have a right to impartial hearings and appeals, if necessary, in case of disagreements.
5. Children in their school situations are assessed only on concurrence of school officials and parents.
6. School records of children are fully open to review by parents.
7. Most parent conferences with exceptional children are arranged to include regular teachers as primary participants. (p. 189)

Administrators would do well to use these preferred practices. In conjunction with the active support of classroom teachers in their efforts to provide instructional programs appropriate for LBP adolescents, these factors will ensure that the interactive school-teacher-parent triad is a meaningful one.

TRENDS AND ISSUES

It always is difficult to judge what is a trend and what is an issue. More often than not, the issue of today will become the trend of tomorrow. The whole concept of mainstreaming was an issue in the early 70s but has become a trend accommodated by the "least restrictive placement" construct of P.L. 94-142. Therefore, the following trends and issues are predicated on the events of today (the early 1980s) but at best must be viewed as speculative. Educational processes and procedures, philosophies, and structures, all of which are subject to frequent change, will influence what occurs at the junior and senior high school level in relation to programming for LBP adolescents.

The implications of the movement toward competency testing, the desire to return to basics, and the revitalization of the traditional school are unclear. Undoubtedly, these events and/or trends will have some impact on the educational programming for handicapped adolescents placed in the mainstream.

With full awareness of the evolving events and of the past, which has observed the concept of mainstreaming range from a focal point in 1953, only to be largely forgotten in the 60s, but remembered again in the 70s, the trends and issues below are suggested for the 80s.

Trends

1. Regular education at all levels will become more like than unlike special education in its programming, orientation, and instruction.

2. The development of programming at the secondary levels for LBP adolescents' problems will continue to expand in both quality and quantity.
3. The expansion of support services at the secondary level to facilitate the "least restrictive placement" intent of P.L. 94-142 will continue.
4. The term "special needs" will be broadened to include both those who experience difficulty in learning as well as the mildly handicapped who manifest learning and behavior problems.
5. Greater attention will be given to the "how-to" aspect of inservice training of teachers of secondary school LBP adolescents.
6. All teachers and related personnel prepared for service at the secondary level of education will be provided concentrations in the effective instruction of LBP adolescents. The one-course approach will disappear in favor of an 18- to 24-credit hour block of intensive course concentration emphasizing instruction.
7. A greater research effort will be focused on the education of the adolescent handicapped in contrast to the present emphasis on early preschool and childhood.
8. The term "mainstreaming" will disappear from use as it moves from its trend status into accommodation under the construct of P.L. 94-142.

Issue(s)/Questions To Be Resolved

1. What determinants are operative in relation to the types of behavioral problems that can be accommodated in the regular classroom at the secondary level?
2. What constitutes a reasonable class size for a teacher at the secondary level who has instructional responsibility for one or more LBP adolescents?
3. Are nonhandicapped adolescents penalized (from an academic viewpoint) when LBP students are placed in regular classrooms? And is the degree to which the content is reduced in scope or intensity analogous to a "regression toward the mean" phenomenon?
4. Will adequate funding accompany programmatic efforts to better serve the handicapped adolescents or will it be business as usual—stretching existing resources to cover the additional costs?

These trends and issues (questions) are based on an analysis of the state of the art as of mid-1982. The trends do point the way, if they are accurate, to a much better future for all students, handicapped or not, adolescent or not. But trends become realities only when educators, and those who impact upon them, determine the new elements to be worthy of incorporation. Progress has been made toward each of those discussed; only time and the decision makers will determine whether their evolution continues. The prospects, however, are better now than ever.

SUMMARY

The moral and ethical basis for the mainstreaming of handicapped adolescents continues to lack clarity. There are those who continue to argue that the inclusion of the handicapped in the mainstream does indeed reduce the quality of education for the nonhandicapped. Some in this group assert emphatically that the real disadvantaged youths in today's educational setting are the ones referred to as average. The advantaged ones, these individuals contend, are those who are different and for whose benefit the bulk of the school's supportive services are deployed.

Whether or not these voices are correct is not the issue. The real issue remains that it is morally right to provide each student with the most appropriate education possible in the least restrictive setting for that individual. The laws are clear; now, the process of moral adjustment and infusion of solid ethical practice must follow. Provisions for adequate programs need not be contingent upon the ultimate realization of the adjustment and infusion process; however, it is unlikely that the desired goal envisioned by the advocates of mainstreaming ever will be realized until the moral and ethical issues are better resolved than they are at present.

The implications of mainstreaming for regular education are huge. Regular classroom teachers, administrators, and even school boards have become accustomed to dealing with LBP adolescents through a process of external placement. The practice of returning more and more of these youths to a regular classroom, along with its attendant problems, causes these students both chagrin and uneasiness.

All kinds of arguments can be formulated as to why mainstreaming should not occur. These arguments can be formulated by both regular and special educators with equal sincerity. Like the efficacy studies regarding special classes for the mentally retarded, research on mainstreaming has produced results that are both pro and con. It is important that the concept of mainstreaming be reviewed and its advantages and disadvantages listed so that educators can make choices as to whether or not retention or placement of LBP youths in the regular classroom is appropriate or inappropriate.

Thanks to P.L. 94-142, programming for adolescents at the secondary level finally has been given a priority, but as this chapter has tried to make clear, the realization of this priority will not be automatic. Much remains to be accomplished. Teachers must be better prepared, curricula must be adaptive and accommodative, support services must be provided, and the total junior and senior high school structure must become sensitive to the needs of LBP adolescents. Mainstreaming provides the conceptual base for this effort; only educators—special and regular—can make the concept a reality in practice.

Chapter 12

Parallel Alternative Curriculum for LBP Adolescents

L. Kay Hartwell, Douglas E. Wiseman, and Anthony Van Reusen

INTRODUCTION

Professionals involved in the education of adolescents with learning and behavioral problems are mandated by law to plan and provide appropriate instructional programs. While some attempt has been made to provide alternate programming for low achievers at the elementary level, little attention has been directed toward this problem at the secondary level (Cullinan & Epstein, 1979; Kronick, 1975; Marsh, Gearheart, & Gearheart, 1978; McDaniels, 1971; Panushka, 1971; Scranton & Downs, 1975).

Professionals have recognized that many programs for secondary age students with learning and behavior problems do meet the mandate of the law. However, these programs have been found lacking in consistency of identification, limited inservice alternatives, and a need for increased understanding between special and regular educators (McNutt & Heller, 1978). In addition, there are untold numbers of gifted and nonhandicapped students who are failing to succeed in the regular classroom or are not being accommodated to meet their fullest potential (Dunn, 1973). Many of these nonachievers share the common denominator of the discrepancy between the demands of the school and their ability to respond or achieve at the levels dictated by the school and the community (Wiseman, 1971).

One attempt to meet the challenge of this discrepancy at the secondary school level is the Parallel Alternate Curriculum (PAC) presented in this chapter. This chapter discusses the development of a parallel alternate curriculum approach to meet the instructional needs of teachers and the learning needs of low-achieving students at the secondary school level. In addition, the rationale for providing a parallel alternate curriculum, historical and current trends in providing alternative programs, and a detailed outline of the Arizona Child Service Demonstration Center (CSDC) Parallel Alternate Curriculum are analyzed. This center serves LBP adolescents and low-achieving high school students.

RATIONALE FOR A PAC

Problems of Low Achievement

Considerable interest and concern have developed since the mid-1970s over adolescents who are having problems of achievement in the secondary schools (Bailey, 1975; Deshler, 1978; Lerner, 1976; Mann, Goodman, & Wiederholt, 1978; Wiseman & Hartwell, 1978). There are several reasons for this concern:

1. Students identified and served in the elementary schools have progressed through programs without substantial change in their learning and behavior problems.
2. Adequate programs for adolescents with severe problems have not been available on a widescale basis.
3. The reading level of the adult population is low. Ruddell (1974) estimates that 40 percent of the adult population reads at or below the sixth grade level and 15 percent below fourth grade.
4. National standardized tests on achievement in basic skills areas have shown a decline in overall school achievement.
5. Statistics increasingly correlate problems of achievement and the incarceration of juvenile offenders.
6. There has been a trend toward increased years in school.

Other reports on students of secondary school age attribute their underachievement to a lack of motivation, poor teaching, low reading levels, and a lack of alternatives for learning content through means other than reading (Hartwell, Wiseman, Krus, & Van Reusen, 1979; Martin, 1976). Solutions being proposed to improve generally low school performance usually ignore the special needs and qualities of adolescents with learning and behavior problems. Many of the popularly identified problems have a direct influence on the achievement, or lack of it, of this population.

For example, some administrators, teachers, and supportive faculty are not trained to make educated decisions about the low-achieving youths for whom they are responsible. Textbooks used in many regular courses have a difficulty or readability level far in excess of the intended grade level population. Students with poor achievement, therefore, suffer from inappropriate materials, procedures, and content.

Emphasis on Reading

A further complication in serving LBP adolescents is that many of them also are poor readers. The problem is compounded by the traditional attitudes and procedures dictating that reading can be stimulated successfully by the practice of doing so while concurrently working on course content.

Proficient readers can and often do improve in that and other basic skills while completing course content. Poor readers, conversely, find that combining reading instruction with course content is a major hurdle. Therefore, without proficiency in the basic skills, poor readers find their attention is divided between the task of decoding words and comprehending the content of the reading material being presented.

Wiseman, Hartwell, and Krus (1978) find, after examining the reading performances of 740 tenth grade students from a comprehensive high school (grades 10-12) that served a middle-class population, that 59 percent performed at a ninth grade level or below and 15 percent at the fifth grade level or lower.

With the emphasis on reading as the primary source of learning in secondary schools, failure will continue to play a devastating role in adolescents' development, affecting self-concept, peer and adult interaction, and aspirations for social and economic mobility. Other alternatives for learning content, such as those proposed by Hartwell, Wiseman, and Van Reusen (1979), Weinberg and Mosby (1977), are incorporated in the Parallel Alternate Curriculum section of this chapter. Also, the reader is directed to review Chapter 7.

Lack of Individualization in Instruction

Another area of importance is the lack of individualization of instruction in secondary schools. Generally, secondary teachers in regular classrooms are not taught techniques of meeting the instructional needs of students with problems of low achievement. The large variance in these students' academic abilities has always been recognized. The attempts to provide instruction for those with differing levels of performance have produced programs that in the past have tended to segregate students on the basis of ability. The emphasis on mainstreaming or serving LBP adolescents in regular classrooms has brought attention to the need for individualizing instruction for secondary level students (Goldberg, 1977).

Individualization at the secondary level is a complicated task and presents unique problems for teachers because of the following features:

1. Most content area teachers are responsible for 130 to 175 students every day. Individualization can be an overwhelming task.
2. Reading levels in any one class can vary from nonreaders to grade 15 (i.e., college level).
3. Secondary teachers are hired primarily for content specialty such as biology, English, mathematics, etc. Most are not trained to work with low-achieving or handicapped students in their content specialty.

4. Educators are primarily responsible for meeting the instructional needs of average and above-average students.
5. The majority of class content uses reading as the primary source of information gathering.
6. Most secondary school texts have readability levels that exceed most students' grade level in that subject.

The Parallel Alternate Curriculum (PAC) instructional method as discussed in this chapter deals with individualization problems by developing alternative methods of teaching. It allows teachers to handle the large variance in students' academic abilities while maintaining a high level of academic expectancy.

Other approaches in developing learning alternatives for adolescents with achievement problems as well as other support programs also are presented. The Parallel Alternate Curriculum used by the Arizona State University Demonstration Resource Center is discussed in detail later in this chapter.

TRENDS IN PROVIDING ALTERNATIVE PROGRAMS

Historical Approaches

The history of providing alternative programs to support the handicapped in special settings is both rich and encouraging. The history of efforts to educate adolescents with learning and behavioral problems in mainstream settings has received infrequent and little public emphasis. The lack of attention to programs for the adolescent mildly handicapped population stems from several very practical reasons.

Little was known of these students in the public schools so a bright pupil who did not achieve to capacity was labeled lazy or unmotivated. The emphasis of the comprehensive high school also has been heavily influenced by the academically elite. Consequently, there was little understanding or interest for low-achieving students, particularly the mildly handicapped. Low-achievers were not expected to matriculate into public high schools but rather to attend vocational schools or to join the labor market.

In recent years, however, the trend of leaving school for the work world has changed. Now, more low-achieving students regularly attend and stay in school. Those enrolled in required courses in secondary schools have become increasingly diverse in ability, encompassing a multistrata group that spans gifted, regular, low-achieving, and mildly handicapped students. Neither programs nor teachers were prepared to accommodate this varied population, but some efforts were explored to meet this new challenge.

Initially, innovative programs were devised by individual teachers or schools but received little attention on a national scale. The scholarly approach to education was generally accepted by the lay and professional populations so exploratory efforts to develop alternative programs to accommodate low-achievers were slow in developing. Some far-sighted attempts were reported that departed from traditional educational efforts (McDaniels, 1971; Panushka, 1971; Silberberg & Silberberg, 1969; Wiseman, 1971).

The St. Paul (Minn.) public schools initiated a pilot study to educate low-achieving students with severe reading problems (McDaniels, 1971; Panushka, 1971; Wiseman, 1971). The experiment called for a comprehensive program to (1) increase basic skills such as reading, spelling, arithmetic, and writing; and (2) teach educational content such as science, social studies, etc., using a predominantly nonreading format. The rationale was that reading was not a necessary prerequisite for acquiring a well-rounded education and that after close examination it was found that little educational content depended on reading as the primary information medium. As Wiseman (1971) said in a speech to St. Paul secondary principals, "Productive thinking, intelligent problem solving, and creativity do not come from a vacuum. Knowledge is King! The scholarly approach to learning is an idealistic refuge perpetuated by highly educated but poorly trained educators. The truth is, it is not how you learn that matters, but rather that you learn."

Other efforts to accommodate LBP adolescents resembled a patchwork quilt rather than a comprehensive educational design. Classes and resource rooms for these teenagers were begun in the secondary schools with the dual purpose of teaching basic skills and academic curriculum content. Some self-contained special classes taught required course work while resource rooms tutored the students to help them pass the regular courses in which they were enrolled. The dilemma, of course, was that emphasis on tutoring course work detracted from instruction in basic survey skills that would be needed in life after school.

Some schools explored training consultants to assist regular class teachers in modifying content and materials to assist learning disabled students. Diagnostic/prescriptive centers were opened to provide comprehensive diagnostic data on LBP youths that led to extensive instructional prescriptions for both special and regular education teachers. The diagnostic/prescriptive centers frequently were greeted with ambivalence by secondary educators, who felt students in such places did not belong in their classes.

Special schools, both public and private, were opened to provide comprehensive educational services for youths with learning and behavioral problems. The Marianne Frostig School and the John Arena School in California, the Pathway Schools in Pennsylvania and Florida, and the Franklyn Groves Learning Center in Minnesota are examples of private schools that led this field.

Vocational programs have enjoyed a long but clouded history in the education of students with achievement problems. Both the public schools and the private sector have addressed the problem of educating LBP students to the world of work, unfortunately with mixed success. Vocational schools designed for the regular population frequently required high level reading skills, so LBP adolescents were excluded from many of their programs. Vocational schools for the handicapped usually had target populations that included mentally retarded and physically disabled youths, groups with which more capable adolescents had difficulty identifying. Many vocational schools had programs well suited to the more seriously handicapped but of questionable value for those with learning and behavioral problems.

Some notable efforts in the public school sector occurred in St. Paul and in Mesa, Ariz. In St. Paul, the vocational high schools had special education paraprofessionals assigned to each vocational class to assist in teaching and supervising the mildly handicapped students. The St. Paul Public School District also opened vocational centers. Students were bused to the centers to receive their training. The programs were designed initially to accommodate the mildly handicapped along with regular students; instruction was by teachers and paraprofessionals with special education training and experience.

The Mesa Public Schools developed a vocational high school with built-in provisions for students with mild learning problems. The school, Mesa Central High, offers academic and vocational classes for students who attend all day. Others attend other schools for academic courses but are bused to Mesa Central High for vocational training. Special education teachers and paraprofessionals are part of the faculty. Students enrolled in a districtwide comprehensive career education program learn about vocational choices and school training opportunities.

A regrettable trend in vocational education has led to a movement to raise the standards—in essence provide instruction that is more academic than hands-on. This emphasis has resulted in the exclusion of many students with learning and achievement problems from otherwise appropriate vocational education placements.

Contemporary Approaches

The extent of the problem of educating adolescents with low achievement in traditional academic secondary schools gradually became sufficiently visible to create special programs at the federal level. The Bureau for Education of the Handicapped, now the Office of Special Education, instituted a Child Service Demonstration Center (CSDC), Title VI E and G, Model Program Grant, to encourage development of exemplary programs for the learning disabled. Many of these projects resulted in the development of secondary level model programs, and led to the development of many public, private, and agency efforts that have broken from traditional emphasis to provide comprehensive programs for the secondary learning disabled.

Following are examples of comprehensive CSDC programs appropriate for urban, suburban, and rural public schools.

Arizona Demonstration Resource Center

Faculty members from Arizona State University and the Mesa public schools combined to develop a comprehensive program for secondary learning disabled and other low-achieving students. The emphasis of the program was bifurcated to include (1) special education students, faculty, and parents in resource rooms, and (2) a mainstreaming model. The project encompassed the following six goals:

1. Design and implement a cost-efficient screening and identification procedure that would result in selective placement and education for learning disabled and other low-achieving students.
2. Develop a basic skills remediation program in the learning disability resource room that emphasized direct teaching to mastery.
3. Develop a mainstream program to permit students to acquire academic course work utilizing a nonreading format. (The Parallel Alternate Curriculum is discussed in detail later in this chapter.)
4. Design an inservice program model to help individual secondary schools train new and experienced faculty and staff members, particularly in relation to low achievers.
5. Design and implement a model for involving parents of learning disabled adolescents, including a parent center, newsletter, and in-staff training programs for parents and students taught by PAC teachers and/or coordinators.
6. Develop and implement a program to teach academic survival skills, including a study skills class emphasizing textbook usage, organizational skills, test taking, strategies for memorizing, note taking, etc.

Lawrence, Kans., Project Strategies To Increase Learner Efficiency (STILE)

The Lawrence Unified School District #497 (CSDC) developed and implemented a program to teach strategies to secondary students to learn more efficiently in the regular classroom. Since many secondary regular education teachers resist altering their curriculum to meet the needs of the learning disabled, it was hypothesized that teaching coping skills to the students would help them compete successfully in regular course work. The learning disability resource room teacher presents learning strategies in listening, reading, thinking, speaking, writing, spelling, mathematics, and personal and social behavior.

Close interaction with the regular teachers assists the specialist in identifying defective learning skills. The project has developed informal assessment procedures to augment the identification or diagnosis of learning skills that can be implemented in a resource room.

Franklin County, Mo. (CSDC)

The Franklin County Special Education Cooperative in Union, Mo., developed a mainstreaming model based on a developmental bypass approach. This compensatory model accents student mastery of curriculum content. The regular curriculum of the school is taught using instructional procedures that bypass students' basic skill deficits. For example, students with inadequate reading skills learn content from cassette tapes or other audiovisual means. Students with poor writing skills dictate reports to a tape recorder. Tests are modified to bypass where students have difficulties in basic skills, permitting a testing of content without interference from other learning problems.

The school resource room assists through tutorial assistance, modifications of course material, and individualized assessment. A district-based psychoeducational/medical diagnostic team works cooperatively with school faculty to design individualized education programs (IEPs). The team, regular teachers, and resource room staff jointly prepare instructional materials for the schools. The team and the resource staff also help train regular teachers in assessing student skills and the modification of instructional materials.

Houston Synergistic Classroom Model

The University of Houston (CSDC) is a multigoal demonstration-research program encompassing both cognitive and affective emphasis. Through a resource room, students are given guided experiences in coping with intellectual and social demands that so frequently plague the secondary learning disabled. Upon entering the program, each adolescent participates in a carefully controlled High Intensity Learning Experience that emphasizes instruction in reading and self-concept development. Social/behavioral skills are developed through communication, assertiveness training, techniques for assuming responsibility, and practice in problem solving.

From this program students selectively matriculate into an Essential Skills Program or a Content Mastery Program. The Essential Skills Program emphasizes remedial reading instruction and instruction in fluency. The Content Mastery Program teaches survival skills necessary for the regular instructional program, emphasizing coping abilities and methods to bypass deficit situations.

A support system utilizing personnel from the learning disability resource room was developed to assist the students and the regular classroom teacher. Heavy emphasis is placed on an involvement program that attempts to encourage parents to be active participants in educational planning. The major thrust of the project is to teach the adolescent learning disabled to work effectively with other people while overcoming their problems.

PARALLEL ALTERNATE CURRICULUM (PAC)

The Parallel Alternate Curriculum (PAC) of the Arizona Child Service Demonstration Center (CSDC) is designed to provide secondary teachers with alternative methods for meeting the education needs of all students. It is a content-centered instructional method in which teachers of nonreaders or very poor readers can substitute or supplement the students' reading and information-gathering requirements with a variety of other communication vehicles.

PAC relies on methods other than reading as its primary source of gathering information. Students using the PAC no longer are denied the acquisition of subject matter because of their low reading levels; rather, they acquire full academic content through nonprint media. An array of auditory, visual, and hands-on methods is used in various combinations. Students may acquire subject matter from recorded materials, lectures, television, movies, group discussions, etc. Students' examinations may be given using a nonreading format. Tape libraries are developed for reading assignments. It should be kept in mind that reading instruction is not forgotten in this program but is presented in a separate program by specially trained teachers. The PAC affords students with learning problems an opportunity to participate and comprehend secondary content material without being subject to a watered down curriculum.

Essentially there are four options that have practical applications for a content class:

1. Total PAC: all content and assignments are presented to students in a nonreading format.
2. Mini PAC: only low-achieving students use PAC materials in the regular class.
3. Partial PAC: only a particular topic or unit is presented in a PAC format.
4. Preference PAC: students are presented with a choice of instructional procedures; the classroom is divided into learning style stations such as reading, discussion, listening, etc.

Total PAC

In a total PAC class, content and assignments are presented in a nonreading format to all students. None of them are permitted to rely solely on reading the materials or tests. Examinations are administered orally—read aloud by the teacher or on tape. The course content and expectancies are identical to regular classes, thus avoiding a watered down curriculum.

Mini PAC

The Mini PAC is used with a small percentage of students in the regular classroom. It is designed for classes that include many levels of ability and skill. Low-achievers are identified as PAC participants; regular students do not take part. In essence, there are two instructional systems operating simultaneously in a classroom. Both cover the same content and class assignments, but the PAC participants are taught by a nonreading format. Tests are modified for PAC participants only. Every effort is made to avoid separating them from the rest of the class.

Partial PAC

The partial PAC provides the instructor an option of presenting a particular topic or curricular unit through a PAC format rather than the traditional format. This option is designed to be used selectively when needed for difficult content or for variety. These units are used later for individualization, small groups, or review activities. With this option, the instructor may or may not want to evaluate and identify low achievers.

Preference PAC

This provides a choice of instructional procedures for both regular and low-achieving students. The classroom is divided into learning style stations. When assignments are given by the teacher, the students select the presentation style they prefer to complete the task. For example, if the teacher assigns a chapter in the text to be read, the following options may be used: listening to tapes of the chapter, listening to the teacher read aloud, reading silently, or listening to a narrative of the content in a small group. For lecture sessions and group discussions, the entire class participates as a group.

SPECIFIC PROCEDURES FOR PAC DEVELOPMENT

The procedures for implementing each of these four options are as follows:

Step 1. Learning outcomes are identified; the knowledge to be acquired by the students.

Step 2. Possible alternatives for presentation are identified and considered for use; for example, taped textbooks.

Step 3. Available materials and equipment are identified for possible use.

Step 4. Students are evaluated for learning style, learning preference, and/or achievement level.

Step 5. Alternatives for presentation (i.e., taped books, discussion methods) are decided upon and matched with student learning styles or preferences.

Step 6. Software materials are developed for future use (i.e., slides are collected, transparencies are made, or textbooks are taped).

Step 7. Presentation is implemented.

Step 8. Student progress is evaluated in a traditional and/or alternative manner such as oral or multiple choice tests.

Step 1: Learning Outcomes

The initial procedure for developing Parallel Alternate Curriculums as with most learning tasks is to identify what is to be taught, including skills, behaviors, and knowledge the students will be expected to have at the end of a lesson unit or entire course of instruction.

Instructional objectives have been used by regular and special educators for many decades. They are most valuable in determining programs of study. Written objectives also provide a clear understanding for both teacher and students of what is to be achieved. But most important, objectives provide measuring points or criteria for evaluating student performance. Many studies, books, articles, etc., have been devoted to the use of behavioral objectives. Glaser (1968) and Gronlund (1973) offer excellent guidelines for the development, implementation, and evaluation of instructional objectives.

When developing instructional objectives for a PAC, tasks and their learning outcomes must be taken into consideration. The types of learning tasks and outcomes at the secondary level usually are complex. Gronlund (1973) identifies two different levels of learning outcomes that have implications for secondary use: mastery and developmental. The mastery level outcomes include sequenced instruction of basic skills such as reading or grammar. The developmental level outcomes are written for a higher cognitive level while utilizing basic skills such as problem solving, concept application, or analysis.

The definition of learning outcomes for use in a PAC format is: A learning outcome is a specific statement of what the student will be expected to know or demonstrate when the learning task or unit of instruction has been completed. The PAC format advocates identifying learning outcomes at both the mastery and developmental levels or a combination of the two. This would depend on the course content.

In writing learning outcomes, three points should be included:

1. identification of the general objectives
2. identification of specific objectives—mastery and developmental

3. establishment of criteria for acceptable performance based on the general and specific objectives

An example of a general instructional objective or learning outcome for a unit on economics would be: The learner will be able to identify, match, or list vocabulary, principles, and characteristics associated with the study of economics and the four major types of economic systems—market, traditional, command, and mixed.

Once the general learning outcome or instructional objective is developed, the teacher can identify and list the specific types of results (mastery and developmental) that the students are to demonstrate at the end of a unit or lesson of instruction. Examples of specific mastery learning outcomes for a unit on economics would be:

Example A Identify vocabulary associated with economics with 80 percent accuracy.
    1.1 Scarcity
    1.2 Human Wants
    1.3 Production Resources
    1.4 Capital
Example B Identify principles and characteristics associated with the four major types of systems with 80 percent accuracy.
    1.1 Market
    1.2 Traditional
    1.3 Command
    1.4 Mixed

Examples of specific developmental learning outcomes would be:

Example A Compare and contrast principles and concepts associated with the study of economics with 75 percent accuracy.
    1.1 Principle of scarcity as it relates to economic systems
    1.2 Traditional economy vs. common economy
    1.3 Human wants as they relate to the principle of scarcity
    1.4 Capital as it relates to a common economic system
Example B Identify vocabulary, principles, and characteristics associated with the study of economics and the four major types of economic systems. Compare and contrast the four major systems.
    A. Identify Vocabulary
        1.1 Scarcity
        1.2 Human Wants
        1.3 Capital

As stated earlier, the PAC format advocates the development of learning outcomes at both mastery and developmental levels, or a combination of the two. The learning outcomes for a unit on economics that includes (1) identification of the general objectives, (2) identification of specific learning outcomes (mastery and developmental), and (3) establishment of criteria for acceptable performance, would be:

Example A Identify vocabulary, principles, and characteristics associated with the study of economics and the four major types of economic systems, and compare and contrast the four major systems.
    1.1 Market
    1.2 Traditional
    1.3 Command
    1.4 Mixed

Example B Identify principles and characteristics associated with the four major types of systems.
    1.1 Market
    1.2 Traditional
    1.3 Command
    1.4 Mixed

Example C Compare and contrast the four major economic systems.
    1.1 Market
    1.2 Traditional
    1.3 Command
    1.4 Mixed

Establish criteria for an acceptable standard of performance related to the above unit.

1. Identify vocabulary	80%
2. Identify characteristics of four systems	80%
3. Compare and contrast principles and concepts	75%

Once the instructor has developed the learning outcomes for the unit or instruction, it is necessary to identify the sequence in which the content will be presented. Both the learning outcomes and content outline should be shared with the students. This is an example of a content outline:

Example Economics PAC
    Content Outline
        A. Overview of the study of economics
            1. Cover vocabulary on the study of economics
            2. Cover the steps in the scientific method used in economics

B. Principles and characteristics of the four types of systems
    1. Scarcity as the major economic problem
C. Importance of the study of economics
    1. Responsibility in a democracy

Step 2: Possible Alternatives

The instructor identifies how the content will be presented in alternative forms or a combination of traditional and alternative forms.

Example Economics PAC
A. How will content be presented?
    1. Contracts for Unit #1
    2. Learning Centers
    3. Reading
        A. Listen to chapters on tape
        B. Peer tutor reads the chapter aloud to the student
        C. Material is paraphrased by the teacher or advanced student and read by the low achiever

Step 3: Materials and Equipment

The instructor makes a list of equipment available in the school.

Example Economics PAC
A. How will content be presented?
    1. Unit #1 will be taught through audiovisual materials (videotapes, films, filmstrips, transparencies, etc.).
    2. Equipment available for use: video monitor, 16 mm film projector, carousel slide projector, overhead projector, clear acetate sheets, etc.

Step 4: Student Evaluations

To evaluate learning style or preference, a survey may be given to the students to complete.

Example Survey Directs Student To
A. teacher-led discussions or presentations
B. movies, slides, videotapes
C. reading books silently
D. reading books silently while listening to the materials on tape
E. laboratories
F. tutoring

Another example of activities to survey student learning styles might be to evaluate achievement levels and entry skills (ability to read text, write, spell, or analyze materials, etc.) (Exhibit 12-1). The following testing procedures are recommended for group and/or individual assessment:

1. Use standardized achievement tests measuring reading, math, spelling, and language to give indications of future performance in class.
2. Use informal teacher-made tests based on course materials and expectancies.

   - Reading Comprehension: Have the student read several paragraphs in text and respond in writing to both fact and inference questions.
   - Note Taking: Direct a minilecture and have students hand in notes.
   - Writing: Analyze writing skill from test questions and note taking.
   - Dictionary Skills: Present several course-related vocabulary words and have students provide dictionary definition.
   - Arithmetic Skills: Provide problems related to course expectancies, if these are necessary.
   - Organizational Skills: Present an assignment that requires students to organize the content into meaningful and appropriate units.

3. Develop course-related cloze tests to provide indications of vocabulary development, reading comprehension, spelling and writing.
4. Develop and administer a test to measure the proposed content for the course. This can serve as a pretest-posttest measure to evaluate what the student knows at entry in comparison to knowledge at completion of course.

Step 5: Students' Learning Styles or Preferences

In an economics PAC, student preference surveys have shown that 75 percent of the class prefers to read the text assignments while listening to them on tape. The remaining 25 percent of the class would prefer to have the teacher read aloud and discuss the material afterwards.

Therefore, the teacher arranges the room with the appropriate number of desks around listening stations with tape players with the remaining desks in other parts of the room to allow for oral reading, discussion, or silent reading options.

Step 6: Coding and Development of Materials

Alternative presentations have been decided upon and matched with student preferences as in Step 5, in which students preferred to listen to taped lessons from

Exhibit 12-1 Classroom Assessment

TEACHER'S NAME: _____
STUDENT'S NAME: _____
COURSE AND HOUR: _____

Assessing Entrance Levels
_____ Sample of oral reading from text
_____ Sample of silent reading from text (with questions)
_____ Level of listening comprehension
_____ Sample of copying
_____ Sample of writing sentences
_____ Sample of writing paragraphs
_____ Spelling (if relevant for course)
_____ Necessary math skills for course
_____ Ability to obtain facts from text
_____ Ability to draw inferences from text
_____ Sample of note-taking ability
_____ Ability to paraphrase
_____ Assessing study habits
_____ Organization of ideas
_____ Understands objectives of course/unit
_____ Interview with student

Homework Assignments - First Week
_____ Completed
_____ Adequate quality
_____ Will examine student cumulative folder. Would like to discuss student with
counselor, psychologist, or special education teacher
_____ Indications of negative attitudes

the text. The instructor or advanced student now can begin to tape the text. After this is completed, the tapes are labeled and arranged for storage and easy retrieval. Tape players are arranged for and labeled for use in the classroom.

Step 7: Implementation of Presentation

The method of alternate presentation and student preference has been decided, materials have been developed, and the classroom has been organized to facilitate the PAC. Thereafter, instruction begins, using the same content but employing a more varied management or presentation procedure.

Step 8: Student Progress Evaluations

Tests evaluating student progress are administered in a traditional and/or alternate manner. The tests should include only items that measure the identified objectives that have been developed from Step 1. Students' preferences for expressing themselves during an evaluation exercise can be as varied as their choices for data acquisition. A test preference survey questionnaire could be included with the learning preference survey at the beginning of the semester. Alternate test methods should be left to the discretion of the teacher.

Example Economics PAC
   A. Students prefer to complete test while listening to questions being read on tape.
   B. Teacher tapes test, then arranges classroom accordingly to administer test.
   C. Some students prefer to read test and write answers; others need to listen to questions and respond orally.

Following these eight steps for implementation, suggestions for content presentation and alternatives for testing are discussed.

CONTENT PRESENTATION

Options for content presentation vary according to each teacher's preference and the availability of choices. Suggestions for content presentation are:

1. Lecture/discussion approach: develop brief outline of planned material and present to class before the lecture
2. Audiovisual presentation: use movies, slides, filmstrips, video, radio, transparencies, records
3. Guest speakers
4. Small group discussion
5. Individual discussion with instructor
6. Programmed learning: utilize reading or a combination of audiovisual and reading
7. Reading: silently, simultaneously with taped version, listening to teacher or other student read aloud, listening to a paraphrased version of the material and following with charts, diagrams, or printed material
8. Field trips

9. Projects: use "hands-on" approach to making a model, other art projects that can aid in establishing academic concepts, facts, etc.
10. Peer tutoring: use outside the classroom
11. Buddy system: use within the classroom
12. Contracts: set up students' prior expectations for achievement for grades
13. Work-study experience: allocate limited time in classroom, majority of time in field
14. Independent study: establish agreement between teacher and student
15. Minicourses: break up content units into smaller learning components; students not responsible for large units of information at one time but are for smaller units
16. Open classroom: arrange large teaching area utilizing team teaching approach
17. Learning centers: set up smaller area of classroom where individual concepts are taught through self-motivating materials (possibly audiovisual)
18. Note taking: have high achievers take notes with carbon paper so copies may be given to low achievers
19. Course syllabus
20. Discovery learning: give students problem situation where no procedures are established; they must develop their own method for finding solutions, facts, or drawing hypotheses
21. Supplementary texts and other written material: provide high-interest and low-vocabulary reading material

TESTING OPTIONS

As in options for content presentation, the selection of testing options will vary by teacher preference and the amount of time and support available. Suggestions for alternate testing procedures are:

1. Open test: have students use textbooks, notes, study guides, etc.; short answer and essay responses are most appropriate with this format
2. Closed test: require students to rely on skills, concepts, and facts they have learned or mastered without the use of notes or textbooks; multiple choice, true/false, and matching type items are most appropriate with this format
3. Teacher reads test: have students respond orally, in writing, or both
4. Reduced reading level of tests: present tests at level more comprehensible to lower achievers
5. Taped tests: direct students to listen to prerecorded tape of the test and respond on answer sheets

6. Small group tests
7. Student-made tests
8. Take-home tests
9. Alternative projects
10. Oral tests or oral reports
11. Taped tests: have students answer questions on tape recorder for teacher to correct later
12. Student-administered tests: ask competent peer to administer test orally and either write down student responses or have students write their own; format recommended for use with individuals or small groups

In addition to identifying content presentation and testing options available to the teacher, assessment of learner preferences in these areas is of major importance when attempting to individualize instruction.

STUDENT ASSESSMENT

To individualize instruction and modify curriculum to meet varied achievement needs, the classroom teacher's assessment of student learning styles, the learning and testing options the youths prefer and methods of assessing entry level skills and student progress all are important considerations.

The types of instruction available will depend on the PAC option selected by the teacher, availability of resources, and assessment information to match student learning styles to instructional alternatives. A *Student Learner Preference Profile Form* (Exhibit 12-2) is one example of an assessment activity that can be conducted by the teacher to assist in individualizing instruction. The profile includes student preferences for testing, motivational factors affecting learning, learning activity, and instructional grouping. Each student completes the preference profile and the teacher compiles a folder for each teenager that includes several assessment information forms, informal tests, and other profiles giving information for individualizing instruction.

An additional assessment designed primarily for teacher use evaluates student entry level skills in the classroom. It involves:

_____ A sample of oral reading from text
_____ A sample of silent reading from text (with questions)
_____ The level of listening comprehension
_____ A sample of copying
_____ A sample of writing sentences

_____A sample of writing paragraphs

_____Spelling (if relevant for course)

_____Math skills necessary for course

_____The ability to obtain facts from text

_____The ability to draw inferences from text

_____A sample of note-taking ability

_____The ability to paraphrase

_____An assessment of study habits

_____Organization of ideas

_____An understanding of objectives of course/unit

_____An interview with student

Homework Assignments—First Week

_____Completed

_____Quality adequate

_____Examination of student cumulative folder; teacher discusses student with counselor, psychologist, or special education teacher

_____Negative attitudes indicated

Other types of assessments developed by teachers include informal listening and reading inventories. In developing an informal listening inventory, the content should be based on textbook information not covered previously in the course and should be read to the students. The teacher asks three or four questions about the content, making sure that they relate to factual information, vocabulary meanings, inferences, and the use of context clues.

An informal reading inventory can be developed in the same way, using other textbook content not learned previously in the course. An example of an informal reading inventory is provided in Exhibit 12-3. The teacher should develop the same type of questions as in the listening test, then analyze the informal tests as to the type of question missed by the students and the total percent correct. These informal assessments are useful as screening devices.

A final assessment might include an analysis of performance levels by the special education, remedial reading, or remedial math teacher if the student is receiving a support service. By requesting the support teacher to give information as suggested below, the regular teacher will have additional helpful material for individualizing instruction for students previously identified as having learning or achievement problems.

After receiving assessment information on student learning strengths and preferences from a variety of sources, the teacher can develop checklists (Figure 12-1 and Exhibit 12-4) for individualizing instruction based on classroom assessment. The checklist can be attached to the student's IEP forms.

Exhibit 12-2 Student Learner Preference Profile Form

NAME _____DATE _____CLASS _____PERIOD _____

DIRECTIONS: Check the ways that you learn best below. You may check more than one, if you wish. Please be honest.

Evaluation Tests Preference Factors
_____Paper/pencil objective tests (multiple-choice), true-false, matching
_____Paper/pencil essay/short answer
_____Oral objective tests (multiple choice), true-false, matching
_____Oral essay/short answer
_____Project evaluation (project)
_____Take-home/open-book tests
_____Oral performance (speech, report)
_____Standardized test
_____Demonstration of skill (i.e., assembling a carburetor). Test should include only items that measure the desired behavior or skill
_____Teacher identification objectives
_____Test should measure only student-identified objectives
_____Items identified by teacher and students

Motivational Preference Factors
_____Teacher-led discussions/presentations
_____Student-led discussion/presentation
_____Movies, slides, filmstrips, video
_____Guest speakers, experts
_____Individual discussion with instructor
_____Small group discussions
_____Reading
_____Listening and viewing
_____Observing situations

Information Gathering or Learning Activity Preference Factors
_____Avid reader (usually can understand and express what I've read)
_____Learn best by listening
_____Like to write or take notes
_____Learn by viewing (movies, filmstrips, pictures, videotapes)
_____Like to tape-record lessons
_____Prefer to talk over ideas
_____Listen to required reading material on tape
_____Discussion—student led
_____Discussion—teacher led
_____Work on independent research or reports
_____Prefer to talk over ideas or information
_____Tutoring
_____Like to listen to a recording of the material to be read while reading it
_____Field trips, visitations

Exhibit 12-2 continued

Instructional Grouping Preferences

_____Large groups for lectures, discussions, movies, etc.

_____Small groups (of 3 to 10 persons)

_____Paired learning (2 or 3 persons learn together)

_____Tutorial—teach or help another person

_____Independent—by myself

Exhibit 12-3 Informal Reading Inventory

ENGLISH

To help follow and remember a lengthy argument, good readers outline and summarize it in their mind as they read. To make sure that their papers are well organized, good writers outline the major steps. Every so often, they stop to sum up for themselves what they have covered. Remember this point when making use of written outlines and summaries:

A rough working outline, adjusted and revised as the paper takes shape, helps writers marshal their ideas. Few experienced writers ever write a page without first jotting down a few major ideas in a tentative order.

1. What could good readers do to help themselves remember the key points of a long article?

2. What might good writers wish to do to help organize a paper?

3. What does the word *marshal* mean in this paragraph?

4. What are two major objectives of an outline?

Figure 12-1 Skills Evaluation of Student

To:

Student's Name:_____ Grade:_____

Special Education Placement:_____

Resource Room Teacher:_____ Date:_____

   The checklist below is designed to give you an overview of your student's areas of relative strength and weakness. Hopefully this will give you an understanding of the academic performance you may expect. As individuals respond very differently to different subjects and teachers the profile is not to be seen as a final statement, but rather as a guide.

   Please contact me if you encounter any serious problems and together we can seek solutions. Also it is important to recognize problems promptly and thus avoid the cycle of failure so many students have experienced.

Schedule	Date:_____
	Course	Teacher
A	
Period 1	
Period 2	
Period 3	
Period 4	
Period 5	
Period 6	

	Skill undeveloped-needs alternative instruction	Minimal skill development - peer tutoring or alternate instruction	Adequate for small group or buddy system work	Skill adequate for independent work at grade level - extra time necessary	Skill adequate for independent work at grade level in usual time	Skill in area of proficiency- could act as peer tutor
Following Directions Oral						
Detecting Facts - Oral						
Detecting Main Idea Oral						
Makes Inferences Oral						
Following Directions Reading						
Detect Facts Reading						
Detecting Main Idea Reading						
Inferences Reading						
Writes Short Answers						
Writes Paragraphs						
Write Reports						
Analyze Charts, Graphs Tables, Etc.						
Math Computation						
Math Concepts						
Memory						

Exhibit 12-4 Individualized Education Plan Checklist

Teacher's Name

Student's Name

Course and Hour

Individualizing Instruction for
_____ Requesting assistance
_____ Total PAC
_____ Partial PAC
_____ Mini PAC
_____ Preference PAC
_____ Reduced reading level
_____ Teaching study habits
_____ Peer tutoring program
_____ Using buddy system
_____ Providing class notes
_____ Tape-recording lectures
_____ Meeting on weekly basis with student
_____ Providing special assignments
_____ Making oral reports
_____ Making group reports
_____ Accepting tape-recorded themes or assignments
_____ Increasing communication with home/parents
_____ Reducing quantity and difficulty level of content
_____ Substituting projects for written assignments
_____ Permitting student to redo assignments

Examinations
_____ Oral exams, oral response (taped, buddy, special teacher)
        Paper and pencil
_____   Short answer
_____   Essay
_____   Multiple choice
_____   True-false
_____ Matching
_____ Fill-in
_____ Individually with teacher (oral or written)
_____ Open-book exams
_____ Take-home exams
_____ Small group tests
_____ Student-made tests
_____ Permission to retake exams
_____ Reduction of test difficulty
_____ Project assignment as alternative for exam
_____ Keeping track of assignments and completed activities
_____ Communication with parents
_____ Meeting on weekly basis with student in feedback sessions

---

OTHER INSTRUCTIONAL CONSIDERATIONS

The PAC format, as noted, provides a structure for organizing course material so that both high and low achievers can benefit from instruction. However, even though specific steps for PAC implementation are provided, other variables must be addressed if successful instructional learning is the expected outcome. These important variables relate more to knowledge and skills in teaching than to course content.

Additional instructional considerations, some of which have been discussed previously but are mentioned again for emphasis, are included in the following list:

1. Compile alternative ways for presenting materials and content for low-achieving students, including taping of textbooks, hands-on projects, etc., rather than term papers. (A table listing various alternatives, including active and passive student participation roles, is provided in Exhibit 12-5.)
2. Identify the audiovisual equipment needed to present the lessons and determine its availability.
3. Identify the entry level achievement skills of students, such as reading, writing, spelling (if relevant to the class), and note-taking ability.
4. Use an established readability formula to determine the readability level of handout materials, the course text, and examinations. Most course textbooks are written at a higher readability level than is necessary to express the content.
5. Identify and match the students' preferred style of learning to the different presentation methods that will be used. For example, if a poor reader prefers learning textbook material auditorily, cassette tapes of the required chapters should be provided.
6. Prepare the desired software before the class begins and have the materials readily available. Software could include tapes of text chapters, transparencies of class notes, videotapes, movies, filmstrips, and study guides. A central storing place in the classroom should be available for easy retrieval.
7. Compile a list of alternative methods for presenting course content such as class discussion, lecture, panels, reading text aloud, cassette tapes of class lectures, methods and comprehensive outlines for introducing films and videotapes, methods for reviewing films, discussions, and lectures.
8. Compile a list of alternative methods for evaluating student growth such as: reading tests aloud to the class, individuals, or small groups of students; tests administered by peer tutors; substituting hands-on projects for tests; and giving tests either open book or from notes.

Exhibit 12-5 Alternative Instructional Considerations

		ACTIVE		PASSIVE
AUDITORY	Talk	Discussion Oral Reading Interviewing Intercom/PA System Telephone Variable Speech Control (VSC) Radio Recorder-Record-Tape Language Labs Lecture Debate		Listen
	Arrange	Travel-Field Trip Guest Speakers Production-Plays Conference Seminar		Observe
VISUAL	Write	Books-Periodicals Chalkboard-Paper Computers-Terminals Typewriter-Duplicator Microfilm-Microfiche Papers-Reports Note Taking		Read
	Show	Movie Projector-Film Filmstrip Projector Teaching Machines Television-Videotape Opaque and Overhead Projectors Color Transparency Slides Camera-Photographs Demonstration Displays		Look
KINESTHETIC	Make	Maps-Globes Paints-Drawings Sculptures-Models Food Charts-Posters-Bulletin Boards		Use
	Handle	Laboratory Equipment Calculators Tools Machinery		Store

Exhibit 12-5 continued

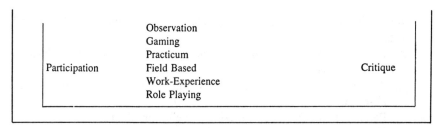

| Participation | Observation
Gaming
Practicum
Field Based
Work-Experience
Role Playing | Critique |

9. Evaluate and teach the study skills necessary for the class such as structures and usage of the text, note-taking skills, organizing materials, and strategies for memorizing and learning vocabulary.
10. Identify volunteers to tape textbook content on audiotapes. Parents, student volunteers, community service club members, or church groups are possible sources.
11. Develop an informational handout sheet for parents, administrators, and students outlining the instructional and learning alternatives to be used in the course.
12. Plan for a student and parent evaluation of the course to determine attitudes and perceived value of the instructional and learning alternative for the adolescents with learning and behavioral problems.

These considerations offer additional ideas to secondary school content teachers who are expected to supply instructional programs to accommodate a large population of students with learning problems. To meet the needs of this population within the existing secondary school structure, content teachers must be aware of and skilled in providing instructional procedures, materials, and evaluation strategies that will benefit all students.

MONITORING STUDENT PROGRESS, PERFORMANCE

The continual monitoring of student progress and performance in class assignments is an important educational obligation. Historically, secondary programs frequently monitor only during grading periods, which often is too late for revising procedures and materials to help students succeed. A parallel would be the importance of regular auditing in business. The business that does not have an organized and regular procedure for auditing its books can be in considerable danger of incurring losses or worse.

Procedures that can be used by the regular class teacher include:

1. Reviewing attendance records of students with learning and behavioral problems.
   a. Excess absences may indicate a general problem or it may be isolated to the one class.
   b. A personal interview should be held with student to discuss reasons for absence.
   c. Parents should be called for conference on problem.
   d. Problems should be discussed with school counselor.
   e. Strategies should be developed for encouraging regular attendance:
      1. parental pressure
      2. contract with student, parent, and teacher
      3. social recognition—before the behavior of others can change, the teacher's must change
2. Reviewing note-taking performance and assignment completion in class on a periodic basis.
   a. Assignments can include a notebook that includes notes taken in class, notes taken during reading assignments, etc.
   b. Class notes and assignments of LBP students should be reviewed periodically in terms of:
      1. completeness
      2. quality
      3. regularity
3. Reviewing grade scores on assignments, quizzes, and tests periodically.
   a. A class notebook to include completed assignments, tests, etc., should be assigned.
   b. Gradebook should be perused regularly.
   c. Performance should be reviewed with student and methods and procedures to improve grades discussed.
4. Maintaining a file on students' completed assignments.
   a. Recording and file-keeping is time consuming, so problematic students should be selected for filing duties.
   b. Class notebook should be assigned.
5. Analyzing type and degree of peer interaction.
   a. A simple sociogram should be observed.
   b. The teacher should observe LBP students as to their:
      1. participation in class discussion
      2. participation in group work and projects
      3. behavior toward peers, both negative and positive
      4. social skills with adults
      5. friends in class

6. Initiating contact with parents.
   a. Parents may be great allies.
   b. Once contact has been established, the teacher should determine whether this link should be regular, periodic, or no longer necessary.
   c. The relationship between parents and student should be determined (the teacher may be the only adult who cares).
7. Initiating and maintaining contact with students with learning and behavioral problems.
   a. Problems should be discussed with each student in private.
   b. Problem areas should be listed with student cooperation and strategies jointly developed for dealing with them.
   c. The student should be part of the decision-making team.
8. Initiating discussion with regular and support faculty.
   a. Counselor
   b. Reading center
   c. Peer tutoring program
   d. Special education staff
   e. School psychologist
   f. Nurse
   g. Administration
   h. Career and vocational education staff
   i. Other regular teachers
9. Developing contracts and sign-off sheets with special education students having special problems.
   a. Problems should be discussed with the special education teacher.
   b. A three-way discussion among the student, special education teacher, and regular teacher should be initiated.
   c. Problems and possible solutions should be listed, with each participant receiving a copy.
   d. A check-off sheet or card should be developed for the student to present to the special teacher each day to assess the youth's performance during the class session. The check-off sheet should be returned to the special teacher at the close of each day.
   e. Times should be established for periodic meetings to review progress and reassess intervention strategies.

Any one or more of these suggestions can assist the teacher in monitoring student progress and performance. Figure 12-2 is a sample Student Monitoring Form that could be used to maintain current and past data on performance. An Instructions for Student Monitoring Forms Sheet (Exhibit 12-6) explains how the form is to be completed.

Figure 12-2 Sample Student Monitoring Form

Last Name ID #	Pretest	Posttest	Unit Tests	Study Sheets	Labs	Projects	Unit Quizzes	Oral/Written Reports	Attendance	On-Task Rating	Academic GPA	Progress Report	Nine-Week Report	Semester Grade

Exhibit 12-6 Instructions for Student Monitoring Forms

1. STUDENT'S NAME:	Report student's last name, initial, then Student I.D.
2. PRETEST SCORE:	Report in grade form (1-5). Convert to a grade if you don't usually use grades.
3. POSTTEST SCORE:	Follow Pretest Score procedure outlined above.
4. UNIT TESTS:	Report in grade form (1-5). Twenty spaces are provided. Double up if you need additional spaces.
5. STUDY SHEETS OR STUDY GUIDES	Report either in grade form (1-5) or in Pass(P)/Fail(F) form. Twenty spaces are provided. Double up if you need additional spaces.
6. LABS:	Same as study sheets.
7. PROJECTS:	Same as study sheets.
8. UNIT QUIZZES:	Report in grade form (1-5). If more than one quiz per unit of study, then total and average.
9. ORAL/WRITTEN REPORTS:	Same as study sheets.
10. ATTENDANCE:	Report total days absent for the semester.
11. ON-TASK RATING:	Report one of the following numbers that best describes the student's overall behavior for the semester.

1	Always on Task	(100% of time)
2		(75% of time)
3	Sometimes	(50% of time)
4		(25% of time)
5	Never on Task	(0% of time)

12. ACADEMIC GPA:	Obtain GPA using only grades from academic courses.
13. PROGRESS REPORT:	Indicate whether a report was sent by checking in the appropriate space.
14. NINE-WEEK GRADE:	Report in grade form (1-5).
15. SEMESTER GRADE:	Report in grade form (1-5).

A teacher wishing to keep a record of the type and frequency of instructional options used in a specific class can use the Instructional Option Form (Exhibit 12-7). This form also is a useful device for department heads to use in helping new teachers or those having difficulty in class.

For teachers wishing to obtain data on the use of equipment and special materials, options and assignments completed, and general feedback on the efforts of class instruction from the students, the Student Feedback Form may be useful (Exhibit 12-8).

Exhibit 12-7 Form for Analyzing Use of Options

(Weekly Teacher Sheet)   TEACHER _____
                                                COURSE _____
                                                WEEK NO. _____ DATE _____

INSTRUCTIONAL OPTION FORM

Check How Many Times This Week the Following Options Were Offered (0-5 possibility):

_____ tapes
_____ peer tutoring
_____ learning center
_____ work on a contract
_____ class notes (lecture material)
_____ reading text
_____ lecture
_____ discussion
_____ audiovisual equipment (films, slides, videotape recorder, etc.)
_____ alternate projects (different options for meeting assignment requirements)
_____ student reports (oral or written)
_____ group projects
_____ study guides
_____ hands-on activities, lab, or experiences
_____ guest speakers
_____ alternative test procedures (taped, oral, etc.)
_____ field trip

Check the PAC Option Used Most This Week:

_____ Total
_____ Partial
_____ Mini
_____ Preference
_____ No PAC at all

EVALUATION CONSIDERATIONS

After the teacher has implemented an alternative instructional approach such as the PAC, consideration should be given to evaluating its effectiveness by students, parents, and the instructor. Some evaluation questions to be answered are:

- Are student grades improving?
- Is a larger percentage of students improving?

Exhibit 12-8 Form for Equipment Usage and Reactions

(Student Sheet-Weekly)   NAME _____
                                           CLASS _____
                                           DATE _____

STUDENT FEEDBACK FORM

During Class This Week How Many Times Did You: (circle the appropriate number)

use tapes	0 1 2 3 4 5
study with another student	0 1 2 3 4 5
use the learning center	0 1 2 3 4 5
fill out a contract	0 1 2 3 4 5
read provided class notes	0 1 2 3 4 5
read the class's textbook assignment	0 1 2 3 4 5
fill out the unit study guide	0 1 2 3 4 5
write your own class notes	0 1 2 3 4 5
come to class with the required materials (books, pens/pencils, paper, etc.)	0 1 2 3 4 5
complete a unit test	0 1 2 3 4 5

I Spent a Total of _____ Hours/ _____ Minutes Studying for This Course Out of Class.

True Or False   (use + for true and 0 for false)

_____ 1. I learned something in this class this week.
_____ 2. The work was too hard for me.
_____ 3. I can explain what I've learned this week.

- Are the gains significant when pretests and posttests are given?
- What are the students' attitudes about the alternative instructional materials?
- Did students perform according to the learning outcomes?
- Was the appropriate option used to meet student needs?
- Was the alternative approach practical for the teacher?
- Were parents aware that instructional alternatives were being provided for the students?
- Was there a decrease in student absenteeism?

These samples of PAC questionnaires are provided as examples of formats for evaluation activities. Included are sample evaluation forms for the student, the parent, and the teacher (Exhibits 12-9, 12-10, and 12-11).

Exhibit 12-9 Sample Evaluation Form for Student

Dear Student:

In the past semester you have been using Parallel Alternate Curriculum (PAC) methods in your _____ class. Will you please help us decide how good this method is by answering the following questions?

Fill in the letter that best describes how you feel. The letters go from

"A" meaning you strongly disagree, to

"C" meaning you feel neutral, to

"E" meaning you strongly agree

Skip the question (leave it blank) if you do not do it in class.

How Do You Feel about the Following:

	Strongly Disagree	Neutral	Strongly Agree
WORKING WITH OTHER STUDENTS	A	B C D	E
1. Using a peer tutor to help you with assignments in class	A	B C D	E
2. Using a buddy in class to work with and complete assignments	A	B C D	E
3. Breaking into groups for completing assignments	A	B C D	E
4. Working by yourself	A	B C D	E
TAPES			
5. Using tapes to read assignments	A	B C D	E
6. Checking out tapes of the textbook to take home and listen to	A	B C D	E
TESTS			
7. Using tapes to take tests	A	B C D	E
8. Taking tests in other ways (take-home, open notes, having teacher read it aloud, group quizzes)	A	B C D	E
TEACHER AND MATERIALS			
9. Watching films and filmstrips	A	B C D	E
10. Playing simulation games (Example: budget games, acting out how a bill is passed)	A	B C D	E
11. Taking notes while teacher writes main ideas or outline of lecture	A	B C D	E

Exhibit 12-9 continued

	Strongly Disagree	Neutral			Strongly Agree
12. Listening to lecture only part of the period and then doing other activities	A	B	C	D	E
13. Doing assignments in class	A	B	C	D	E
14. Doing assignments at home	A	B	C	D	E
15. Choosing a grade by contracts	A	B	C	D	E
16. Seeing assignments and due dates written on the board	A	B	C	D	E
17. Breaking into different learning stations (one group listens to tapes, one group listens to teacher read aloud, one group reads silently)	A	B	C	D	E
18. I would like to take another PAC class	A	B	C	D	E
19. I learned a lot from this class	A	B	C	D	E
20. I would like to have this teacher for another semester	A	B	C	D	E
21. I would like to go back to the regular class next semester	A	B	C	D	E
22. I liked the amount of reading required in this PAC class	A	B	C	D	E
23. This course made me feel good about myself	A	B	C	D	E

Exhibit 12-10 Sample Evaluation Form for Parents

Dear Parents:

For the past semester, your child has been using Parallel Alternate Curriculum (PAC) instructional materials in his/her _____ course. These materials rely heavily on a nonreading format utilizing tapes, audiovisuals, and special teacher lectures. This class covered the same content, and the grading requirements were the same as other classes. We would appreciate it if you would answer some questions. This is an anonymous survey, and you can return it to us in the enclosed, stamped envelope.

Directions: Place an "X" in the column showing whether you agree or disagree.

	Agree	Disagree
1. I was aware that my child was using PAC materials.		
2. I want my child to take more PAC courses.		
3. My child felt better about school last semester than before.		
4. I have noticed an improvement this past semester in my child's attitude toward school.		
5. I attended the dinner or one of the parent meetings sponsored by the Mountain View Staff.		
6. My child's grades have improved this past semester.		

Please Fill in the Blanks

7. I would like more information about _____.

8. What my child needs in school is _____.

9. PAC sounds like _____.

10. How do you feel about Mountain View's efforts to help students who are having difficulty in academic courses? _____.

Thank you very much for providing us with feedback about PAC.

Exhibit 12-11 Sample Evaluation Form for Teacher

Dear Participating Teacher:

  We are trying to evaluate the worth and effectiveness of PAC instruction from a teacher's point of view. Will you please mark the degree to which you agree or disagree with the following statements?

	Strongly Disagree		Neutral		Strongly Agree
1. PAC is effective with regular students	1	2	3	4	5
2. PAC is effective with learning disabled students	1	2	3	4	5
3. I plan on using PAC again	1	2	3	4	5
4. I would like to see more PAC courses developed	1	2	3	4	5
5. I let PAC students use alternate testing formats (take home, open notes, tests on tape, reading tests verbally, etc.)	1	2	3	4	5
6. I believe that low-achieving students made better grades on alternate test formats as opposed to traditional formats	1	2	3	4	5
7. I believe I spend more time in preparation for PAC classes than a regular class	1	2	3	4	5
8. After PAC is developed in my class, I feel that I will spend as much time in daily planning as I did prior to the development of the PAC	1	2	3	4	5
9. The tapes were easily utilized	1	2	3	4	5
10. The tapes helped students learn more easily	1	2	3	4	5
11. I feel that the students liked the PAC format	1	2	3	4	5
12. I liked teaching with the PAC format	1	2	3	4	5
13. I referred frequently to the PAC curriculum model	1	2	3	4	5
14. I feel that too much audiovisual equipment is needed	1	2	3	4	5
15. I feel that the PAC format lends itself to student acquisition of study skills (note taking, etc.)	1	2	3	4	5

Please Fill in the Blanks

16. I think PAC should be used with _____% of my low-achieving students
17. What PAC needs is _____
18. The best thing about PAC is _____
19. The worst thing about PAC is _____
20. My three favorite instructional methods for learning disabled students are
    (1) _____
    (2) _____
    (3) _____

SUMMARY

This chapter has presented information on the need for alternative programming for adolescents with learning and behavioral problems in the secondary schools. The problems of low achievement, those schools' emphasis on reading as the primary means of learning content, and lack of skills in individualizing instruction on the part of content teachers have played important roles in educators' efforts to provide alternate programs for an increasing number of skill-deficient secondary students.

Descriptions of federally funded demonstration programs offering alternative approaches have been provided. One of these projects, the Arizona State University Demonstration Resource Center, developed an approach for designing, implementing, and evaluating secondary content instructional units in conjunction with required textbook activities.

This approach, the Parallel Alternate Curriculum (PAC), was designed to be used in classrooms that include students with learning and behavioral problems. It permits teachers of students who either do not read or who are very poor readers to substitute or supplement the reading and information-gathering requirements of their courses with other communication vehicles such as audiovisual materials, lectures, demonstrations, group discussions, and learning centers.

Four PAC options were presented for teachers, along with a detailed outline of steps for implementing the PAC approach. Finally, the advantages to be considered in using an alternative approach for students with learning and behavioral problems were presented:

1. The teacher can provide different or varied options for course content, based on a match between the students' best learning style and preferences.
2. Mainstreaming secondary students with learning and behavioral problems into content classes utilizing the PAC format can provide increased time for remediation activities in other supportive services.
3. Class attendance by these secondary students usually increases because they have options available for learning content.
4. Learner efficiency is increased by the teacher's identification of goals, objectives, vocabulary, and learning outcomes.
5. Student progress is monitored in a structured fashion as it relates to identified outcomes and objectives for the content to be learned.
6. Both adolescents with learning and behavioral problems and nonlearning handicapped students are scheduled into PAC classes, thus facilitating mainstreaming efforts.
7. Preparation time for succeeding semesters is decreased once the initial teacher completes arrangements for implementing the PAC format.

8. PAC options provide meaningful learning of academic content for students who cannot read at the grade level of the classroom text.

The PAC approach described in this chapter is a viable system of education for LBP adolescents. This approach provides the practitioner with another option for instruction.

Chapter 13

Career and Vocational Education for LBP Adolescents

Bruno J. D'Alonzo and William S. Svoboda

INTRODUCTION

As students with learning and/or behavior problems (LBPs) progress through the educational system, schooling becomes the great difference maker instead of equalizer for them. Their performance on cognitive tasks, in self-control, and in more advanced reading, writing, computational, and spelling skills generally results in wider discrepancies between actual and predicted school performance each year they are in attendance. The diversity of needs manifested by LBP adolescents requires persons responsible for their education to provide a wide variety of program options.

Interestingly enough, programs at the secondary level have been virtually devoid of such options for students in career and vocational education. The lack of this emphasis has been an outgrowth of and can be directly attributed to a dependence on traditional elementary education models carried over to secondary schools.

The elementary remedial model emphasizes mastery of the basic skills such as reading, writing, and computation. Emphasis on basic skill acquisition for adolescents who have experienced repeated academic failure denies them learning experiences in career and vocational education. Indeed, their futures may depend on learning experiences that can best be provided in the career and vocational education arena preparing them for adult life.

Special education programming at the secondary level—curricula for LBP students—appears to be pointless when not linked to a vocational program for their needs. In comparison to the total number of special education programs in existence, relatively few offer secondary students a vocational or career education option. However, helpful trends should be noted, such as:

1. legislative acts that have increased funding to such programs
2. an increase in special conferences and programs that focus on career and vocational education topics
3. newsletters and publications from the field
4. information retrieval centers
5. the establishment of professional organizations (e.g., the Division on Career Development of The Council for Exceptional Children; the National Association for Vocational Education Special Needs Personnel of the American Vocational Association)
6. preservice and inservice preparation of teachers
7. an increase in the number of secondary programs for students with learning and/or behavior problems
8. better accessibility to career and vocational education program opportunities
9. an increase in positive attitudes toward the handicapped in the community and specifically by employers

All of these trends help make the educational and occupational outlook much brighter for adolescents enrolled in special education programs.

The initial impetus for career education by U.S. Commissioner of Education Sidney P. Marland (1971) arose because of (1) the large numbers of adolescents dropping out of school, (2) the apparently irrelevant curricula they had to pursue, (3) the large numbers of them leaving school without the salable skills necessary for entry into the work force, (4) the virtual void in career education for various special groups, including the handicapped. The 1970s were a period during which the career education movement gained momentum and set the stage for the 1980s.

This chapter defines career and vocational education, analyzes the theories that influenced the delivery of career education and its development, and discusses student goals and competencies and the essential components of programs for LBP adolescents. An overview of vocational education and its relationship to career education, and several service models, are presented.

DEFINITIONS OF CAREER EDUCATION

Defining career education (development) is not easy, and there are nearly as many definitions as definers. Hoyt, Evans, Mackin, and Mangum (1974) say "Career education is the total effort of public education and the community to help all individuals become familiar with the values of a work-oriented society, to integrate these values into their personal value systems, and to implement these values in their lives in such a way that work becomes possible, meaningful, and satisfying to each individual" (p. 15). Hoyt (1975) gives the following definition of career education: "the totality of experiences through which one learns about and prepares to engage in work as a part of her or his way of living" (p. 4).

Many interpreted this as a focus on job preparation, even though unpaid work (volunteerism, homemaking, productive leisure and recreational time) was considered part of productive work life. But its primary emphasis was the preparation of students for paid employment following their formal school experience.

Hoyt (1977) redefines career education as "an effort aimed at refocusing American education and the actions of the broader community in ways that will help individuals acquire and utilize the knowledge, skills, and attitudes necessary for each to make work a meaningful, productive, and satisfying part of his or her way of living" (p. 5). He describes work as paid employment for some and the productive use of leisure time, volunteerism, or homemaking for others. Thus, it appears that Hoyt's position, though still emphasizing paid employment, recognizes more clearly the other roles that constitute a total pattern of life.

Goldhammer (1972) identifies several "life careers" in which individuals engage as members of society: "(1) producer of goods and renderer of services; (2) member of a family group; (3) participant in social and political life; (4) participant in avocational pursuits; and (5) participant in the regulatory functions involved in aesthetic, moral, and religious concerns" (p. 129). The Executive Committee of the Division on Career Development presented a definition for approval to the board of governors of The Council for Exceptional Children in 1977. This definition was approved in 1978. Their definition of career education follows:

> Career education is a totality of experiences through which one learns to live a meaningful and satisfying work life. Within the career education framework, work is conceptualized as a conscious effort aimed at producing benefits for oneself and/or others. Career education provides the opportunity for children to learn, in the least restrictive environment possible, the academic, daily living, personal-social and occupational knowledge and specific vocational skills necessary for attaining their highest levels of economic, personal and social fulfillment. The individual can obtain this fulfillment through work (both paid and unpaid) and in a variety of other social roles and personal life styles including his/her pursuits as a student, citizen, volunteer, family member and participant in meaningful leisure time activities. (Official Actions of the Delegate Assembly of the 56th Annual Council for Exceptional Children International Convention in Kansas City. *Exceptional Children,* Vol. 45, p. 46, 1978.)

Brolin and Kokaska (1979) define career education as the "process of systematically coordinating all school, family, and community components together to facilitate each individual's potential for economic, social, and personal fulfillment'' (p. 102). They endorse the Council for Exceptional Children's (1978) definition.

Brolin and D'Alonzo (1979) and Brolin and Kokaska (1979) agree that a suitable definition of career education should include the many roles and positions occupied by handicapped individuals during their lifetime. This distinguishes career education from vocational education and emphasizes the important knowledge, skills, and attitudes students and other individuals need for their various life roles and settings, including that of paid work.

For the majority of handicapped individuals, paid employment will be a major part of their careers if they receive the necessary occupational guidance and preparation to permit them to earn a decent living. For many others, paid employment will not necessarily be a major part of their career. These individuals, being limited in their vocational activity, may have a successful career and productive life by learning how to function adequately in avocational, family, and civic pursuits. Career education thus is for everyone, the focus depending on each individual's unique set of abilities, needs, interests, and ultimate potentials.

Further clarification is needed, particularly as to professional agreement about a universal and operational definition of career education so that programs can be developed in a systematic manner. Mori (1979) supports this position when he states: ''an operational definition and working model of career education should be developed so that all parties are working from a common ground'' (p. 5). The authors of this chapter believe that the career education movement has suffered from the lack of an operational definition. Furthermore, if it had been so defined by Marland (1971) when he was U.S. Commissioner of Education, it is likely that many of the problems encountered in implementation, development, and research would not have occurred.

In the early stages of the career education movement, professionals were inclined to agree with Marland that the concept should evolve through the efforts of education professionals, parents, business executives, and labor to meet the needs of the nation's children and youths. Unfortunately, this resulted in a lack of direction and commitment by many professionals, confusion, and little if any comprehensive programming.

The authors believe that a structure for career education similar to that of vocational education is needed. The career education sequence would commence much earlier than high school, preferably when the child begins formal schooling. This is not to advocate a total infusion approach as urged by most career educators. As usually is the case with most new educational efforts, the time, the place, the amount of financial support, and the prevailing circumstances will influence and often dictate the approach a given school system will pursue.

THEORIES ON CAREER EDUCATION DELIVERY

There are many theories about how career education should be delivered to students in the schools. Several of the most popular ones are discussed briefly. These should be viewed as complementary rather than mutually exclusive. That is, a combination or blending of the ideas into a scheme that will work in a particular situation should prove more useful than looking for the one theory that will solve all problems.

Womb to Tomb

This idea was succinctly addressed by Hoyt (1975) when he stated that "Since both one's career and one's education extend from the preschool through the retirement years, career education must also span almost the entire life cycle" (p. 3). Although the phrase "womb to tomb" is overstated, it nevertheless points up the idea that career education is much more than a career fair in the ninth grade and a career week in high school. A program to deliver career education in the school needs to be continuous and planned. Even though schools can most directly influence adolescents while they actually are students, it is envisioned by advocates of career education that others will become involved and that concepts and skills will be retained and used beyond class and even passed on to younger people.

While it is agreed that career education is a lifelong pursuit, this book focuses on what schools can do for adolescents with learning and behavioral problems. The structured components of career education for many of these students will have to be achieved while they are in school. Their past cannot be changed; their present and future have to be the areas of concentrated effort.

Clusters and Exploration

Perhaps the most agreed-upon strategy in career education is the exploration of occupational clusters. The U.S. Office of Education (1971) has identified 15 occupational clusters, each of which consists of similar types of jobs. They range the full scope of technicality and education but are related because they include similar teachable skill and knowledge requirements. Other groupings are used, but career education literature and materials most often refer to this U.S. Office of Education list of occupations:

Agribusiness and Natural Resources
Business and Office
Communications and Media
Construction
Consumer and Homemaking

Environment
Fine Arts and Humanities
Health
Manufacturing
Marine Science
Marketing and Distribution
Personal Service
Public Service
Recreation, Hospitality, and Tourism
Transportation

The career clusters provide students with a convenient source of available occupational alternatives. The adolescents are not forced to choose specific types of jobs; instead, they can explore groupings of occupations. They can look at the skills and education required in these groupings. Then they can gradually narrow their choices—based on increasingly specific comparisons of areas such as personal aspirations, skills, interests—with the clusters and then with their subareas until a final selection is made and acted upon. This process should increase the probability that more youths will enter occupations in which they will be productive and satisfied.

Another use of the career clusters that would have more far-reaching effects would be to have tracking in the schools done on the basis of career clusters rather than on college preparatory/vocational or normal/remedial bases. This seems especially relevant the last year or two of high school.

Collaboration

The ideal delivery plan for a career education program would have many segments of the community actively involved in the original planning and through all the phases, including implementation and evaluation. Although the term "cooperation" is heard often, it is used here to emphasize more of a sense of commitment to the goals. Another way of viewing this basic idea is expressed by Hoyt et al. (1974) when they use the term "interactive network":

> Interest and personal commitment are the two most basic qualifications for participating in the planning and organization of local programs of career education. However, the design, development, and expansion of this new program will not achieve its full potential if local school systems or state education agencies work in isolation from each other or if the school functions apart from other groups or agencies in the community. The cross-fertilization of ideas and concepts and the transfer of successful methods and similarities of experiences are essen-

tial. . . . All of this support and momentum must be coordinated and fully used. (p. 168)

Whatever the process is called, the community needs to be involved. The school cannot deliver a realistic or reasonable career education program only within the confines of its building and its books. Students need more first-hand experiences with the world of work and the people who function there. This needed collaboration could best be built on a realistic and mutually advantageous set of priorities such as those presented in Exhibit 13-3. A successful career education program not only increases the potential for individual fulfillment but logically should have a positive effect on many parts of the community such as business, industry, welfare, crime, and mental and physical illnesses.

Infusion

The concept of infusion is the basic mode of introducing the specifics of career education into the curriculum. Infusion is a process by which all course content is studied as a means to fulfill students' career needs. Traditional academic and vocational content are not altered nor will they be replaced by career education. Infusion is merely teaching any subject content, adding in necessary career education concepts. For example, a social studies class discussing the concept of racial, sexual, or other types of discrimination would at least include examples of discrimination in occupations. This might lead to discussions of discrimination based on societal values about job status, comparing personal work satisfaction with a task's perceived social status, or comparing occupational status with financial compensation or the potential contribution an incumbent in that position can make to society.

Regardless of how much infusion has been advocated, it is limited in its usefulness. The infusion process demands a great deal from teachers, many of whom already are overburdened. It demands that teachers not only have a mastery of the content but also of the concepts of career education. They then must use a methodology that they have never seen modeled. This blending of content to fit the traditional subject matter goals and career education objectives is extremely difficult. Given the history of change and innovation in the public schools, this approach does not seem to have a positive future, yet in principle it has extreme merit. The infusion model has been advocated by Brolin and Kokaska (1979). A model for implementing career education through infusion into curricula has been developed by Brolin (1974), e.g., *Life Centered Career Education: A Competency Based Approach.* This model program was implemented into 12 school districts in the United States.

The biggest problem with the infusion process is that it cannot maintain continuity of the type that is demanded through the sequence of self-awareness, occupational awareness, educational awareness, career cluster analysis, and decision making about occupations. Unless programs are outlined clearly and specify that a certain teacher or group of teachers is responsible for the program, it is left to chance. Far too many infusion programs consist of a broad statement of career education goals and philosophy, a set of unrelated career education activities, and encouragement to be successful. Everyone is expected to teach career education, but no one is given specific responsibility to carry out a specific task.

It is proposed that the infusion process be used for types of career education goals that are not directly related to occupational choice. Broad goals of career education such as "learning to live" and "learning to learn" seem appropriate to the infusion process.

For example, the State of Arizona has three broad goals of career education: "learning to live," which means the developing of students' self-awareness of their capabilities and the ability to deal with leisure time and society in general; "learning to learn," which means teaching students skills that they can use to learn throughout life after they have left formal school; and "learning to make a living," which means preparing students to be able to support themselves economically in occupations that are self-fulfilling to them personally and productive for society.

A general understanding of the intent of these goals can serve as relatively compatible means of planning and implementing infusion of career education goals into the regular school program. Self-awareness, leisure, human relations, and learning skills can be related to some aspects of nearly all classes rather easily. For some classes, the relationships may be more difficult, but there is no overall sequenced strategy that must be articulated among the many subjects.

Separate Program Approach

Advocates of this approach point out that career education, or at least some parts of it, warrants a separate place in the school curriculum. While some assert that a separate approach is adding more to the curriculum, the writers believe this actually is a strength. If career education is as valid as its advocates suggest, it warrants being in the secondary school curriculum. It is time that school personnel begin looking for more relevant approaches to helping adolescents. New approaches such as career education should not be added to the curriculum but should replace content that has been judged to be less worthy. In educators' efforts to please everyone, they have shirked their responsibilities to make hard decisions. Career education should not be relegated to only an infusion process of delivery, but some aspects should be considered as a separate part of the curriculum.

The most appropriate use of career education as a separate part of the curriculum would be in that part mentioned earlier as "learning to make a living." This is the aspect that is common to all definitions. It involves the overall developmental process of matching people with appropriate careers. This process needs the coordination and proper sequencing of a series of activities that involve the LBP students' understanding themselves, being aware of occupational opportunities, comprehending the costs involved if one wishes to pursue a particular occupational field, and systematically narrowing choices and preparing educationally until they enter a job.

The separate program could be implemented in many ways. A counseling staff could be given major responsibility to carry it out. A series of required or voluntary courses could be made available that would lead adolescents through the occupational choice part of the career educational program or at least would make the systematic and sequenced opportunities available. A team of counselors, teachers, and business persons could be assigned responsibility for the program.

CATEGORIES OF CAREER DEVELOPMENT

The stages and processes of career development fall into six distinct but overlapping categories. Therefore, they should be viewed as flowing together, part of a continuing process, and having strong interrelationships.

Self-Awareness

Adolescent students with learning and behavioral problems gain information about themselves. This includes identification of values, desired life styles, strengths, limitations, interests, and all similar types of personal information that might be important in consideration of career alternatives.

Career Awareness

The students gain information about the broad world of work. This includes general knowledge about the roles of work, the variety of jobs, and career clusters or areas.

Career Orientation

The students begin to draw relationships between themselves and the world of work. This includes matching self-knowledge with more in-depth investigation of specific career clusters. Students should increasingly realize the important role that occupations play in self-fulfillment. They can begin to take advantage of opportunities to control and plan for this part of their lives.

Career Exploration

Students increase the depth of investigation of occupations and begin to make some basic decisions. This includes narrowing occupational alternatives based on increased knowledge. Some sort of plan should be developed that combines the knowledge of self, available occupations, and the realities of obtaining or using entry level skills.

Career Preparation

Students should be involved in carrying out their career plans. This usually involves acquiring entry level skills in one of the occupational clusters or continuing to take prerequisite courses for further education.

Maturation

This usually does not involve students in secondary schools. Persons in this category already have entered the world of work. They are involved in maintaining, improving, or changing their job status. Although few students will be actively involved in any one of these stages in school, they should be aware of their importance and include them in their career plans.

CAREER DEVELOPMENTAL TASKS IN SCHOOL

Although there is no hard-and-fast rule concerning the development of the different categories of career education, some usual patterns receive emphasis at the different school levels. (For a detailed and somewhat different discussion of career development, see Bailey and Stadt, 1973.) For example, the primary school normally is a place where the child is acquiring a broad idea of self and careers. A positive self-concept should be a prime consideration at this level, although its importance cannot be minimized at any time. Children also should grasp the idea that work provides things—that a home, food, luxuries, are the consequences of work. Examples from the home usually are the most effective at these early stages and should expand as the students' awareness grows.

The upper elementary grades offer basically a development of the broad ideas that were begun in the primary grades. Students should begin to see relationships among occupations. The functioning of the school often is used to show how different people have different roles and how they combine to provide the totality of what is called school. The community provides a larger example that can be studied systematically. Further examples from the state and the nation are used to show interrelationships such as the many vocations involved in the production of some common products with which the students are familiar. The concept of job satisfaction and personal satisfaction of doing something well can be introduced in this phase.

The junior high school level begins the crucial stage of examining occupational choices in a more deliberate and systematic manner. Occupational clusters are introduced, and usually a few are studied in detail. Drawing from self-studies, students can isolate the broad categories of work that seem to best fit their desires, abilities, and preferred futures. They should be viewing occupations as means to achieving hoped-for ends. They should be using systematic decision-making skills that stress consequences and responsibility for behavior. Formal counseling, often including the administration of interest inventories, is one important aspect of the program. Although junior high school is a time when students are making some initial decisions about work, they involve broad concepts of career clusters and are not restricted to specific occupations.

Secondary school also is where students face some of the actualities of the real world as it relates to work. Three kinds of alternatives represent major decisions for secondary school adolescents. The first is that no decision concerning an occupation is made. Some students simply cannot make such a decision at this time. Depending on their circumstances, adolescents usually pursue a program of continued exploration. It is important to note that students are encouraged to make career choices but only when they are ready and are comfortable with the fact that the decision is theirs. A legitimate decision might be that a student needs more time and information even though formal secondary education soon will be ending.

The second alternative involves students who have made relatively specialized occupational choices. This group will be investigating one or more of the career clusters in depth. Ideally, the choices of occupational areas become narrower as graduation nears. The more students know about themselves and occupational and educational areas, the more they can see these variables coming together as viable career choices. Some will narrow the choices to one group of occupations or even to a single type of job.

Students who have made occupational choices that require additional formal academic training should be planning their high school courses with the deliberate intention of obtaining the proper prerequisites. Many work toward obtaining entry level job skills for a cluster even though their goal is a higher level occupation within the cluster. These young people have made cluster choices but will not enter the actual job market until they have obtained considerably more formal training.

The third alternative involves students who have made more specific choices and are ready to enter the world of work immediately. Entry level for skills is of more immediate importance. Many of these youths will be in work/study programs, attending school part of the time and spending the rest of the time in an actual work situation. Their needs are more immediate in areas such as job skills, social skills, economic considerations, long-range predicting, and other realities that they no longer can defer.

PRINCIPLES OF CAREER DEVELOPMENT PROGRAM

The principles of a career development program are based on an overriding idea or assumption that people want to know how to make their lives productive and happy. Career education is a concept that attempts to promote students' general welfare by using the inherent motivation and importance of careers as the basic foundation for curriculum development. A successful career education curriculum should produce a large number of persons who achieve their potential because their work better suits such factors as individual needs, values, or talents. Society also should profit as social problems associated with job dissatisfaction and low productivity are lessened. School programs for career development should be planned carefully if these lofty goals are to be met. They should be based on principles that can be used by the curriculum planner or implementor. Career development programs should:

- be for all individuals, regardless of the minority to which they might belong
- help students achieve positive but realistic self-concepts
- begin early in the elementary grades and continue throughout formal schooling
- develop vocational skills
- develop positive attitudes toward the necessities for and the values in work
- help students acquire social skills necessary for vocational success
- involve parents, business, and industry as much as possible
- help students see the tremendous impact their vocational choices can have on their physical and mental health
- allow students to select from a variety of alternatives in pursuit of the options they desire
- provide greater relevancy for schoolwork and vocational fulfillment through exploration of the world of work
- increase personal fulfillment through paid vocational experiences and satisfactory avocational avenues as well

School personnel using these basic guiding principles should be better prepared to provide the programming necessary to enhance the students' career development.

STUDENT GOALS AND COMPETENCIES

It is important to establish goals and competencies so the career education program will have direction and structure. Educational personnel then can systematically instruct and provide learning experiences to assist students in reaching these goals and acquiring the necessary competencies. The evaluation of the career education program becomes easier because achievement of these goals and competencies can be measured. This in turn provides a system that can be monitored and for which accountability can be established.

The U.S. Office of Education (1975) developed a list of learner outcome goals for persons leaving the formal education system at the completion of specified levels of education. To meet the following career education goals, which are commensurate with those traditionally advocated by special educators involved with the education and training of LBP adolescents, the students should be:

1. competent in the basic academic skills required for adaptability in a rapidly changing society
2. equipped with good work habits
3. capable of choosing (and have chosen) a personally meaningful set of work values that foster a desire to work
4. equipped with career decision-making, job-hunting, and job-getting skills
5. equipped with vocational/personal skills at a level that will allow them to gain entry into and attain a degree of success in the occupational society
6. equipped with career decisions based on the widest possible set of data concerning themselves and their educational/vocational opportunities
7. aware of means available to them for continuing and recurrent education once they have left the formal schooling system
8. successful in a paid occupation, in further education, or in a vocation consistent with their current career education
9. successful in incorporating work values into their total personal value structure in such a way that they are able to choose what is for them a desirable life style

CAREER EDUCATION COMPONENTS

The following discussion of the components of a typical career education program for adolescents with learning and behavioral problems is designed to provide those interested in helping these young people with a better sense of the organization involved and of the alternatives available.

Clearly Stated Student Outcomes

Any program needs specific and clearly stated goals. Career education as a broad movement does not have one clear definition or set of goals. This makes it even more imperative that the local school or system spell out specifics. Based on these specifics, more details of method, materials, and evaluation can be developed.

A reasonably clear and precise set of student outcomes has been produced by the Arizona Department of Education in its *Career Education Matrix* (1976). This matrix recommends that to attain the broad outcomes expected from career education, students be able to:

- achieve an increased awareness and understanding of interests, aptitudes, and responsibilities as these relate to various careers
- demonstrate increased interests and achievement in the educational program, emphasizing communications and basic skill areas
- understand the world of work and its impact on society
- make decisions related to career areas being explored
- possess career entry-level skills upon exiting from the formal educational program
- develop an understanding of and appreciation for the value of continual learning, the arts, and leisure qualities of life

With these as the expected outcomes, a matrix is constructed. The horizontal axis consists of eight elements of career education: self-awareness, educational awareness, career awareness, economic awareness, decision making, beginning competency, employability skills, and appreciations and attitudes. The vertical axis consists of the four levels of the public schools: primary, intermediate, junior high, and senior high. The 32 cells created by this matrix provide 14 goal statements and 204 enabling objectives for all levels of school under the eight educational elements of career education. This results in 318 rather specific student outcomes from which teachers can plan, materials can be developed, and programs can be developed more efficiently.

For example, an intermediate school goal for career awareness is "the students will identify and classify local jobs." Preciseness and clarity such as this are required in developing a sound career education program. Following is an example of one cell of the Arizona matrix (1976) from the High School Level and Decision Making axes:

DECISION MAKING

The students will understand that decision making includes responsible action in identifying alternatives, selecting the alternative most consistent with their goals, and taking steps to implement a course of action.

- The students will understand that a given set of facts can support different decisions.

- The students will predict and analyze the immediate, intermediate, and long-term effects their decisions will have on themselves, family, and society.

The students will become proficient in using resource information to make career decisions.

- The students will understand how school and work experiences meet the needs of occupational preparation.
- The students will continue to acquire information in the continuing evaluation and development of their educational plans.

The students will identify personal goals as part of making career decisions.

- The students will analyze their career goals and the subsequent decisions that are required by such goals.
- The students will make tentative plans for developing their long-range career responsibilities and what is required to achieve them. (p. 1)

Teaching Staff

Most of the actual implementation of a total career education program will require some kind of involvement of classroom teachers. They seldom have formal undergraduate training in career education concepts. A large part of their training has been undertaken in short-term institutes and workshops or other inservice approaches. Although future training activities will vary, the teacher outcomes are relatively clear. Hoyt (1976) states that inservice programs should be helping teachers:

- understand and accept the career education concept
- learn how to think of the goal of education as preparation for work in relationship to (1) other basic goals of education and (2) the process and content goals to which they are already accustomed
- learn both about (1) the nature of the world of paid employment outside of education and (2) how that world operates
- learn about the multiple career implications of their subject matter
- learn how to use community personnel as resource persons in the classroom
- learn how to use the community as a learning laboratory for helping students learn more subject matter of the course

- learn the basic principles of career development to an extent that ensures the process will be taken into account correctly in planning classroom activities
- learn how to thread career education skills, knowledge, and attitudes into the teaching/learning process in ways that will retain the basic importance of the teacher's subject matter

Of the many designs and activities that can be used to augment staff development, Svoboda and Wolfe (1974) mention several of the basics for bringing about changes such as those necessary for a traditional teacher to begin to voluntarily utilize ideas from the area of career education. They believe that change should be built on the desire of the person who will have to implement it. Desire usually comes when the status quo is found to be undesirable. For A simply to tell B that B must change has little chance for success unless A, who is dictating the change, is willing to constantly police the activities of B, who has to carry out the mandate.

Persons implementing a change must have the knowledge and skills to bring it about. Change will occur only if great effort is expended. Even if an individual has the desire, knowledge, and skills, and is willing to expend effort, there may be some areas of the environment that will not allow change to take place.

Workshops must help teachers deal effectively with environmental constraints such as time, money, schedules, incompatible imposed testing, facilities, etc. Whenever possible, a pilot test of a change in some small and controlled environment could be conducted to solve unforeseen problems with a minimum of potential harm to students.

These ideas are appropriate as a basis for action that can be used before, during, and after inservice activities. Those who are sponsoring and/or conducting staff development programs should determine first that the general environment does not have obvious constraints that would make career education infeasible. If there seems to be no gross impediment, then the actual inservice program should be planned in such a way that the teachers will be involved in comparing the status quo and the probable benefits of the innovation. If improvement is seen and if teachers desire to investigate this part of career education further, they must be helped to attain the necessary knowledge and skills. They also must be prepared for the usual expenditure of extra effort and must be part of an evaluation of the possible restrictions on implementation of new programs in the school and community.

A career education workshop should provide the information and activities that at minimum respond to the teachers' desire for career education, knowledge about it, willingness to expend effort to implement it, and the degree to which their specific class environments will allow such a program to be implemented. Teachers must demand that staff development programs contain these factors. More in-depth knowledge of inservice workshop programs is provided in workshop programs developed by Brolin (1978), Raymond (1978), and Schwartz (1980).

Community and Parent Involvement

Since career education programs are focusing on the world of work, which for the most part is outside the school, it is necessary to involve the community. Based on an understanding that a successful career education program is valuable not only to the students but also to the community, opportunities for the members of the latter to be involved would include:

- serving on advisory councils
- assisting in staff training
- serving as guest speakers
- providing sites for field trips
- providing sites for internships and job-shadowing experiences, e.g., spending variable amounts of time observing employees at work
- being involved in curriculum development
- developing and donating materials on the world of work
- assisting in the development of public awareness of career education
- providing work experience sites
- projecting future job needs

Parents probably are not as conspicuously necessary in this aspect of the program as are members of business and industry groups of the community, but their influence is enormous. Basic ideas about work, prestige, life styles, success, happiness, responsibility, and other value-laden concepts can be greatly influenced in the home. This probably is the weightiest contribution parents can make. Other roles in which they may become involved include:

Serving as resource persons or as volunteers
Assisting in school resource surveys or on field trips
Serving on parent discussion groups
Demonstrating their hobbies
Assisting with school newsletters
Being involved with P.T.A. programs
Serving on advisory committees
Assisting with special projects (Preli, 1978, p. 9)

Any school program can be improved by the involvement of the parents and the larger community, but the career education effort is especially vulnerable to an apathetic community or to school officials who want to remain aloof from their constituents.

Resource Centers

Career education programs need resources that are comprehensive, up to date, and easily available. These resources also should include the counseling and guidance personnel in the school or community. Career education resource centers sometimes are unified, as in a large community or school district where resources are pooled in one location and made available to everyone. These centers act as clearinghouses where information is readily available. These large clearinghouse-type centers are especially useful because they can specialize in quantity, quality, and up-to-date information. Their main drawback is that they serve large areas, and the public (including potential users) often does not know they exist or they are not readily accessible.

The usual type of resource center that adolescents will encounter is likely to be much smaller, located in the school building, much less comprehensive in material coverage, and may be a part of the library or of the counseling center. Wherever it is located, the center should include a wide variety of occupational information at a reading level that students can understand. The materials should be up to date and should be selected with the particular school population in mind. The center should be easily accessible, pleasant, and convenient. It should be open at times when students can drop in, and should have personnel who can help to interpret information as well as locate it. Although the center is sure to be used as a result of structured career education activities, much of the students' investigations will be done on the spur of the moment when they need to check out a job's rewards, entry skill level, or future, so material availability becomes a top priority.

Of special importance in any kind of resource center is the staff. Obvious qualities such as competence in obtaining, maintaining, evaluating, and circulating resources are important, as are the general traits of positive human relations, kindness, and a desire to help others. Since the functions of career education centers invariably involve counseling and guidance, some of the staff should be formally trained in those fields, especially in career guidance.

Resource Units

An effective career education program is no different from any other effort in the need for quality content and methodology. Both the infusion and separate program approaches could be improved by some type of resource unit presentation. A resource unit, for example, gives direction but still leaves the creative teacher room in which to operate. These units can be purchased, produced by specialists, or developed by individuals or teams of classroom teachers.

The typical format of a resource unit begins with the identification of a specific concept (big idea) or a skill (way to do something). This is followed by a rationale that explains the merits of the unit in terms of value to the students. Specific objectives then are listed. An outline of content necessary to achieve the objectives is included. This is followed by a series of activities, each designed to use the content to achieve one or more of the objectives. Suggestions are offered for evaluating the instruction, and a comprehensive list of resources is made available to the person(s) who would be teaching or learning from the unit.

All teachers can be required to meet the objectives of the unit, but the means of achieving those goals can be completely at the discretion of the individual teacher. One teacher can choose to use the suggested content, activities, evaluations, and resources; another can use any means desired as long as the objectives are achieved. In this way the objectives are clear, accountability is possible, and the program is given a chance without placing undue restrictions on the teaching professionals.

If a unit approach is not used, it still is imperative that the systems chosen to develop curriculum and methodology must result in teachers' getting clear ideas of what is expected of them in specific terms. They should have suggestions available that include many optional ways to achieve the objectives and to evaluate the degree of learning that takes place. Appropriate materials not only should be made available but their presence must be made known to the teachers.

Since most schools seem to be taking the infusion approach to career education, it is of utmost importance that the planning be done with more care and precision than in the past. There are few career education textbooks on which teachers can rely when they are told to implement career education. Initially, few teachers will be as committed to that program as they are to their subject matter fields. They simply will not give time to some fuzzy idea that someone calls career education. If career education is important enough to be advocated, it is important enough to be given a fighting chance by using some principles of change and curriculum development in a deliberate and specific process.

Five sources are suggested to assist in career and vocational curriculum and program development for LBP adolescents: Brolin, 1978 and 1982; Brolin and Kokaska, 1979; Meers, 1980; and Miller and Schloss, 1982.

VOCATIONAL EDUCATION

Although vocational education has been an integral part of the American educational system since around World War I, handicapped youths have had limited opportunities to be involved until legislation during the 1960s and 1970s recognized the need to provide vocational and career education and employment opportunities to the disabled. These legislative changes are forcing school districts that had not been operating vocational programs for the handicapped to make such classes available to them.

440   EDUCATING ADOLESCENTS WITH LEARNING AND BEHAVIOR PROBLEMS

The next sections cover (1) definitions of vocational education, (2) stages of vocational education, (3) program adjustments needed to assist students in vocational education, (4) vocational placement options, and (5) the role of vocational educators.

Definitions of Vocational Education

Professional workers in vocational education have not suffered from the lack of an operational definition that has afflicted those involved with career education. Several definitions have emerged in the more than 60 years that vocational education has been in existence. The most recent definition and the one used in this chapter is from Title 45 U.S. Code of Federal Regulations (1979):

> The term "vocational education" means organized educational programs which are directly related to the preparation of individuals for paid or unpaid employment, or for additional preparation for a career requiring other than a baccalaureate or advanced degree; and, for purposes of this paragraph, the term "organized education program" means only, (a) instruction related to the occupation or occupations for which the students are in training, or instruction necessary for students to benefit from such training, and (b) the acquisition, maintenance, and repair of instructional supplies, teaching aids and equipment, and the term "vocational education" does not mean the construction, acquisition, or initial equipment of buildings, or the acquisition or rental of land. (p. 166)

Most definitions include components such as an organized program of instruction, vocational guidance and counseling, structured learning experiences in prevocational instruction, related academic instruction, work-related experiences, and follow-up.

A certain amount of confusion still exists among professional groups regarding the definition of vocational education and its relationship to career education. Because of this confusion, the distinction between vocational and career education developed by Brolin and Kokaska (1979) is presented in Exhibit 13-1.

Much of the confusion about career education can be attributed to the attempt by professionals to distinguish it from vocational education. According to Evans (1975), "the easiest way to describe the relationship between career education and vocational education is to point out that all of the latter is part of the former." (p. 1)

Stages of Vocational Education

A considerable number of LBP students suffer not only from social and academic lag but also from vocational developmental discontinuity. Unlike aver-

Exhibit 13-1 Differences between Career Education and Vocational
Education

Career Education	*Vocational Education*
Focuses on paid and unpaid work (e.g., volunteer, leisure and recreation, homemaking)	Focuses on paid work (although unpaid work is referred to in the Vocational Education Amendments)
Emphasizes general career skills	Emphasizes occupational preparation
Promotes cognitive, affective, and psychomotor skill development	Promotes psychomotor skills for entry into occupational society
Meets the needs of the learners	Meets the needs of the labor market
Is a systemwide effort, not specific courses or an instructional program	Is defined in terms of courses and is an instructional program
Is taught by all educators	Is generally taught by vocational educators
Focuses on all instructional programs at all levels of education	Focuses on the secondary and post-secondary levels
Involves family, agencies, and business/industry	Involves primarily business/industry

Source: Reprinted with permission from *Career Education for Exceptional Children and Youth* by D.E. Brolin and C.J. Kokaska, The Charles E. Merrill Publishing Company, Inc., 1979, p. 102.

age students who are enrolled in regular or vocational programs, LBP adolescents often are denied or excluded from programs. The longer the interruption from vocational education, the more critical will be the long-range educational and vocational problems that the students face. Consequently, the development of an integrated academic vocational program must be viewed as a means through which related learning experiences are introduced and taught. The integration of the two formerly separate curricula can be an effective mechanism for acceleration (Brolin & D'Alonzo, 1979).

Besides failing to provide a system that integrates all of the curricular experiences, the majority of programs proceed inadequately through the essential steps for orienting LBP adolescents to the world beyond home and school. Orientation must be supervised and structured toward exposure to the full range of opportunities that will better prepare them for the adult world of work.

The following four stages of experiences are recommended for the handicapped, commencing at the elementary grade levels.

Occupational Awareness

This experience provides for self and career awareness of academic needs and career availability in the community. The experiences can be accomplished through field trips, movies, videotaping, printed materials, cassette slide presentations, guest speakers, simulation, and role-playing activities. This stage of experiences is designed for grades K-6.

Occupational Exploration

This is a limited involvement program that provides students an opportunity for formal observation of a career setting or settings. The youths' involvement may include visual observation, verbal interaction, and/or limited task performance. The observational experience is provided in a community business or industrial environment as an integral part of the classroom instruction. The emphasis is placed on students in grades 7 to 9 but does not exclude other grade levels.

Occupational Work Experience

This is designed to provide direct experience at a learning center in actual or simulated work situations. These programs may be one of two kinds: (1) exploratory in terms of learning about a variety of careers, or (2) employability skill training to learn attitudes, responsibility, cooperation, and skill application in an occupational area. School personnel assist students in the determination of learning objectives to be attained, job placement, and supervision. The worksite or training station may be at a retail store, industry, or rehabilitation workshop. The related academics usually are directly related to the work experiences but occasionally may have more global application to daily life experience. This type of program is designed for students grades 9 to 12 (D'Alonzo & Barrett, 1977).

Cooperative Vocational Education

This is the most refined form of work education, blending related classroom instruction, on-the-job-training, and coordinated follow-up involving home, school, and employer. Occupational skill development, skill application, and/or internships characterize this program. While working in the community, the students are closely supervised on the job by a person designated by the employer or employing agency and by a staff member assigned as coordinator from the school. This program is designed for students grades 10 to 12.

These work-oriented programs and the related academics comprising the curriculum require a sophisticated organizational system to implement them effectively into school, community, and business-industrial settings. Organizational areas that need to be considered to ensure the effective placement of students in the least restrictive educational environment are:

1. Who will provide the supervision of the student?
2. How will the student be transported?
3. How will the school schedule be arranged?
4. What related classes are needed?
5. How will graduation credit be given for these experiences?
6. During what time of the school day will the student be assigned to these phases?
7. What type of student involvement is recommended in each of these phases?
8. What is the end product (student) at the completion of these phases?
9. What type of evaluation system will be used and who will conduct the assessment of the program components?

Program Adjustments

Before LBP adolescents are integrated into vocational programs, several adjustments may have to be made in the overall effort. Teachers must receive inservice training and be prepared to accept the students, not only physically but psychologically. Another fundamental element is the understanding that these students have a right to vocational programs if they can benefit from them. Other important adjustments to be made, if they are not already an integral part of existing vocational programs, include:

- inservice education for all personnel involved with the student
- individualization of instruction
- flexibility in scheduling
- additional time for the students to complete assignments and develop vocational skills
- follow-along personnel to tutor and help the students adjust
- special education consultants to the vocational educator
- orientation periods during the academic year and special summer programs so the students can get a feel for vocational education and the vocational educator for them
- modification of textbooks, technical manual content, instruction, machinery, equipment, or methods
- peer tutoring, buddy systems, programmed learning, minicourses, instructional packages
- extended school day and year programs, evening and weekend courses

- extensive use of audiovisual equipment and materials, e.g., movies, overhead projectors, filmstrips, cassette slide projectors, videotaping, television, radio, record players, cassette tape recorders, opaque projectors, Tutorgram
- alternate grading and testing procedures

Vocational Placement Options

In addition to institutional routine and curriculum adjustments, a variety of placement options must be available in the institutions serving LBP adolescents to guarantee least restrictive placement for them. Davis and Ward (n.d.) list alternative placements that must be available to implement individualized education programs for handicapped students in vocational education:

Placement in regular vocational classroom:
  Consultative assistance for teacher
  Provision of direct services to students by itinerant specialists
  Resource room help for students

Placement in separate vocational classroom:
  Student is in regular class part-time
  Self-contained class in regular education facility
  Self-contained class in special education facility

Placement in a sheltered environment:
  Residential
  Hospital
  Other institution
  Sheltered workshop
  Work activities center

Placement in work study or cooperative education program

Homebound instruction. (p. 42)

An example of one area vocational school's placement options was reported by Linari in 1974:

Full-time programming at the vocational/technical facility with resource assistance as required

Cooperative education at the vocational/technical facility with work arrangements for seniors

One-half day at the vocational/technical facility and one-half day in public school

One or two year training programs at the vocational/technical facility

Prevocational experience arrangements for eighth and/or ninth grade students on a part-time basis for exploration purposes

After-school training programs at the vocational/technical facility with academic instruction at the area public schools

Satellite-community programs in which students participate in community-based vocational instruction and receive limited academic work at the vocational/technical facility

Substantially separate programs at the vocational/technical facility.

Students who remain unserved by the vocational/technical facility should receive vocational education through other options made available by the home school.

Role of Vocational Educators

Vocational education teachers who have special students enrolled in their classes must be able to perform a variety of tasks to ensure the appropriate delivery of services to these youths. A General Accounting Office (1976) report reveals that in 78 percent of the school districts sampled nationally, vocational educators were insufficiently trained in special education skills. Only 2 percent of the school districts reported that nearly all of their vocational staff (81 percent to 100 percent) were sufficiently trained. In a national survey, Phelps and Clark (1977) list the 12 highest ranked of 49 tasks that vocational education special teachers must perform to be effective with handicapped students, including those with learning and/or behavior problems. These top 12 tasks require these teachers to:

1. Identify instructional techniques appropriate for special needs learners.
2. Provide reinforcement for learning.
3. Evaluate and upgrade the effectiveness of instruction.

4. Analyze students' occupational interests.
5. Plan a sequence of modules or units of instruction according to the learners' needs.
6. Coordinate with instructional planning in academic areas for students with learning problems (reading, math, and other academic areas required for graduation).
7. Develop instructional materials for special needs learners.
8. Provide career counseling and guidance.
9. Select or modify instructional materials appropriate for different special needs learners.
10. Develop individual student performance goals and objectives.
11. Collaborate with other educators, specialists, and parents in evaluating the learners' educational needs.
12. Identify available assessment instruments appropriate for special needs learners. (p. 43)

Special and vocational educators working collaboratively must at least have an understanding of the general structure of each other's discipline even if they do not know the details of its application. This gives each group an interpretive knowledge and enhances the services provided for the students. Increased integration of the handicapped is needed and new approaches must be initiated if they are to be given equal educational experiences that are relevant, possible, meaningful, and satisfying and that lead them to productive roles in society.

CAREER AND VOCATIONAL SERVICE MODELS

Adolescents with learning and behavior problems usually have more program options available to them in the secondary schools than they had at the elementary level. The options most frequently available that are related to career and vocational education at the secondary school level are:

1. career education
2. career and vocational counseling
3. cooperative vocational education
4. vocational classes
5. special needs vocational education programs
6. industrial arts
7. in-school work experience
8. community-based work experience
9. career and vocational evaluation
10. vocational rehabilitation

Most conceptual models that professionals have advocated include these components. Examples are models developed by Bailey and Stadt (1973); Brolin (1974); Brolin and Kokaska (1979); Clark (1979); and D'Alonzo (1978a, 1981). These models primarily involve school-based and community-based career and vocational education experiences. The original career education models formulated by the U.S. Office of Education (1971) incorporate four major service areas: (1) the School-Based Comprehensive Career Education Model; (2) the Employer-Based Career Education Model, later changed to the Experience-Based Career Education Model; (3) the Rural-Residential Model; and (4) the Home-Based Career Education Model.

Each of these was designed to give professionals a wide range of options in delivering career and vocational experiences to individuals.

School-Based Model

The School-Based Comprehensive Model contains a sequenced program of experiences as the student progresses from kindergarten through 12th grade. The student acquires through these experiences an understanding of self and others; occupational awareness; positive attitudinal development toward school, work, and society; the relationship and relevance of school to work; personal development skills; and a salable skill for employment after completion of formal schooling.

Experience-Based Model

This model emphasizes provisions for a system of comprehensive delivery of service to curriculum alternatives for disadvantaged, alienated, potential drop-out, or unmotivated adolescents traditionally found in drop-out prevention and alternative school programs. Many of those students enrolled in special needs vocational programs also would be served through this type of model.

Rural-Residential Model

This model provides a structure to serve rural families who were underemployed or unemployed. Services offered are educational, basic skill acquisition, and remedial as well as standard schooling opportunities. Counseling and essential family and homemaking skill development are incorporated to help the family members become more functional and independent in their communities.

Home-Based Model

The conceptual framework for this model is designed for adults who have completed, or dropped out of, school or are not employed. The major emphasis areas are to use the home and community for training and counseling, develop more career and work-related opportunities, and provide for personal, social, and life-role development.

CAREER EDUCATION MODELS

Career education models have been developed as an optimal service delivery system for the handicapped by Brolin and Kokaska (1979), Clark (1979), and D'Alonzo (1978a). Each of these models expands the options that traditionally have been available to adolescents in special education programs. These programs primarily have involved occupational education or prevocational experiences and work-study programs. These program options usually were available only to the mentally retarded in special education programs based in public schools (D'Alonzo, 1977). The authors listed above are in agreement as to the components needed to deliver effective programming to the handicapped in career and vocational education.

Brolin and Kokaska Model

This model is developed around 22 major competencies—Number (1) on the Model—and 102 subcompetencies, clustered in three primary domains: (1) Daily Living Skills, (2) Personal-Social Skills, and (3) Occupational Guidance and Preparation—Number (4) on the Model. The 22 major competencies are:

1. Managing family finances
2. Selecting, managing, and maintaining a home
3. Caring for personal needs
4. Raising children, family living
5. Buying and preparing food
6. Buying and caring for clothing
7. Engaging in civic activities
8. Utilizing recreation and leisure
9. Getting around the community (mobility)
10. Achieving self-awareness
11. Acquiring self-confidence
12. Achieving socially responsible behavior
13. Maintaining good interpersonal skills

14. Achieving independence
15. Achieving problem-solving skills
16. Communicating adequately with others
17. Knowing and exploring occupational possibilities
18. Selecting and planning occupational choices
19. Exhibiting appropriate work habits and behaviors
20. Aquiring physical-manual skills
21. Obtaining a specific occupational skill
22. Seeking, securing, and maintaining employment

This three-dimensional model contains an interface with the 22 competencies, the stages of career development (Awareness, Exploration, Preparation, and Placement/Follow-up)—Number (3) on the Model—and School, Family, and Community Experiences—Number (2) on the Model.

The model is designed for professional and lay personnel to alert them to the various elements to be considered in a student's career development. Brolin and Kokaska's model is called "A Competency-Based Model for Infusing Career Education into Curriculum" (Figure 13-1).

Clark Model

This model is based on four content-area components with instruction and learning experiences beginning at the kindergarten level and continuing through adulthood. The four components that are the foundation of the model are: (1) Values, Attitudes, and Habits; (2) Human Relationships; (3) Occupational Information; and (4) Acquisition of Job and Daily Living Skills. These components change in scope and sequence as pupils pass through the grades or as mastery of the objectives is achieved. Clark calls his model "A School-Based Career Education Model for the Handicapped" (Figure 13-2).

D'Alonzo Model

The basic premise of this model is that if educators are to be able to advance students effectively from the point of initial school entry to the completion of formal classes, a system for movement between these two points must be in operation. The belief is that if the learning experiences provided in the school system in the form of a curriculum are sequential, developmental, goal directed, published for districtwide dissemination, and evaluated for efficacy and modification, the first prerequisite of a comprehensive program is available. The second and equally important prerequisite is the system through which these students are transported, such as the physical plant, teaching stations, and learning environments.

Figure 13-1 Competency-Based Infusion Model

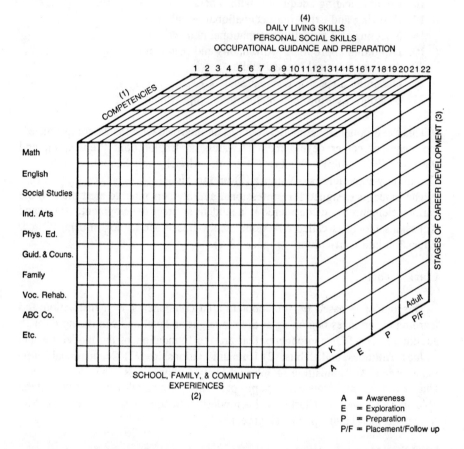

Source: Reprinted with permission from *Career Education for Handicapped Children and Youth* by Donn E. Brolin and Charles J. Kokaska, The Charles E. Merrill Publishing Company, Inc., © 1979.

This model contains seven basic environments, each separate but necessary to the development of the others. Training of personnel that will be involved in career and vocational education is the focus of the first two environments. The next four contain the components for a series of structured learning experiences either through separate programming, infusion, or a combination of both. (This is accomplished in the various continuum-of-service options described in Chapter 5.) The last environment contains the postschool opportunities available to the handicapped. D'Alonzo calls his effort "A Career Educational Model" (Figure 13-3).

Figure 13-2 School-Based Career Education Model

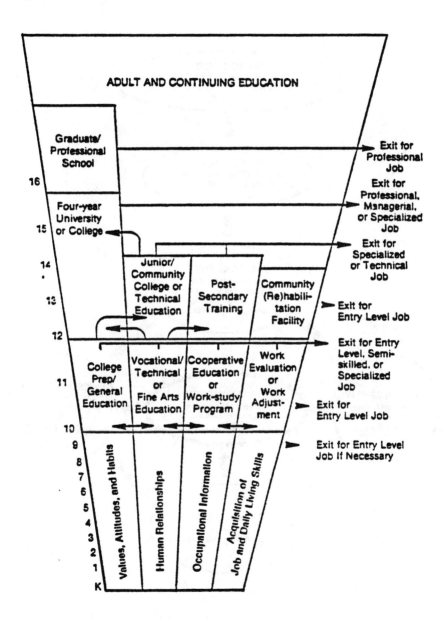

Source: Reprinted with permission from *Career Education for the Handicapped Child in the Elementary Classroom* by Gary Clark, Love Publishing Company, © 1979.

Figure 13-3 Career Education Model

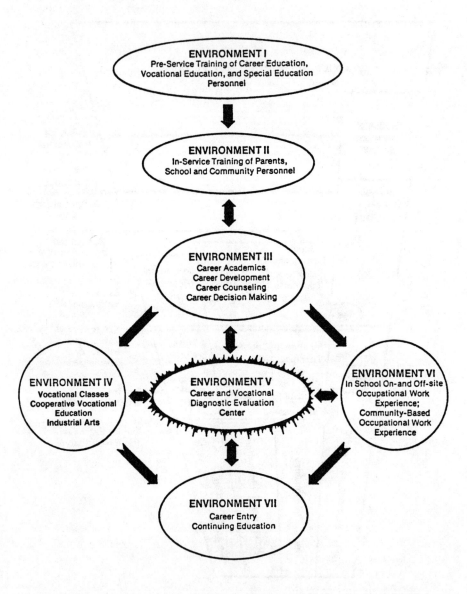

Source: Reprinted with permission from "Career Education for Handicapped Youth and Adults in the 70's" by Bruno J. D'Alonzo, *Career Development for Exceptional Individuals,* 1978a, 1-9.

OTHER OPTIONS

The authors of this chapter advocate combining the components of the School-Based Comprehensive Model with the Experience-Based Career Education Model. These combined approaches will enable students to pursue their career development in a more effective way. Exhibits 13-2 and 13-3 contain the components of a comprehensive delivery of service system that includes those of both models. The matrix in Exhibit 13-3 was developed by the members of the National Panel on High School and Adolescent Education (Martin, 1976). This matrix contains structured components and learning situations that can be made available to students through integrated school-based and community-based collaborative learning experiences. The National Panel encourages community-based government-supported programs that generate resources, provide citizen commitment, and are performance based.

Among the panel's many recommendations is the creation of a community-based career education center. Each center would serve as a clearinghouse and vehicle for new forms of community-based vocational education, work experiences, on-the-job-training, job-finding resources, and career information activities. To enhance these opportunities for adolescents the panel urges the removal of regulations other than minimum wage or safety and health requirements, including tax and insurance penalties that the panel feels impede and restrict the employment of these youths. The panel further recommends that federal and state subsidies for high school vocational classes be made transferable at local options to various on-the-job-training, job placement, and job subsidy programs. Unfortunately these recommendations have not been implemented except indirectly through legislated monies or because of professionals independently taking the initiative to change their existing programs.

This decentralized approach is not intended to replace the formal education structure at the high school level but can provide diverse learning experiences in a community for the students. The panel provides this word of caution:

> For out-of-school learning opportunities to be most educationally significant for their participants, they have to be designed and operated as independent but integral parts of the total educational environment of adolescents. Thus, effective experience-based learning opportunities and programs must operate neither as a replacement for the existing high school nor as a mere adjunct to it. For community-oriented experiences to be viable components of the adolescent education system, the emphasis in their development should be on opening up alternative educational structures and experiences, not on offering diversity for its own sake or as a substitute for structure in general. Such an approach is necessary if out-of-school learning experiences are to be more than game-playing or officially sanctioned truancy. (Martin 1976, p. 57)

Exhibit 13-2 School-Based and Experience-Based Career and Vocational Education Model

Grade Level	General Education	Career Education	Vocational Education	Special Education	Vocational Rehabilitation
Postsecondary	Adult Continuing Education University-College Community College Technical School-College Apprenticeship Programs Employment Program (CETA/YEDPA)[1] Career Resource Centers	Adult Continuing Education University-College Community College Technical School-College Apprenticeship Programs Employment Program (CETA/YEDPA) Career Resource Centers	Adult Continuing Education University-College Community College Technical School-College Apprenticeship Programs Employment Program (CETA/YEDPA) Career Resource Centers Mobile Occupational Education Unit	Adult Continuing Education University-College Community College Technical School-College Apprenticeship Programs Employment Program (CETA/YEDPA) Career Resource Centers Mobile Occupational Education Unit Vocational Rehabilitation Facility	Adult Continuing Education University-College Community College Technical School-College Apprenticeship Programs Vocational Evaluation Center Vocational Rehabilitation Facility Agency or Association Workshop
Secondary 9-12	Academic Subjects in General-College Preparatory Industrial Arts Extracurricular Activities Career Resource Centers Employment Program (CETA/YEDPA)	Career Preparation 11-12 Career Orientation 9-10 Employment Program (CETA/YEDPA)	Apprenticeship Programs Mobile Occupational Education Unit Cooperative Vocational Education Vocational Education Centers Vocational Education Special Needs Occupational Work Experience Occupational Exploration Occupational Awareness Extracurricular Activities Employment Program (CETA/YEDPA)	Vocational Education Special Needs Mobile Occupational Education Unit Vocational Evaluation Work-Study (Community/School) Industrial Arts Prevocational Skills Special Subjects Basic Skill Subjects Extracurricular Activities Employment Program (CETA/YEDPA)	Vocational Rehabilitation Facility Agency or Association Workshops Vocational Evaluation Cooperative Agreement for Clients 16 Years+

Junior High	Academic Subjects Industrial Arts Extracurricular Activities	Career Exploration	Prevocational Skills In-School Work Special Subjects Basic Skill Subjects Extracurricular Activities
Elementary **K-6**	Academic Subjects Basic Skill Subjects Extracurricular Activities	Career Awareness	Prevocational Skills Special Subjects Basic Skill Subjects Extracurricular Activities

[1]Comprehensive Employment and Training Act (CETA)
Youth Employment and Demonstration Projects Act (YEDPA)

Exhibit 13-3 Matrix of Experience-Based Learning Situations and Structural Components

STRUCTURAL COMPONENTS \ LEARNING SITUATIONS	Regular Jobs	Community Service Activities	Schools-Without-Walls	Internships in Public Agencies	Apprenticeships	Artistic Performance Opportunities	Action Learning* (with associated academic study)	Public Action Activities	Curriculum-Based Learning Projects Involving Concrete Experiences	Structuring Experience-Based Learning Opportunities for Other Youth
1. PAYMENT										
a. No pay										
b. Partial or subsidized payment										
c. Full payment										
2. ADMINISTRATIVE SUPERVISION										
a. Full school supervision										
b. Joint institutional supervision										
c. Full supervision by non-school institution										
3. FUNDING SOURCE										
a. School										
b. Joint institutional funding										
c. Non-school institution										

4. ACADEMIC CREDIT

a. Full credit

b. Partial credit

c. No credit

5. AMOUNT OF PARTICIPANT INVOLVEMENT

a. Part-time

b. Full-time

6. DEGREE OF PROGRAM AUTONOMY

a. Integrated with academic curriculum

b. Related to academic curriculum

c. Independent of academic curriculum

7. PROGRAM CONTROL

a. Student-controlled

b. Joint student-adult controlled

c. Adult-controlled

8. PROGRAM IDENTIFICATION

a. Participant identification with and responsibilities to the program itself

Exhibit 13-3 continued

STRUCTURAL COMPONENTS \ LEARNING SITUATIONS	Regular Jobs	Community Service Activities	Schools-without-Walls	Internships in Public Agencies	Apprenticeships	Artistic Performance Opportunities	Action Learning (with associated academic study)	Public Action Activities	Curriculum-Based Learning Projects Involving Concrete Experiences	Structuring Experience-Based Learning Opportunities for Other Youth
8. PROGRAM IDENTIFICATION (cont.)										
b. Participant has no special status in the non-school setting which derives from the program										
9. PROGRAM PATTERNING										
a. A general program model										
b. Each experience individually negotiated										
10. CROSS-CULTURAL EMPHASIS										
a. Efforts to provide participants with such contacts										
b. No particular efforts										
11. PERSONAL REFLECTION OPPORTUNITIES										
a. Provision of opportunities for participant reflection on the experience										

Source: Reprinted from *The Education of Adolescents: The Final Report and Recommendations of the National Panel on High School and Adolescent Education* by John H. Martin, U.S. Government Printing Office, 1976, pp. 54-56.

The use of the school and career and vocational centers must be available to students through an extended school day (evenings) and an extended school year (summers). Collaborative efforts in program options with vocational/technical schools and colleges, community colleges, and university-based instructional efforts would be a viable addition to the enhancement of career opportunities for adolescents. These efforts should result in better student orientation and feelings toward continuing education opportunities.

STATE OF THE ART

Hoyt et al. (1974) state that only a few school-based career education efforts reflect an adequate research base. Brolin and Kolstoe (1978) agree that, when comparing traditional programs with career education, there is no proof that the latter are more effective. One document that contains many of the research studies that have been conducted in career and vocational education is by Brolin and Kolstoe (1978).

Hoyt (1982) predicts an especially bright future for career education because of the endorsement and support provided by special educators. Hoyt believes, "The professional expertise and high levels of involvement in both conceptualizing and delivering career education on the part of such experts has played a significant role in the positive evolution of the career education movement" (p. 12).

In summarizing accomplishments by educators who have implemented career education in schools, Hoyt and High (1982) describe these actions succinctly under three major general goals:

1. With respect to the goal of providing persons with 10 general employability skills:
   Strong evidence that career education can deliver:
      Skills in understanding and appreciation of the private enterprise system;
      Skills in self-understanding and in understanding of educational/ occupational opportunities;
      Skills in overcoming bias and stereotyping as deterrents to full freedom of career choice;

   Promising, but not yet conclusive, that career education can deliver:
      Improvement in basic academic skills;
      Skills in developing and using personally meaningful work values;
      Career decision-making skills;
      Job seeking/finding/getting/holding skills;

Evidence largely lacking that career education can deliver:
   Skills in practicing good work habits;
   Skills in making productive use of leisure time;
   Skills in humanizing the workplace for oneself.

2. With respect to the goal of increasing community/school system linkage efforts in the work/education relationships domain, evidence is very strong that career education can and is meeting that goal.
3. With respect to the goal of changing the education system through inserting a "careers" emphasis throughout the K-12 curriculum, evidence is very strong that this can occur and, when it does, it receives very wide support from many diverse segments of the total community.

This listing essentially contains a summary of the occurrences in career education over the last decade or so.

Career and vocational education are viable educational experiences that should be provided to LBP adolescents. However, in view of issues raised in this chapter, a definite need exists to expand the opportunities available in these areas to such persons. Several options have been discussed; others need to be developed, and increased utilization of existing ones should be explored.

Three ways to improve and expand these opportunities would be to (1) include career and vocational education annual goals and short-term objectives in each handicapped student's IEP, (2) include career and vocational education components as an integral part of staff development at all levels of the educational system, and (3) increase the career and vocational education aspects of training educational personnel in teacher education programs.

SUMMARY

The information, strategies, and issues presented in this chapter should provide you with a solid fundamental foundation about career and vocational education. Definitions, information about the various approaches used for the education of LBP adolescents, and strategies presently being advocated for implementation can be found in this chapter as can several models, exemplary programs, and organizational structures to improve upon career and vocational education programs already in existence. Lastly, materials and methods for use by classroom teachers are provided.

It is hoped that this chapter will generate more interest among professionals, parents, leadership personnel, and legislators so that the movement of career and vocational education will continue into all sectors of American life—especially in the schools. This should occur because of the leadership in existence throughout the various levels of educational and governmental agencies.

Chapter 14

Alternate Educational Service Models for LBP Adolescents

Janice M. Schnorr, Bruno J. D'Alonzo, and David A. Sabatino

INTRODUCTION

Public school districts since 1975 have been functioning under tremendous pressure to implement Public Law 94-142. In the past, school administrators merely had to state that they simply could not meet the needs of adolescents with learning and behavior problems, and parents were forced to make one of two decisions: either enroll their children in private schools in order to obtain educational services, or keep them at home. Now that public school district administrators no longer can abdicate service responsibilities, they are attempting to better meet the needs of these students through a variety of service models in their districts. Differing patterns of instructional delivery have implications for the mainstreaming of these youths. Among the more popular of these arrangements is the alternative school.

ALTERNATIVE SCHOOLS

Alternative schools have been used to a large extent as a means of providing greater structure within a specific context that deals with individuals' behavior as well as their need for learning. The instructional strategies of such institutions usually are quite distinct from those in the public schools' general education program. However, while this form of organizing to facilitate learning has the characteristics of a mainstream setting, it also very quickly takes on the properties of a segregated special education.

The educational value of alternative programs is to: (1) the students, (2) society, and (3) the educational community. Once again, a major educational movement has been instituted that is not based on data.

461

Following are analytical comments on the alternative school trend:

1. "Alternative programs were developed because the traditional program was *not* serving all youth satisfactorily" (Coleman et al., 1966).

2. "Alternative programs were developed because 17.1 percent of the secondary school-age youth dropped out or were excluded from attendance" (Washington, 1973).

3. "Alternative programs were developed because 10.9 percent of the secondary school-age youth are known to be handicapped, while 6.9 percent are in fact being served" (National Center for Educational Statistics, 1978).

4. Alternative programs were developed because the attitude of the traditional educator was one of focusing on the general and vocational programs, not student function. General and vocational achievement was viewed as a privilege, not a right; therefore, failure was held by many to be a self-determined act of the student, not a factor beyond that youth's control.

5. Traditional programs treat all students equally, generally lock stepping them into the same curricula, without adjustment, regardless of ability, reading level, motivational factors, or internal adjustment factors.

6. Traditional programs emphasize the development of giftedness or talent in the order of their exaggerated value system, first, for the gifted athlete; second, the academically talented; and third the social role learner with talent to interrupt a democratic (so-called) society.

7. Alternative programs provide for ethnic, cultural, and linguistic differences; their development is an insistence that no one curriculum is suitable for all students all the time. "To insist that there is only one curriculum is to confuse the means of education with the end" (Silberman, 1970, p. 9).

8. Alternative programs provide students with a choice, and frequently they provide the majority (students) with the right to make and enforce the rules, not the majority (school officials). Alternatives are a part of the American heritage, the opportunity to refute tradition, and stand for a more self-fulfilling satisfactory alternative.

9. "Alternative programs frequently are not 'full-blown alternatives' to the traditional program; they merely offer an improvisational and, in many instances, last-resort alternative program to those students who had failed to respond to conventional schooling" (Shanker, 1972).

10. Alternatives are just that—various types of programs—not a specific program. Therefore, when educators talk in general about alternative curricula, they really are discussing alternatives as program types, e.g., schools without walls, minischools, schools within schools, dropout cen-

ters, schools for special learners, open schools, ethnic-centered schools, self-programming opportunities. The term alternative school is generic in the fullest sense of the word.

SELECTED ALTERNATIVE SCHOOL PROGRAMS

Alternative school approaches can be effective, as indicated by the following examples of alternative programs available in various cities across the country.

SAIL Project (Student Advocates Inspire Learning)
Hopkins School District #270
2400 Lindbergh Drive
Minnetonka, Minnesota 55343

SAIL is designed to help students cope academically, socially, and emotionally in an integrated school environment. The youths are assessed as emotionally disturbed, exhibit numerous behavior problems, and often are involved in the juvenile justice system.

Bellefaire School
22001 Fairmount Boulevard
Cleveland, Ohio 27013

The treatment at Bellefaire is an integrated program of group living, education, and psychotherapy designed to meet the unique needs of each child and family. Bellefaire School is an integral part of the Bellefaire Residential Treatment Center. It is an official public school serving adolescents 8 to 18. The students are severely behaviorally handicapped and multiply handicapped. Some have been involved in the juvenile justice system. Generally speaking, they are of average or above-average intelligence.

Longfellow Education Center
3017 East 31st Street
Minneapolis, Minnesota 55406

The Longfellow Education Center (LEC) is designed to serve multiply handicapped youths ages 11 to 16 who exhibit serious emotional disturbances. Its goals are to (1) provide appropriate psychoeducational diagnostic services; (2) provide an intensive, daily self-contained educational program for youths whose emotional disturbance is a primary handicap; (3) maximize their reentry to a less restrictive environment; and (4) provide behavioral training, family support, and counseling and referral services for student and family. LEC is a self-contained, 100 percent special education day placement. As students progress, they are moved into a program designed to integrate them into a less restrictive environment.

SPRING (Special People Realizing Individual New Goals)
892 Vedado Way, N.E.
Atlanta, Georgia 30308

SPRING's first goal is to serve severely emotionally disturbed youths over 14. Its second and third goals are to orient agencies, schools, and decision makers to the needs of these youngsters and to serve a limited number of severely emotionally disturbed adolescents and their families. The purpose of psychoeducational treatment utilizing the SPRING model is to teach emotionally disturbed adolescents how to survive in society outside of institutions and, it is hoped, to make a contribution to society.

The Starr Commonwealth Schools
Alternative Education Program (AEP)
RR #2, Box 84
Van Wert, Ohio 45891

As a comprehensive children's organization, Starr Commonwealth provides alternative day school programs, family and child guidance clinics, and residential programs for emotionally and socially maladjusted young people ages 14 to 18. A socioeducational strategy is designed to create a positive student culture. The goals are (1) positive teacher-student relations, (2) positive peer group relations, (3) positive relations with parents and community, and (4) positive academic achievement and attitudes.

LIFE Center
6701 Fortuna Road N.W.
Albuquerque, New Mexico 87105

This school serves students of high school age with a wide range of academic abilities. The majority are low achievers and all are potential dropouts. About 50 percent have some type of behavior problem. The entire curriculum is based on the alternative schools philosophy that believes strongly in the process of education. Product is not emphasized. Parent, student, and staff all are involved in the IEP, and the final decision is left up to the youths on a contractual basis.

Walbridge Academy
Grand Rapids Public Schools
1024 Ionia, N.W.
Grand Rapids, Michigan 49503

The students enrolled at Walbridge have normal range IQs, are underachievers, have had behavioral and academic problems, and have been labeled potential dropouts. The goals of Walbridge are to (1) increase reading and math skill levels, (2) improve attendance, (3) help students earn credits toward a high school diploma, (4) increase socially desirable behaviors, (5) increase decision-making skills, and (6) improve self-image.

Kansas City Youth Diversion Project
4th Floor, City Hall
Kansas City, Missouri 64106

The Kansas City Youth Diversion Project is a demonstration program designed to compare alternative approaches to delivering youths from the juvenile justice system. The ages of those served range from 10 to 16, of whom 60 to 70 percent have learning disabilities and have been enrolled previously in school but are not attending.

Project CITE (Crisis Intervention Techniques for Education)
Terrell I.S.D.
Department of Special Services
212 West High Street
Terrell, Texas 75160

Project CITE is a hospital program designed to help youths 6 to 21 who have been referred by a local agency. The primary handicapping condition presented is serious emotional disturbance, with a secondary handicapping condition being learning disabilities. Some of CITE's objectives are to improve social interaction, to facilitate change in maladaptive behavior, and to develop therapeutic relationships with students and family to facilitate growth and change in youth and family response.

Open Education

Another variation in delivering instruction to LBP adolescents is the concept of Open Education. This is predicated on an informal structure that believes that students by nature are learners with the potential to be self-directive if placed in an environment where resources are available to facilitate their learning. Unlike many alternative schools where structure is very much a part of the organization to promote learning, the Open School enables youths to influence their own learning environment and have input into the structure in which the education will occur.

Year-Round School

Still another concept that is receiving greater and greater support in organizing for the improvement of learning is that of the year-round school. This has a particular implication for individuals with learning and behavior problems because it affords the school an opportunity during the summer months to provide adolescents with a variety of experiences other than the usual academic type. Jensen (1969) offers several suggestions about the year-round-school concept that should be kept in mind in light of the U.S. Court of Appeals decision—*Armstrong v. Kline*, 476 F. Supp. 583 (E.D. Pa. 1979) on the 180-day rule which resolved in favor of summer school for profoundly mentally retarded persons when regression can be demonstrated. Some of Jensen's suggestions are that: (1) more teachers will have the opportunity to be employed for 12 months; (2) the curriculum can be restructured to become more flexible, effective, and relevant; and (3) delinquency and school vandalism that historically crest during the summer months should be reduced.

Other court decisions have focused the attention of professionals on year-round programming for the handicapped (*Armstrong v. Kline*, 1979; *Battle v. Commonwealth of Pennsylvania*, 1980; *Bernard v. Commonwealth of Pennsylvania*). Teachers and parents historically have expressed concern about the disruption of instruction and student regression in summer. It becomes imperative that special educators do their homework by developing appropriate strategies for year-round educational programming. Key points in the development of programs for the extended school year are made by Larsen, Goodman, and Glean (1981):

1. The need for clear eligibility criteria.
2. The need to base eligibility determinations on valid and reliable student performance data.
3. The need to reduce the number of students who need extended school year programs through effective instructional programs and parent/home involvement.
4. The need to explore the use of alternative service models to encourage instruction in naturalistic settings.
5. The need to clearly identify funds and funding mechanisms for extended school year programs and to operate programs cost effectively. (p. 262)

It will become necessary for local school districts and state education agencies to take the initiative to develop appropriate policies and guidelines to implement these policies for year-round schooling.

PRIVATE SCHOOL PROGRAMS

Under some circumstances, appropriate placement within the district is not feasible, so contracting with private facilities is undertaken. Since there is a paucity of information on private schools, a major portion of this section seeks to fill the gap by addressing issues regarding selection and evaluation criteria for those schools. The section is divided into three major parts: (1) the purpose and characteristics of private schools, (2) criteria that can be used to evaluate their services, and (3) lists of private schools in the United States (and three in Canada) along with some demographic data.

As mentioned, private schools for years served as the only educational opportunity for students who were excluded from public education prior to the adoption of P.L. 94-142. With that act, and the subsequent proliferation of services in public schools, it might be concluded that private schools would lose enrollment and be forced to close. This, however, does not appear to be the trend. Four factors appear to influence a reversal:

1. Many small rural districts are unable to meet the needs of handicapped students in their community so they frequently contract with private schools and/or larger districts for services.
2. School districts, irrespective of size, usually make every effort to meet the needs of students in their boundaries first. Where this cannot be accomplished, contracts with private schools are solicited to ensure that students receive the required services.
3. Parents become disenchanted with the educational services available to their teen-agers and request that the school district pay for services in private facilities.
4. Some districts are using a voucher system that allows parents to choose the school they prefer.

These factors indicate that private schools will continue to be available to meet future needs and that public school personnel will have to become cognizant of the types of services provided by each private facility. Public schools also have to be able to determine the efficacy of those services so they can make appropriate recommendations to parents and district personnel. The characteristics of private schools, and procedures to evaluate them, are described in the next two sections. Professionals can use this information to assist parents in making placement decisions about their adolescents.

CHARACTERISTICS OF PRIVATE SCHOOLS

The growth of private schools for LBP adolescents has paralleled federal legislation. This movement started with the advent of the field of learning disabilities. In 1963, after the term "learning disability" was coined by Dr. Samuel Kirk at the annual meeting of the Conference on Exploration into the Problems of the Perceptually Handicapped Child, a series of events occurred that gave impetus to private school involvement with LBP adolescents.

During the same period a special steering committee was planning and delineating the objectives of three task forces on minimal brain dysfunction (Clements, 1966), a term that now has been replaced by the term learning disabilities. Upon completion of the reports in 1969, U.S. Senator Ralph Yarborough of Texas introduced what became the Children with Specific Learning Disabilities Act of 1969 and became law in 1970 as part of the Elementary and Secondary Educational Amendments of 1969 (P.L. 91-230). This act amended Title VI (known as the Education of the Handicapped Act of 1967) of the Elementary and Secondary Education Act of 1965 by providing authority to the U.S. Office of Education to fund programs for the learning disabled.

A few private schools were organized during the 1960s, but the most dramatic increase occurred in the 1970s, in part because of federal financial incentives. These, plus federal insurance programs, e.g., Civilian Health and Medical Program of the Uniformed Services (CHAMPUS), led to a surge of private schools to be opened during the early 1970s. CHAMPUS is a federal insurance program that pays for educational services required by handicapped children and adolescents of military personnel. Numerous private schools formerly solicited such individuals almost exclusively. CHAMPUS provided a valuable service to LBP adolescents prior to P.L. 94-142. However, a reorganization of CHAMPUS and the implementation of P.L. 94-142 have dramatically affected the enrollment of these types of schools because the responsibility for education and financial assurances has been mandated to the public schools.

Financial Considerations

The financial component of such private schooling generally puts a strain on the family budget; however, concerned parents are willing to make such sacrifices for their children because they feel compelled to provide an educational experience of some sort. Tuition and fees at private day schools range from $1,000 to $7,000 a year and in private boarding schools from $8,000 to more than $30,000. Some schools, categorized as tax-exempt corporations, grant full or partial scholarships to a limited number of families in order to maintain that tax advantage. Such benevolence is relatively rare, however. The expenses of private schools continue to increase just as do those of public schools. Economically, private schools must be self-sustaining or they go bankrupt. Private schools, particularly for the severely handicapped, always will be more expensive than public education. Traditionally, schools organized by parents attempt to provide maximum services at minimum cost. At the other extreme are private schools, usually operated by professionals, that provide quality services for a seemingly exorbitant amount of money. Although the tuition and fees may seem outrageous at first glance, an inspection of the financial records usually documents them as valid expenditures.

Tuition and fee schedules vary greatly. Clinic schools that provide tutoring on an hourly basis tend to charge the least. Day schools that offer a full day of educational instruction rank the next higher, and residential schools that provide a live-in academic setting are the most expensive. Table 14-1 summarizes tuition and fee schedules for the 1978-79 academic year taken from a nationwide sample of private schools by Schnorr (1978).

In some cases, private schools are supported at least in part through contracts with public school districts that cannot and/or prefer not to provide such services. Leary School, Inc., of Falls Church, Va., is one such facility. More than half of its enrollment is reserved for handicapped children from the Fairfax County Public Schools System (Marsh, Gearheart, & Gearheart, 1978).

Contracting of services with private schools and facilities is becoming more prevalent now that school districts have been charged with providing for all

---

Table 14-1 Tuition and Fee Schedules of Selected Private Schools

(1978-1979 Academic Year)

Tuition Range	Day Schools	Residential Schools
1,000 - 1,999	3	0
2,000 - 2,999	4	0
3,000 - 3,999	9	0
4,000 - 4,999	14	0
5,000 - 5,999	5	0
6,000 - 6,999	2	0
7,000 - 7,999	0	2
8,000 - 8,999	0	0
9,000 - 9,999	0	3
10,000 - 15,999	0	2
16,000 - 20,999	0	2
21,000 - 29,999	0	2
30,000 +	0	1

Note: The median cost is $4,000 for day schools and $9,925 for residential schools.

handicapped children. In many states, such contracting is common now in educating the trainable mentally retarded who in the past were simply institutionalized. In some cases, particularly in small school districts, it is financially infeasible to attempt to initiate an entire program for one or two students, so outside agencies are hired.

Occasionally the expenses for private schooling are paid directly by parents who have become dissatisified with the services their public school district has provided. If they are financially able to afford the expenditure, they simply pay the costs and do not request reimbursement from the public schools.

Growth of Private Schools

The number of private schools and facilities for the handicapped has been increasing dramatically in recent years. Public awareness and concern for the disabled have spurred a desire to create a better life for them. This increase in humanitarianism, coupled with federal legislation and financial support, has acted as an incentive in the development of a number of private schools.

The general pattern of growth is similar in all sections of the United States. Initially, LBP adolescents were simply identified. In most districts, programs for them did not exist so parents banded together to voice their concerns. In some cases, clinics were formed to meet the needs of these students to keep operational costs at a minimum. These clinics usually were managed by special education personnel, remedial reading teachers, and school psychologists who wished to supplement their incomes. Adolescents usually attended their local high school during the day, then reported to the clinic for an additional hour or so of tutoring in a specific problem area. Clinic programs have been very popular and probably will continue to thrive as long as parents feel that only a little extra assistance is necessary.

Private day and residential schools also have increased in numbers, the reverse of the trend for private preparatory schools, many of which have been forced to close for financial reasons, especially during high inflationary years. Other preparatory schools have attempted to capitalize on the individualized education concept by opening their doors to all students, including the handicapped, as long as the problems are not severe. LBP adolescents enrolled in such settings probably would be readily identified and often ostracized by other students.

Grading Philosophy

The school's grading philosophy may dramatically affect services that LBP students receive. If the school has a reputation for scholastic excellence, students may be required to meet minimum proficiency standards that they are unable to attain. Under these circumstances, most schools provide special tutoring to all who need it. Youths who benefit from the program are encouraged to remain in school while those who fail are advised to complete the last year or two of their program at some other school. From this standpoint, tuition and fees from the LBP students provide supplemental financial support necessary for operating but allow the school administration to effectively disown all failures before the senior year in order to uphold their academic tradition.

Enrollment Considerations

Some prep schools have opened their doors to LBP adolescents and are providing supportive services as needed. This type of arrangement is quite common among recreationally oriented schools. These are in areas of the country that foster participation in specific recreational activities such as skiing, horseback riding, or camping. Many of these schools have suffered drastic enrollment declines since the late 1970s.

Prep schools are not the only ones so afflicted. Special education schools catering to highly specific groups also have encountered this problem. In some cases, the schools were founded to serve learning disabled students but, during a period of declining enrollment, often included other handicapped types. This generally was done without making major changes in the existing staff. These schools now serve a wider range of handicapped students than they intended originally.

Of the 150 facilities listed in the *Directory of Educational Facilities for the Learning Disabled* (1978), 67 responded to a survey instrument (see Exhibit 14-1). Twenty-five indicated that they served learning disabled students exclusively, ten handled those with behavior and learning problems, and the remaining 32 provided for youths with handicaps including mental retardation and physical disabilities (Schnorr, 1978).

Enrollment figures of private schools and facilities generally reveal two facts: (1) that the total per school and/or facility is smaller than in most public schools, and (2) that the student-to-teacher ratio is lower. Tutoring clinic enrollments range from three or four students per week to 300 or more in large metropolitan areas. The student-to-teacher ratio usually ranges from one-to-one to 10 students to one teacher in residential and day schools.

Curricular Considerations

Curricular emphases vary considerably from school to school. Most private schools stress academic subjects such as reading, writing, and mathematics. During the last year or two of schooling, the curricular emphases may more directly reflect daily living skills. These include the mechanics of balancing a checking and savings account, planning and managing a budget, and using credit.

Such programs are designed to prepare students to function adequately in the world upon graduation from high school without the need for additional training.

Many schools and facilities are incorporating a vocational component in their program (see Chapter 13). Students are exposed to information on vocational choices and are encouraged to participate in work/study programs. Specific vocational skills are taught, and academic skills are practiced as they relate to vocational needs. From this standpoint, these students usually are more highly motivated than they would be in a traditional academic program.

Another curricular emphasis is recreation, particularly at prep schools that have solicited LBP students in order to remain solvent. In these instances, academic instruction takes place during the school day, and numerous recreational opportunities are available outside the classroom. The environmental advantages are stressed heavily.

Accreditation Considerations

No matter what the curricular emphases might be, most reputable private schools establish credentials with a recognized accrediting agency such as the NAPSEC (The National Association of Private Schools for Exceptional Children). In addition, since the passage of P.L. 94-142, most schools also have obtained state accreditation.

Private schools generally seek state accreditation only if federal and state subsidy programs for the handicapped will become available to them if they gain such certification. They then qualify for state reimbursement based on the average daily attendance (ADA) of handicapped students. They must employ teachers who are certifiable in such curricula.

Private schools also must adhere to all state guidelines regarding placement and services. An appropriate educational plan must be included before an LBP student is placed in a private school. An in-depth evaluation and educational plan must be delineated for parents so they will be cognizant of the scope of the services to be provided. The factors presented in Exhibit 13-2 (supra) that may influence placement decisions are described next.

EVALUATION CRITERIA FOR PRIVATE SCHOOLS

When evaluating a private school for possible placement, it is crucial to analyze all facets of the operation. A mere visit to a school, and resulting initial impressions, should not be the only criteria for placement. Rather, an in-depth analysis should be undertaken. Once the analysis is completed, a comparison can then be made to determine which school might best serve the needs of a particular student. Exhibit 14-1 lists 49 questions that can be used in evaluating a private facility.

Exhibit 14-1 Evaluation Criteria for Private Schools

A. *Accreditation*
  1. Has the facility been approved by an accrediting agency?
     Yes   No
     If *yes*, list the agency _____
  2. What criteria does the agency utilize?
     _____
     _____

B. *Ownership and Control*
  1. Who are the owners? _____
     _____
  2. Who is the director? _____
     _____
  3. Does the facility have a board of directors?
     Yes   No
     If *yes*, list their names and relationships:
                                             Child enrolled in school
     _____   Yes   No
     _____   Yes   No
  4. If you as a parent have a complaint to register, with whom should you discuss it?
     _____
  5. If your child has a complaint, with whom should it be discussed?
     _____
  6. Who has responsibility for disciplinary action? _____
  7. What type of disciplinary action is taken against students who break rules? _____
     _____

C. *Financial Stability*
  1. How much is the annual budget? $_____
  2. What percentage of the annual budget is utilized for administrative overhead? ____
  3. What is the salary schedule for teachers?
             First-year teachers _____
             Second-year teachers _____
             Experienced teachers _____
             Other categories _____
             Total budget _____
  4. What is the average salary for public school teachers? _____
  5. How many years has the school been in operation? _____
  6. What portion of the total budget is financed through tuition and fees paid by parents and/or school districts? _____
  7. What portion of the budget is financed through gifts? _____
  8. Is the facility a tax-exempt organization? Yes   No
     If *yes*, how much does it allocate toward student scholarships? _____

D. *Staff Credentials*
  1. Does each teacher possess a Bachelor's Degree in the area of teaching responsibility?
     Yes   No

Exhibit 14-1 continued

(List each teacher's name, teaching responsibility, and degree(s))
Teacher   Degree
_____
_____
_____

2. How many teachers are in their first or second year of teaching? _____
3. How many teachers have at least three years of experience? _____
4. How many teachers possess advanced degrees? _____
5. How many teachers possess state certification credentials in the area of their teaching responsibility? _____
6. Does the facility have a licensed school psychologist or counselor on staff? Yes   No
   If *yes*, indicate services provided:
   Testing   Yes   No
   Group Counseling   Yes   No
   Individual Counseling   Yes   No
   Family Counseling   Yes   No
7. Does the facility have licensed medical personnel on staff? Yes   No
   If *yes*, indicate personnel below:
   Medical Doctor   Yes   No
   Registered Nurse   Yes   No
   Practical Nurse   Yes   No
   Physical Therapist   Yes   No
   Occupational Therapist   Yes   No
   Others _____
8. If medical services are not available, what provisions are made? _____
   _____
9. Where is the closest hospital? _____
10. Does the school carry liability insurance? Yes   No
    If *yes*, specify amount _____

E. *School Accommodations*
   1. What type of facility is it?
      Clinic _____
      Day School _____
      Residential school _____

F. *Cost of Services*
   1. How much does the service cost?
      Per hour _____ group _____ individual _____
      Per semester _____
      Per year _____
   2. How much do additional services cost?
      Weekly allowance? _____
      Recreational expenses? _____
      Testing costs? _____
      Private tutoring? _____
   3. When are payments to be made?
      Beginning of each semester _____

Exhibit 14-1 continued

    Month by month _____

    Other _____

  4. If you withdraw your child from the school, how much of your payment will you receive as a refund? _____

    When will you receive the refund? _____

G. *Characteristics of the Student Population*

  1. How many normal or nonhandicapped students are enrolled in the school? _____

  2. How many handicapped students are enrolled in the school? _____

  3. How many handicapped students in each category are enrolled in the school?

    Learning disabled? _____ Blind? _____

    Behavior problems? _____ Deaf? _____

    Mentally retarded? _____ Physically

    Other? _____ handicapped? _____

  4. How many years has the school been serving these categories of handicap? _____

  5. How many girls are enrolled in the school? _____

  6. How many students fall into each age range below?

    6-9   _____

    9-12   _____

    12-15   _____

    15-18   _____

    18-21   _____

H. *Educational Plan*

  1. Does the school advocate that a staffing be held prior to placement?

    Yes   No

  2. Does the school advocate that an Individualized Education Plan (IEP) be developed prior to placement?   Yes   No

  3. Does the school advocate that you, as the parent, participate actively in the IEP?   Yes   No

  4. Does the school advocate that public school personnel participate actively in the IEP?   Yes   No

  5. Does the school provide you with a copy of the IEP?

    Yes   No

I. *Daily Schedule*

  1. In what subjects will your child be enrolled, how much time will be devoted to each, and how many other students will be enrolled in each?

Subjects	Time per week/day	Student Enrollment

J. *Program Emphases*

  1. Based on the daily schedule above and other recreational opportunities available, what emphases seem to be stressed?

    Academic subjects? _____ Social skills? _____

    Vocational skills? _____ Self-help skills? _____

    Recreational skills? _____ Daily living skills? _____

Exhibit 14-1 continued

K. *Orientation to the School*
1. Does the school recommend that you visit it before enrolling a student?
   Yes   No
2. Does the school recommend or allow you to speak with parents who have students enrolled in the school?
   Yes   No
   If yes, do the parents recommend the services?
   Additional Comments: _____

   _____

3. Does the school recommend or allow you to speak with students who are enrolled in the school?
   Yes   No
   If yes, do the students like the atmosphere and do they feel that they are benefiting from the service?
   Yes   No
   Comments: _____

   _____

4. Does the information printed in the school brochures agree with information obtained from your personal interviews?   Yes   No   Discrepancies _____

   _____

Accreditation

First, it is absolutely necessary to determine whether the school has been approved by any accrediting agency. If so, it is essential to verify the credential and the criteria for approval.

Ownership and Control

Knowledge of ownership and administrative control is of paramount importance because those factors reflect curricular emphases and other school policies. Some private schools are operated as tax-exempt corporations managed by a board of directors composed of parents who originally desired services for their children. In some of these corporations, the board establishes the policies, which a director administers. From this standpoint, the board may mandate academic emphases to the exclusion of other activities. If one individual is the sole owner of the school, the curricular emphases probably reflect that person's personal educational philosophy.

Administrative control in small private schools is relatively easy to analyze because all teachers are accountable to the director. However, in larger schools, the chain of command may not be clear. If the school has a large faculty, it is important to ascertain various roles and responsibilities so as to ensure effective delivery of services. Thus, if problems do develop, the causes can be pinpointed and rectified easily. It is helpful if students can become familiar with the chain of command also so they can learn to deal effectively with the social problems they might be expected to encounter.

Financial Stability

The annual budget should be examined for the following pieces of information:

- What percentage of the budget goes for administrative overhead? If more than 20 percent is spent in this area, the private school should be asked to justify the expenses. An inflated administrative line may indicate that certain persons are being paid a disproportionately high income in relation to the services they provide. That can cause tuition fees to be excessive and/or prevent the school from obtaining trained personnel because of budget limitations.
- What are the salaries of the faculty? These should be compared to those of public school personnel in the area. If they are higher in the private school, the administration can hire highly qualified persons from nearby public schools if it so desires. On the other hand, if the administration is unable to pay higher salaries, it might be forced to employ less acceptable teachers because many would prefer to work for the public schools. This is particularly important during periods of economic uncertainty.
- How long has the private school been in existence? The longer its survival, the easier it is to evaluate it because it will have stood the test of time.
- What is the school's financial base? It is important to know how much of the budget is supported through tuition and fees paid by parents and/or school districts. Most private schools are supported almost entirely by this means. Such institutions are required to give scholarships to deserving students.
- Does the school have a large proportion of handicapped students and meet state accreditation standards? If it does, it may qualify for state ADA support. With large enrollments, this could form a considerable portion of the capital needed for the yearly budget.

Additional sources of income for the school might include government grants, trusts, and gifts.

Staff Credentials

Qualified personnel are essential in providing services to LBP adolescents. An untrained parent or regular education teacher simply does not possess the competencies necessary to deal effectively with the educational and behavioral problems that will confront them. As a matter of fact, more harm than good can result in situations where untrained personnel attempt to guide students through a program.

Simply being concerned about students and caring for them does not solve their problems. Specific intervention strategies that only professionals are familiar with will remedy the myriad of problems that most such students face. For this reason, it is of paramount importance that the professionals who provide services to LBP students be trained in a specific area. Several indexes can be used to determine the extent of their preparation.

One method is to review the college degrees of all persons responsible for instructional activities. Do all teachers have at least a bachelor's degree? If so, are they trained in an appropriate area of special education, e.g., behavior disorders, mental retardation, or learning disabilities? Most teachers, after several years in the classroom, return to a university to update their knowledge and skills. A key factor is whether any have other advanced degrees. Those who have several years of teaching experience generally become more effective as time passes. This is not always the rule, however, as some first-year and second-year teachers far surpass even the most experienced practitioners.

State certification or licenses offer another means of evaluating professional expertise. In some states, teaching credentials are difficult to obtain because numerous methods courses must be completed before individuals can be certified in a specific area. As a consequence, some teachers who move to a different state may experience difficulty obtaining a new credential. Even though they may possess a master's degree, they may be required to complete additional courses to qualify for a standard teaching certificate. Schools that solicit state ADA reimbursement usually require that all teaching personnel possess valid state credentials.

When state credentials are examined, each area of certification should be reviewed. Is the teacher qualified to teach LBP students? Is there a certified counselor and/or school psychologist who provides the counseling services? Is the person who is administering various tests qualified to do so? If medical services are provided on site, is the person a registered nurse and/or physician? If no medical services are available on site, what happens when emergencies arise and who is legally liable?

School Accommodations

The types of private school accommodations vary greatly along with cost of the services, which is discussed later. There are three basic types of services: (1) the clinic, (2) the day school, and (3) the residential school.

The clinic offers tutoring services to students on a part-time or hourly basis. The students usually attend a public school for the major portion of the school day, if not the whole day, then report to the clinic for additional assistance with their assignment and/or remedial work in the academic subjects and in perceptual development.

In contrast, the private day school requires full-day attendance, after which students return home.

The residential model is similar to the day school except that students live on campus and do not return home each afternoon.

Cost of Services

As mentioned, the costs of services vary considerably. Therefore, it is important to determine budget constraints, if any, when selecting a program. The most reasonably priced program is the clinic model. Its price may vary from $7 at university operated clinics to $30 an hour at private ones, depending on the type of services and the qualifications of the persons providing them. Group instruction usually is less expensive than individual instruction. The individual tutoring rate also may be less when a student is tutored by a beginner or teacher. After a tutor has several years of experience and/or an advanced degree, the hourly rate generally increases.

Tuition and fees for day and residential schools are considerably higher than those of clinics. Of the two, a day school is less expensive. Residential costs are inflated by ancillary personnel expenses or by capital outlays. As noted in Table 14-1 (supra), based on calculations from 49 private schools throughout the United States and Canada, the median for day schools is $4,000, for residential schools $9,925 (Schnorr, 1978).

Some schools tack on additional charges for extracurricular activities such as horseback riding and backpacking. Other schools require that parents supply $10 or more per week for students to use at their own discretion. Whatever the charges may be, it is important to determine whether any refunds are given to parents for unused services. Thus, if a student is withdrawn from school during the middle of a semester, will the unused portion of the tuition for that semester be refunded? A considerable sum ($5,000 or more) could be involved.

Characteristics of the Student Population

The characteristics of a private school's student population should be examined. A breakdown of specific areas of handicaps might reveal that nearly 75 percent of all students enrolled have no problems and only 25 percent are handicapped. If that is the case, the school might not be prepared professionally to deal with the problems of handicapped adolescents.

In the past, some schools catered to specific handicapped groups; however, during periods of economic instability, enrollment privileges were extended to other disabled populations. Thus, if parents request information about a school that caters to only students who have learning and behavioral problems, they should not be referred to one that includes other handicapping conditions. An analysis of the population by sex enrollment may be necessary, particularly if the student is a girl. Most schools cater to male populations, and placement in such an environment could create additional problems.

Educational Plan

According to P.L. 94-142, every handicapped student must have an individualized education plan (IEP). In most cases, these plans are developed by the public schools. However, over a period of time, if parents become disenchanted with public school progress and transfer the student to a private school, the IEP will have to be rewritten to reflect that change. In such situations, the private institution must communicate with the public school so it can write a plan that can help the student to return eventually to the public school. Parents should participate actively in this process and should receive a copy of the plan for their records.

Daily Schedule

A daily schedule should be a part of the IEP. The subjects offered and the amount of time that will be devoted to each on a daily basis should be ascertained. In addition, the director should be asked how many students will be enrolled in each class. Large enrollments may reduce teaching effectiveness and should be avoided whenever possible.

Program Emphases

After the schedule is examined, the program emphases can be analyzed. If all courses reflect academic subjects, the program obviously is academically oriented. Not all students will benefit from such a program; some may profit more from a vocationally oriented one. If so, a school that incorporates career awareness activities and vocational training into the daily schedule should be selected. The preparation for life orientation is reflected in the development of leisure time skills, e.g., sports and other activities, and social skills. Unfortunately, specific goals and objectives in these areas often are overlooked.

Orientation to the School

Before placement into any program is recommended, the school should be visited first. The parents and the prospective student should spend a minimum of one day on site to develop a feeling for the atmosphere of the learning environment. Most of the questions previously discussed can be posed at that time. In addition, parents should have an opportunity to discuss the program with other parents who have students enrolled in the school to determine whether they are satisfied with the services. They also should have an opportunity to speak with students.

Copies of information brochures regarding the school should be solicited, and the information they contain should be compared with that obtained through other sources. This serves as a validity check on publicity and may indicate a measure of the ethical standards of the school's administration.

Although the information defined in the preceding section may take considerable time and effort to compile, it is crucial that such an evaluation be conducted in order to protect the student and the financial investment. All placement decisions should be weighed carefully in favor of the criteria that are most important for each student. Weightings are expected to vary as are the decisions on schools. One school probably will not be able to meet the needs of all students requiring special placement.

DIRECTORY OF PRIVATE SCHOOLS

Many public school educators are unfamiliar with private schools that may meet the needs of some of their students. One of the best resources available is the *Directory of Educational Facilities for the Learning Disabled* (1978), published by Academic Therapy. One problem with that list is that it provides only limited information regarding the schools' services and other characteristics. In an effort to clarify and expand on that information, a mail questionnaire was sent to 150 of the directory's facilities that appeared to provide services to adolescents with learning and behavior problems. Data from 66 responses to the questionnaire are summarized in Exhibit 14-2. This may assist professionals in identifying or eliminating prospective placements for their students.

Exhibit 14-2 Additional Services Provided by Private Schools That Enroll
Adolescents with Learning and Behavior Problems

	Alphabetically by States	
Name & *Location*	*Handicaps* *Enrolled*	*Curricular* *Emphases*
UNITED STATES		
Gables Academy 3134 Cottage Hill Road Mobile, Alabama 36606	LD	Math, reading, language, social studies, English-writing,[1] science, art, physical education, skills of daily living, career awareness, perceptual therapy, speech therapy, and physical therapy
Devereux Day School & Clinic 6404 East Sweetwater Scottsdale, Arizona 85254	LD, EH, MH	Math, reading, language, English-writing, art, physical education, skills of daily living, career awareness, vocational training
Brighton School & Diagnostic Center P.O. Box 32104 Phoenix, Arizona 85064	LD, EH	Math, reading, language, social studies, English-writing, science, art, skills of daily living, career awareness, psychological therapy
Special Learning Center The College of the Ozarks 415 College Avenue Clarksville, Arkansas 72830	LD	Reading, social studies, English-writing, science, art, physical education, foreign language, skills of daily living, career awareness, social skills, emotional adjustment
Exceptional Children's Foundation 2225 West Adams Boulevard Los Angeles, California 90018	TMR, LD, EH, MH	Math, reading, language, social studies, English-writing, art, physical education, skills of daily living, vocational training
Ellen K. Raskob Learning Institute 3520 Mountain Boulevard Oakland, California 94619	LD	Math, reading, language, social studies, English-writing, science, art, physical education, skills of daily living, music, drama
Hillside Developmental Learning Center 1223 Verdugo Boulevard La Canada, California 91011	LD	Math, reading, language, social studies, English-writing, science, art, physical education, career awareness, visual and auditory perceptual training

Exhibit 14-2 continued

Language Associates 3408 Dearhill Road Lafayette, California 94549	LD	Math, reading, language, English-writing, physical education, career awareness
Poseidon School 11811 West Pico Boulevard Los Angeles, California 90064	LD, EH	Math, reading, language, social studies, English-writing, science, art, physical education, vocational training, and counseling
California School of Learning Systems 5140 Country Lane San Jose, California 95129	EMR, LD, MH	Math, reading, language, social studies, English-writing, science, art, physical education, skills of daily living, career awareness
Clinic for Learning Evaluation and Remediation 834 Mission Avenue San Rafael, California 94901	LD	Math, reading, language, English-writing, skills of daily living, career awareness
The Devereux Foundation P.O. Box 1097 Santa Barbara, California 93102	EMR, TMR, LD, EH, PH, MH	Math, reading, language, social studies, English-writing, science, art, physical education, skills of daily living, vocational training, psychotherapy
Melmed Clinic Inc. 957 Dewing Avenue Lafayette, California 94549	LD, VH, D/SH	Math, reading, language, social studies, English-writing, skills of daily living
Wilshire West School and Learning Center 1145 Twenty-Fifth Street Santa Monica, California 90403	LD, EH	Math, reading, language, social studies, English-writing skills, science, art, physical education, skills of daily living, career awareness, vocational, driver education, typing
Sabin-McEwen Learning Institute, Inc. P.O. Box 6518 Carmel, California 93921	LD	Math, reading, language, English-writing, skills of daily living
Escalon, Inc. 536 East Mendocino Altadena, California 91001	EMR, LD, EH, MH	Math, reading, language, social studies, English-writing, science, art, physical education, skills of daily living, career awareness, vocational training

Exhibit 14-2 continued

Name & Location	Handicaps Enrolled	Curricular Emphases
John Arena School 1314 Lincoln Avenue San Rafael, California 94901	LD, MH	Math, reading, language, social studies, English-writing skills, science, art, physical education, career awareness, vocational training
Almansor Education Center 9 North Alamansor Street Alhambra, California 91801	LD, EH, MH	Math, reading, language, social studies, English-writing, science, art, physical education, skills of daily living, career awareness, vocational training
Bond Street School for Learning Disabilities 4450 Bond Street San Diego, California 92109	LD, EH, PH	Math, reading, language, social studies, English-writing, science, art, physical education, skills of daily living
Aseltine School 4027 Normal Street P.O. Box 33185 San Diego, California 92103	EMR, LD, EH, MH	Math, reading, language, social studies, English-writing, art, physical education, skills of daily living, career awareness
Skill School Residential Treatment Center Route 1 Box 253A Henderson, Colorado 80640	LD, EH	Math, reading, language, English-writing, science, art, physical education, skills of daily living, vocational training
A & D Life Education Center 288 Clayton Street Suite 202 Denver, Colorado 80206	LD, EH, MH	Math, reading, language, English-writing, art, physical education, skills of daily living, career awareness, GED (General Equivalency Diploma) preparation
Denver Academy 320 South Sherman Denver, Colorado 90209	LD, EH, MH	Math, reading, language, social studies, English-writing, science, physical education, history
Benhaven 9 St. Ronan Terrace New Haven, Connecticut 06511	MH	Language, physical education, skills of daily living, vocational training

Exhibit 14-2 continued

Hall-Brooke 47 Long Lots Road Westport, Connecticut 06880	EH, LD	Math, reading, language, social studies, English-writing, science, art, physical education, foreign language, skills of daily living, career awareness
Becket Academy River Road East Haddam, Connecticut 06423	LD, EH	Math, reading, language, social studies, science, physical education, skills of daily living, vocational training
Grove School Box 646 Madison, Connecticut 06443	EH	Math, reading, language, social studies, English-writing, science, art, physical education, foreign language, skills of daily living
Southern Academy 5801 Parker Avenue West Palm Beach, Florida 33435	LD	Math, reading, language, social studies, English-writing, science, art, physical education, skills of daily living
Gables Academy 6503 West Sunrise Blvd. Plantation, Florida 33313	LD	Math, reading, language, social studies, English-writing, science, physical education, skills of daily living, career awareness
Brandon Hall 1701 Brandon Hall Drive Dunwoody, Georgia 30338	LD	Math, reading, language, social studies, English-writing, science, physical education, foreign language, skills of daily living, career awareness
The Howard School, Inc. 1815 Ponce de Leon Avenue, N.E. Atlanta, Georgia 30306	LD	Math, reading, language, English-writing, physical education, career awareness
Cove School, Inc. 1100 Forest Avenue Evanston, Illinois 60202	LD	Math, reading, language, social studies, English-writing, science, art, physical education, skills of daily living, typing
Summit School, Inc. 611 East Main Street Dundee, Illinois 60118	LD	Math, reading, language, social studies, English-writing, physical education, skills of daily living, career awareness

Exhibit 14-2 continued

Name & Location	Handicaps Enrolled	Curricular Emphases
Brough Learning Center 1774 Georgetown Road Danville, Illinois	LD	Math, reading, language, social studies, English-writing, science, art, physical education, foreign language, career awareness, vocational training
Grove School 40 East Old Mill Road Lake Forest, Illinois 60045	TMR, LD, EH, MH	Math, reading, language, social studies, art, physical education, skills of daily living, career awareness, vocational training
The Berkshire Learning Center, Inc. Box 1224 Pittsfield, Massachusetts 01201	EH	Math, reading, language, social studies, English-writing, science, art, physical education, foreign language, skills of daily living, career awareness, vocational training
Riverview School Route 6A East Sandwich, Massachusetts 02537	EMR, LD	Math, reading, language, social studies, English-writing, science, art, physical education, skills of daily living, career awareness, prevocational training
Landmark School Prides Crossing, Massachusetts 01965	LD	Math, reading, language, social studies, English-writing, science, art, physical education, skills of daily living, career awareness, vocational training
The Carroll School Bahu Bridge Road Lincoln, Massachusetts 01773	LD	Math, reading, language, social studies, English-writing, science, art, physical education, skills of daily living
Braintree Saint Coletta Day School, Inc. 85 Washington Street Braintree, Massachusetts 02184	EMR, TMR, LD, MH	Math, reading, language, social studies, English-writing, science, art, physical education, skills of daily living, career awareness, vocational training
Brush Ranch School, Inc. Tererro, New Mexico 87573	LD	Math, reading, language, social studies, English-writing, science, art, physical education, skills of daily living, career awareness, vocational training

Exhibit 14-2 continued

Hebrew Academy for Special Children 1311 55th Street Brooklyn, N.Y. 11219	EMR, TMR, LD, EH, PH, MH	Math, reading, language, social studies, English-writing, science, physical education, skills of daily living, career awareness, vocational training
Summit School 339 North Broadway Upper Nyack, New York 10961	EMR, LD, EH	Math, reading, English-writing, science, art, physical education, skills of daily living, career awareness, vocational training
Bergen Center for Child Development 245 Tenafly Road Englewood, New Jersey 07631	LD, EH, MH	Math, reading, language, social studies, English-writing, science, art, physical education, skills of daily living, vocational training
Six Pence School, Inc. 3589 East Main Street Columbus, Ohio 43213	EMR, LD, EH, D/SH	Math, reading, language, social studies, English-writing, science, art therapy, physical education, skills of daily living, vocational training
Wordsworth Academy Camp Hill and Pennsylvania Avenues Fort Washington, Pennsylvania 19034	LD, EH, D/SH, MH	Math, reading, language, English-writing, physical education, skills of daily living, career awareness, vocational training, career counseling
Hickory Valley 6220 Hickory Valley Road Nashville, Tennessee 37205	LD	Math, reading, language, social studies, English-writing, science, physical education, skills of daily living, vocational training
Community Center for Citizens with Learning Disabilities 106 Wild Timber Drive Kerrville, Texas 78028	TMR, LD, EH	Reading, language, English-writing
Dallas Academy 950 Tiffany Way Dallas, Texas 75218	LD, EH, VH	Math, reading, language, social studies, English-writing, art, physical education, skills of daily living, career awareness
Lake Country Academy 6500 Shadydell Drive Fort Worth, Texas 76135	LD, EH	Math, reading, language, social studies, English-writing, science, art, physical education, foreign language, skills of daily living

Exhibit 14-2 continued

Name & Location	Handicaps Enrolled	Curricular Emphases
Leland Hall 27 Leland Road Norfolk, Virginia	LD	Math, reading, language, social studies, English-writing, science, art, physical education, foreign language, skills of daily living, career awareness, vocational training
Pinewood Academy R.R. 3 Eagle River, Wisconsin 54521	LD	Math, reading, language, social studies, English-writing, science, art, physical education, foreign language, skills of daily living, career awareness

CANADA

Name & Location	Handicaps Enrolled	Curricular Emphases
Reinex Educational Centre, Ltd. 143 Lakeshore Road East Oakville, Ontario L6J1H3	LD	Math, reading, language
The York Centre for Learning Disabilities 11225 Leslie Street R.R. #2 Gormley, Ontario L0H1G0	LD	Math, reading, language, English-writing, skills of daily living
St. Barnabas' School P.O. Box 583 R.R. #1 Fort Erie, Ontario L2A5M4	LD	Math, reading, language, social studies, English-writing, science, physical education, foreign languages, skills of daily living

Key:
D/SH = Deaf and Speech Handicapped
EH = Emotionally Handicapped
EMR = Educable Mentally Retarded
LD = Learning Disability
MH = Multiply Handicapped
PH = Physically Handicapped
TMR = Trainable Mentally Retarded
VH = Visually Handicapped

1. English-writing refers to grammar and expository writing.

SUMMARY

Private school programs will continue to be a viable alternative to public school enrollment for many adolescents with learning and behavior disabilities. Before these young people are placed in such facilities, it is imperative that parents and professionals collaborate in decisions affecting such students when private school enrollment is indicated. The information in this chapter should assist parents and professionals in need of data to support their decisions about private school placement.

Because parents increasingly are becoming disenchanted with the public school education provided to nonhandicapped as well as disabled adolescents, private school programs are growing throughout the United States. This chapter also presented information to help special education professionals in the public schools and those undergoing training become more aware of private schools and career opportunities that they may not have considered previously.

References

Abeson, A. The logic and the law for parent participation in the education of handicapped students. *Journal of Career Education,* 1978, *5,* 35-43.

Abeson, A., & Weintraub, F. Understanding the individualized education program. In S. Torres (Ed.), *A primer on individualized education programs for handicapped children.* Reston, VA.: The Council for Exceptional Children, 1977.

Abrams, J.C., & Kaslow, F.W. Learning disability and family dynamics: A mutual interaction. *Journal of Clinical Child Psychology,* 1976, *5,* 35-40.

Aiken, M.C. Evaluation theory development. *Evaluation Comment,* 1969, *2,* 2-7.

Alexander, A.B., & Parsons, B.V. Short term behavioral intervention with delinquent families. Impact on family process and recidivism. *Journal of Abnormal Psychology,* 1973, *81,* 219-225.

Alexander, R.N., Kroth, R.L., Simpson, R.L., & Poppelreiter, T. The parent role in special education. In R.L. McDowell, G.W. Adamson, & F. Wood (Eds.), *Teaching emotionally disturbed children.* Boston: Little, Brown and Co., 1982.

Algozzine, R.F., Alper, S.K., & Sabatino, D.A. Program and teacher evaluation. In D.A. Sabatino (Ed.), *Learning disabilities handbook: A technical guide to program development.* DeKalb, Ill.: Northern Illinois University Press, 1976.

Allen, K.E., Budd, K., Fowler, S., Peterson, N.L., Rowbury, T.G., & Thompson, B.J. The IEP: A practical priority in early childhood education. In B. Weiner (Ed.), *Periscope: Views of the individualized education program.* Reston, Va.: The Council for Exceptional Children, 1978.

Allen, R.C. *Legal rights of the disabled and disadvantaged.* Department of Health, Education, and Welfare, Social and Rehabilitation Services, SRS, Washington, D.C.: 1969.

Allen, R.C. The retarded offender: Unrecognized in court and untreated in prison. *Federal Probation,* 1968, *32,* 22-27.

Allen, R.C. Towards an exceptional offender's court. *Mental Retardation,* 1966, *4*(1), 3-7.

Alley, G., & Deshler, D. *Teaching the learning disabled adolescent: Strategies and methods.* Denver: Love Publishing Company, 1979.

Alley, G., & Foster, C. Nondiscriminatory testing of minority and exceptional children. *Focus on Exceptional Children,* 1978, *9*(8), 1-14.

Alper, T.G., Newlin, L., Lemoine, K., Perrine, M., & Bettencourt, B. The rated assessment of academic skills. *Academic Therapy,* 1973, *9*(3), 151-164.

491

American Psychiatric Association. *Diagnostic and statistical manual of mental disorders, DSM-III.* Washington, D.C.: American Psychiatric Association (1st ed.), 1952, (2nd ed.), 1968, (3d ed.), 1980.

American psychological association standards for educational and psychological tests. Washington, D.C.: American Psychological Association, 1966.

Anderson, D.R., Hudson, G.D., & Jones, W.G. *Instructional programming for the handicapped student.* Springfield, Ill.: Charles C Thomas, Publisher, 1975.

Arena, J. *How to write an I.E.P.* Novato, Calif.: Academic Therapy Publications, 1978.

Arizona Department of Education. *Career education matrix.* Phoenix, Ariz.: Department of Education, 1976.

Armstrong v. Kline, 476 F. Supp. 583 (E.D. Pa. 1979).

Arnove, R.F., & Strout, T. Alternative schools for disruptive youth. *The Educational Forum, 54,* 453-471, 1980.

Ashlock, R.B. *Error patterns in computation: A semi-programmed approach.* Columbus, Ohio: The Charles E. Merrill Publishing Co., Inc., 1976.

Ayllon, T., & Azrin, M. *The token economy: A motivational system for therapy and rehabilitation.* Englewood Cliffs, N.J.: Prentice-Hall, Inc., 1968.

Axelrod, S., & Palushka, J.A. A component analysis of the effects of a classroom game on spelling performance. In E. Ramp & G. Semb (Eds.), *Behavior analysis: Areas of research and application.* Englewood Cliffs, N.J.: Prentice-Hall, Inc., 1973.

Bailey, E.J. *Academic activities for adolescents with learning disabilities.* Evergreen, Colo.: Learning Pathways, 1975.

Bailey, L.J., & Stadt, R. *Career education: New approaches to human development.* Bloomington, Ill.: McKnight Publishing Company, 1973.

Bailey, S.K. *Disruption in urban public secondary schools.* Syracuse, N.Y.: Syracuse University Research Corporation, 1969.

Bachara, G.H., & Zaba, J.W. Learning disabilities and juvenile delinquency. *Journal of Learning Disabilities,* 1978, *1,* 58-62.

Bachman, J.G., O'Malley, P.M., & Johnston, J. *Youth in transition* (Vol. 6), Ann Arbor, Mich.: Institute for Social Research, 1978.

Bandura, A. *Principles of behavior modification.* New York: Holt, Rinehart & Winston, 1969.

Barlow, D.H., & Hersen, M. Single case experimental designs: Uses in applied clinical research. *Archives of General Psychiatry,* 1973, *29,* 319-325.

Bass, G.V. A study of alternatives in American education. *District policies and the implementation of change* (Vol. 1). Santa Monica, Calif.: The Rand Corporation, 1976.

Bateman, B.D. *The essentials of teaching.* Sioux Falls, S.D.: Adapt Press, 1971.

Battle v. Commonwealth of Pennsylvania, 629 F.2d 269 (3d Cir. 1980).

Bazleton, D.L., Boggs, E.M., Hilleboe, H.E., & Tudor, W.W. Report on the task force on law: The president's panel on mental retardation. Washington, D.C.: United States Government Printing Office, 1963.

Beare, D. Self-concept and the adolescent learning disabled student. Texas Personnel and Guidance Association, *TPGA Journal,* 1975, *4,* 29-32.

Becker, W.C. *Parents are teachers.* Champaign, Ill.: Research Press Co., 1971.

Becker, W.C., Englemann, S., & Thomas, D.R. *Teaching 1: Classroom management.* Chicago: Science Research Associates Inc., 1974.

Becker, W.C., Englemann, S., & Thomas, D.R. *Teaching 2: Cognitive learning and instruction.* Chicago: Science Research Associates, Inc., 1975.

Behan, E.F. A resource room program at the junior high school level. In *Successful programming: Many points of view. Proceedings of the Fifth Annual Conference of the Association for Children with Learning Disabilities,* Boston, 1968.

Behavioral characteristics progression (BCP). Palo Alto, Calif.: VORT Corporation, 1973.

Bendell, D., Tollefson, N., & Fine, M. Interaction of locus-of-control orientation and the performance of learning disabled adolescents. *Journal of Learning Disabilities, 13,* 83-86, 1980.

Bergin, A.E. Some implications of psychotherapy research for therapeutic practice. *Journal of Abnormal Psychology,* 1966, *71,* 235-246.

Bergin, A.E., & Strupp, H.H. *Changing frontiers in the science of psychotherapy.* Chicago: Aldine-Atherton, 1972.

Berman, A. *Incidence of learning disabilities in juvenile delinquents and nondelinquents: Implications for etiology and treatment.* Ann Arbor, Mich.: ERIC Clearinghouse, 1975. (ERIC Document Reproduction Service No. ED 112 620)

Bernard v. Commonwealth of Pennsylvania, 629 F. 2d 269 (3d Cir. 1980).

Besant, L. The Rodman experience with dropouts. *Today's Education,* 1969, *58,* 52-54.

Biklen, D. Myths, mistreatment, and pitfalls: Mental retardation and criminal justice. *Mental Retardation,* 1977, *15,* 51-57.

Biklen, O. *Let our children go: An organizing manual for advocates and parents.* Syracuse, N.Y.: Human Policy Press, 1974.

Blackhurst, A.E. Mental retardation and delinquency. *The Journal of Special Education,* 1968, *2,* 379-391.

Blake, K.A. *Teaching the retarded.* Englewood Cliffs, N.J.: Prentice-Hall, Inc., 1974.

Bloom, B.S., Engelhart, M.D., Furst, B.J., Hill, W.H., & Krathwohl, D.R. *Taxonomy of educational objectives. Handbook I: Cognitive domain.* New York: David McKay Company, 1956.

Bloom, B.S., Hastings, J.T., & Madaus, G.F. *Handbook on formative and summative evaluation of student learning.* New York: McGraw-Hill Book Company, 1971.

Bornstein, P.H., & Querillon, R.R. The effects of a self-instructional package on overactive preschool boys. *Journal of Applied Behavior Analysis,* 1976, *9,* 179-188.

Bracht, G.H., & Glass, G.V. The external validity of experiments. *American Educational Research Journal,* 1968, *5,* 437-474.

Briard, F.K. Counseling parents of children with learning disabilities. *Social Casework,* 1976, *57,* 581-585.

Brolin, D.E. *Programming retarded in career education.* Working paper No. 1, Project P.R.I.C.E. University of Missouri-Columbia: Department of Counseling and Personal Services, 1974.

Brolin, D.E. *Life-centered career education: A competency-based approach.* Reston, Va.: The Council for Exceptional Children, 1978.

Brolin, D.E. *Vocational preparation of persons with handicaps* (2nd ed.). Columbus, Ohio: The Charles E. Merrill Company, Inc., 1982.

Brolin, D.E., & D'Alonzo, B.J. Critical issues: Career education for the handicapped. *Exceptional Children,* 1979, *45,* 346-353.

Brolin, D.E., & Kokaska, C.J. *Career education for exceptional children and youth.* Columbus, Ohio: The Charles E. Merrill Publishing Company, Inc., 1979.

Brolin, D.E., & Kolstoe, O.P. *The career and vocational development of handicapped learners.* Columbus, Ohio: The National Center for Research in Vocational Education, 1978.

494 EDUCATING ADOLESCENTS WITH LEARNING AND BEHAVIOR PROBLEMS

Brolin, J.C., & Brolin, D.E. Vocational education for special students. In D. Cullinan & M.H. Epstein (Eds.), *Special education for adolescents: Issues and perspectives.* Columbus, Ohio: The Charles E. Merrill Publishing Company, Inc., 1979.

Brookover, W.B., Erickson, E.L., & Joiner, L.M. *Self-concept of ability and school achievement III. Relationship of self-concept and achievement in high school.* U.S. Office of Education, Cooperative Research Project No. 2831. Michigan State University, East Lansing Office of Research and Publications, 1967.

Brown, B.S., & Courtless, T.F. *The mentally retarded offender.* (DHEW Report No. (HSM) 72-9039.) Rockville, Md.: National Institute on Mental Health, 1971.

Brown, S.M., & Robbins, M.J. Serving the special education needs of students in correctional facilities. *Exceptional Children,* 1979, *45,* 574-579.

Brown v. Board of Education, 347 U.S. 483, 493 (1954).

Bruininks, V.L. Peer status and personality characteristics of learning disabled and nondisabled students. *Journal of Learning Disabilities,* 1978, *11,* 29-34.

Brutten, M. Vocational education for the brain-injured adolescent and young adult at the Vanguard School. In International approach to learning disabilities of children and youth. *Proceedings of the Third Annual Conference of the Association for Children with Learning Disabilities,* Tulsa, Okla., 1966.

Bryan, T.H. Peer popularity of learning disabled children: A replication. *Journal of Learning Disabilities,* 1976, *9,* 307-311.

Bryan, T.H. Social relationships and verbal interactions of learning disabled children. *Journal of Learning Disabilities,* 1978, *11,* 107-115.

Bryant, T.E. The effect of student failure on the quality of family life and community mental health. *Bulletin of the Orton Society,* 1978, *28,* 8-14.

Burke, N.S., & Simons, A. Factors which precipitate dropouts and delinquency. *Federal Probation,* 1965, *29,* 28-32.

Buros, O.K. (Ed.). *The eighth annual mental measurements yearbook* (Vol. 182). Highland Park, N.J.: The Gryphon Press, 1978.

Bursuk, L.Z. *Sensory mode of lesson presentation as a factor in the reading comprehension improvement of adolescent retarded readers.* New York: City University of New York, York College, 1971. (ERIC Document Reproduction Service No. ED 047-435)

Buscaglia, L.F. Parents need to know: Parents and teachers work together. In J.I. Arena (Ed.), *The child with learning disabilities: His right to learn.* Pittsburgh: Association for Children with Learning Disabilities, 1971.

Bush, W.J., & Waugh, K.W. *Diagnosing learning disabilities.* Columbus, Ohio: The Charles E. Merrill Publishing Company, Inc., 1976.

Buswell, G.T., & John, L. *Diagnostic studies in arithmetic.* Chicago: University of Chicago Press, 1926.

Butler, A.J., & Browning, P.L. Predictive studies on rehabilitation outcome with the retarded. In P.L. Browning (Ed.), *Mental retardation: Rehabilitation and counseling.* Springfield, Ill.: Charles C Thomas, Publisher, 1974.

Byrne, P. PL 94-142 State agency reports of handicapped children receiving special education and related services 1981-1982. Washington, D.C.: Department of Education, Special Education Programs, 1982.

Campbell, D.T., & Stanley, J.C. *Experimental and quasi-experimental designs for research.* Chicago: Rand McNally Co., 1963.

Cansler, O.P., Martin, G.H., & Valana, M.C. *Working with families.* Winston-Salem, N.C.: Kaplan Press, 1975.

Canter, L., & Canter, M. *Assertive discipline, a take-charge approach for today's educator.* Los Angeles: Canter & Associates, 1976.

Cartwright, G.P., Cartwright, C.A., & Ysseldyke, J.E. Two decision models: Identification and diagnostic teaching of handicapped children in the regular classroom. *Psychology in the Schools,* 1973, *10,* 4-11.

Castor, J. What is "mainstreaming"? *Exceptional Children,* 1975, *42,* 174.

Cawley, J.F., Goodstein, H.A., Fitzmaurice, A.M., Lepore, A., Sedlak, R.A., & Althause, V. *Project MATH: Mathematics activities for teaching the handicapped: Levels I and II.* Tulsa, Okla.: Educational Process Corp., 1976.

Charles, C.M. *Educational psychology: The instructional endeavor.* St. Louis: The C.V. Mosby Company, 1976.

Cheek, L.M. Cost effectiveness comes to the personnel function. *Harvard Business Review,* 1973, *51*(3), 99-104.

Clarizio, H., & McCoy, G.F. *Behavior disorders in children.* New York: Crowell-Collier, 1976.

Clark, G.M. *Career education for the handicapped child in the elementary classroom.* Denver: Love Publishing Company, 1979.

Clark, G.M. Career preparation for handicapped adolescents: A matter of appropriate education. *Exceptional Education Quarterly,* 1980, *1*(2), 11-17.

Clark, G.M., & Oliverson, B. Education of secondary personnel: Assumptions and preliminary data. *Exceptional Children,* 1973, *39,* 41-46.

Clements, S.D. *Minimal brain dysfunction in children,* NINCB Monograph No. 3, U.S. Public Health Service Publication N. 1415. Washington, D.C.: U.S. Government Printing Office, 1966.

Clifford, G.J. A history of the impact of research on teaching. In R.M.W. Travers (Ed.), *Second handbook of research on teaching.* Chicago: Rand McNally Co., 1973.

Cobb, H.V. *The forecast of fulfillment: A review of research on predictive assessment of the adult retarded for social and vocational adjustment.* New York: Columbia University Teachers College Press, 1972.

Coffey, A., Eldelfonso, E., & Hartinger, W. *An introduction to the criminal justice system and process.* Englewood Cliffs, N.J.: Prentice-Hall, Inc., 1974.

Cole, N. School habilitation program for secondary students. *Rehabilitation Literature,* 1967, *28,* 170-176.

Colella, H.V. Career development center: A modified high school for the handicapped. *Teaching Exceptional Children,* 1973, *5,* 110-118.

Coleman, J.S., Campbell, E.Q., Hobson, C.S., McDartland, J., Mood, A.M., Weinfeld, F.D., & York, R.L. *Equality of educational opportunity.* Washington, D.C.: U.S. Office of Education, 1966.

Commonwealth of Massachusetts v. Femino, 226 N.E. 2d 248 (Mass. 1967).

Connolly, A.J., Nachtman, W., & Pritchett, E.M. *Key math diagnostic arithmetic test.* Circle Pines, Minn.: American Guidance Service, Inc., 1971.

Cook, L.D. The adolescent with a learning disability: A developmental perspective. *Adolescence,* 1979, *14,* 697-707.

Crawford, D. *A summary of the results and recommendations from the ACLD-R & D Project.* Unpublished paper presented at the meeting of the Federal Coordinating Council, Washington, D.C., December 16, 1981.

Cronbach, L.J. Course improvement through evaluation. *Teachers College Record*, 1963, *64*, 674-683.

Cronbach, L.J., & Snow, R.E. *Aptitudes and instructional methods*. New York: Irvington Publishers, 1977.

Cullinan, D., & Epstein, M.H. *Special education for adolescents: Issues and perspectives*. Columbus, Ohio: The Charles E. Merrill Publishing Company, Inc., 1979.

D'Alonzo, B.J. Perceived role behavior expectations of full-time work-study coordinators. *Education and Training of the Mentally Retarded*, 1974, *9*, 131-133.

D'Alonzo, B.J. Trends and issues in career education for the mentally retarded. *Education and Training of the Mentally Retarded*, 1977, *12*, 156-158.

D'Alonzo, B.J. Career education for handicapped youth and adults in the 70's. *Career Development for Exceptional Individuals*, 1978, *1*, 4-12. (a)

D'Alonzo, B.J. Developing secondary school individualized education programs. In B. Weiner (Ed.), *Periscope: Views of the individualized education program*. Reston, Va.: The Council for Exceptional Children, 1978. (b)

D'Alonzo, B.J. Curriculum adjustments in the area of vocational preparation for emotionally disturbed youth. In D.R. Eyde, F.J. Menolascino, & A.H. Fink (Eds.), *Nebraska Symposium on Current Issues in Education of the Early Adolescent with Behavioral Disorders* (Vol. 1). Omaha: Nebraska Psychiatric Institute, 1981.

D'Alonzo, B.J., & Barrett, J.C. Special education's dilemma: Integration of the handicapped into vocational programs. *Illinois Career Education Journal*, 1977, *34*, 45-47.

D'Alonzo, B.J., & Miller, S.R. A management model for learning disabled adolescents. *Teaching Exceptional Children*, 1977, *9*, 58-60.

D'Alonzo, B.J., & Wiseman, D.E. Actual and desired roles of LD resource teachers. *Journal of Learning Disabilities*, 1978, *11*, 390-397.

D'Alonzo, B.J., D'Alonzo, R.L., & Mauser, A.J. Developing resource rooms for the handicapped. *Teaching Exceptional Children*, 1979, *11*, 91-96.

D'Alonzo, R. *An introduction to the behavior management-discipline programs utilized within the Mesa Public School District*. Mesa, Ariz.: Mesa Public Schools, 1980.

Dauw, E.G. Individual instruction for potential dropouts. National Association for Secondary School Principals *(NASSP) Bulletin* 1970, *54*, 9-21.

Davis, S., & Ward, M. *Vocational education of handicapped students: A guide for policy development*. Reston, Va.: The Council for Exceptional Children (n.d.).

Deno, E. Special education of developmental capital. *Exceptional Children*, 1970, *37*, 229-237.

Deshler, D.D. Learning disability in the high school student as demonstrated in monitoring of self-generated and externally generated errors. (Doctoral dissertation, University of Arizona.) Ann Arbor, Mich.: University Microfilms, 1975, No. 75-4135.

Deshler, D.D. Psychoeducational aspects of learning disabled adolescents. In L. Mann, L. Goodman, & J.L. Wiederholt (Eds.), *Teaching the learning-disabled adolescent*. Boston: Houghton Mifflin Company, 1978.

Designing effective instruction. Palo Alto, Calif.: General Programmed Teaching, 1970.

DeVault, M.V. Research and the classroom teacher. *Teachers College Record*, 1965, *67*, 211-216.

Dillner, M.H. The effectiveness of a cross-age tutoring design in teaching remedial reading in the secondary schools. (Doctoral dissertation, University of Florida). Ann Arbor, Mich.: University Microfilms, 1971, No. 72-15, 671.

Dinkmeyer, D., & McKay, G. *Systematic training for effective parenting.* American Guidance Service, Inc., Circle Pines, Minn., 1976.

Directory of Educational Facilities for the Learning Disabled (7th ed.). San Rafael, Calif.: Academic Therapy Publications, 1978.

Division on Career Development, The Council for Exceptional Children. *Newsletter,* 1977, *1*(1), 1.

Division on Career Development, The Council for Exceptional Children. *Newsletter,* 1978, *1*(1).

Douglass, H.R. An effective junior high school program for reducing the number of dropouts. *Contemporary Education,* 1969, *41*(8), 34-37.

DuBose, R.F., Langley, M.B., & Stagg, V. Assessing severely handicapped children. *Focus on Exceptional Children,* 1977, *9*(7), 1-13.

Duling, F., Eddy, S., & Risko, V. *Learning disabilities of juvenile delinquents.* Morgantown, W.Va.: Department of Educational Services, Robert F. Kennedy Youth Center, 1970.

Dunn, L.M. Special education for the mildly retarded—Is much of it justifiable? *Exceptional Children,* 1968, *37,* 229-237.

Dunn, L.M. (Ed.). *Exceptional children in the schools: Special education in transition* (2nd ed.). New York: Holt, Rinehart & Winston, 1973.

Ebel, R.L. Educational tests: Valid? Biased? Useful? *Phi Delta Kappan,* 1975, *57,* 83-88.

Edwards v. Arizona, 451 U.S. 477 (1981).

Edwards, L.L. Curriculum modification as a strategy for helping regular classroom behavior-disordered students. *Focus on Exceptional Children,* 1980, *12*(8), 1-12.

Erickson, D. Research on educational administration: The state of the art. *Educational Researcher,* 1979, 8(3), 9-14.

Evans, R.N. Career education and vocational education: Similarities and contrasts. *Monographs on career education.* Washington, D.C.: U.S. Department of Health, Education, and Welfare, U.S. Office of Education, 1975.

Evans, S. The consultant role of the resource teacher. *Exceptional Children,* 1980, *46,* 402-404.

Faas, L.A. *Children with learning problems: A handbook for teachers.* Boston: Houghton Mifflin Company, 1980.

Federal Bureau of Investigation. Uniform crime report: Crime in the United States-1978. Washington, D.C.: United States Department of Justice, 1979.

Federal Register. Financial assistance to local and state agencies to meet special educational needs, and financial assistance to local educational agencies for children with special educational needs; Regulations. Part II Department of Education, Office of Elementary and Secondary Education, Washington, D.C.: U.S. Government Printing Office, January 19, 1981, 5135-5236.

Fimian, M.J. *Best practices manual.* Unpublished manuscript. Utah State University, Exceptional Child Center, 1978.

Fox, R.G., Copeland, R.E., Harris, J.W., Rieth, H.J., & Hall, R.V. A computerized system for selecting responsive teaching studies, catalogued along twenty-eight important dimensions. In E. Ramp & G. Semb (Eds.), *Behavior analysis: Areas of research and application.* Englewood Cliffs, N.J.: Prentice-Hall, Inc., 1973.

Freeman, S.W., & Thompson, C.R. The counselor's roles with learning disabled students. *School Counselor,* 1975, *23,* 28-36.

Frith, G.H., Lindsey, J.D., & Sasser, J.L. An alternative approach to school suspension: The Dothan model. *Phi Delta Kappan,* 1980, *61,* 637-638.

Furman, W., Geller, M., Simon, S.J., & Kelley, J.A. The use of a behavioral rehearsal procedure for teaching job interviewing skills to psychiatric patients. *Behavior Therapy,* 1979, *10,* 157-167.

Gallagher, J. The prospects for governmental support of educational research. *Educational Researcher*, 1975, *4*(7), 13-14.

Ganzer, V.J., & Sarason, I.G. Variables associated with recidivism among juvenile delinquents. *Journal of Consulting and Clinical Psychology*, 1973, *40*, 1-50.

Gardner, M. (Ed.). *The annotated Alice*. New York: Bramhall House, 1960.

Gearheart, B.R. *Learning disabilities: Educational strategies*. St. Louis: The C.V. Mosby Company, 1973.

Gearheart, B.R. *Special education for the 80's*. St. Louis: The C.V. Mosby Company, 1980.

Geer, W.C. *Testimony before House of Representatives Subcommittee on Elementary, Secondary and Vocational Education*. Washington, D.C.: U.S. Government Printing Office, March 19, 1975.

General Accounting Office. *Training educators for the handicapped: A need to redirect federal programs*. Washington, D.C.: Comptroller General of the United States, September, 1976.

Gerlach, V.S., & Ely, D.P. *Teaching and media*. Englewood Cliffs, N.J.: Prentice-Hall, Inc., 1971.

Gideon v. Wainwright, 372 U.S. 335 (1963).

Gilhool, T.K. Changing public policies: Roots and practices. *Minnesota Education*, 1976, *2*, 8-13.

Glaser, R. Adapting the elementary school curriculum to individual performance. *Proceedings of the 1967 Invitational Conference on Testing Problems*. Princeton, N.J.: Educational Testing Service, 1968.

Glass, G.V., Cahen, L.S., Smith, M.L., & Filby, N.N. Class size and learning—new interpretation of the research literature. *Today's Education*, 1979, *68*, 42-44.

Glasser, W. Reality therapy. In V. Binder, A. Binder, & B. Rimland (Eds.), *Modern therapies*. Englewood Cliffs, N.J.: Prentice-Hall, Inc., 1976.

Gold, M.W. *"Did I say that?": Articles and commentary on the try another way system*. Champaign, Ill.: Research Press Co., 1980.

Goldberg, Mark, F. Individualized instruction: Myths and characteristics. National Association for Secondary School Principals *(NASSP) Bulletin*. *61*(406), 1977.

Goldfield, M.R., & Pomerang, D.M. Role of assessment in behavior modification. *Psychological Reports*, 1968, *23*, 75-87.

Goldhammer, K.A. A careers curriculum. In K. Goldhammer & R. Taylor (Eds.), *Career education: Perspectives and promise*. Columbus, Ohio: The Charles E. Merrill Publishing Company, Inc., 1972.

Good, C.V., & Scates, D.E. *Methods of research*. New York: Appleton-Century-Crofts, Inc., 1954.

Goodman, L., & Mann, L. *Learning disabilities in the secondary school*. New York: Grune & Stratton, Inc., 1976.

Gordon, T. *Parent effectiveness training: The "no-lose" program for raising responsible children*. New York: Peter H. Wyden, Inc., 1974.

Greenlee, W.E., & Hare, B. A close look at learning disabilities. *Academic Therapy*, 1978, *13*, 345-349.

Gregarus, F.M., Broder, P.K., & Zimmerman, J. *Establishing an operational definition of juvenile delinquency* (Tech. Rep. 13). Omaha: Creighton University, Institute for Business, Law and Social Research, March 1978.

Grinder, R.E. Adolescence in the United States: A review of contemporary research trends and problems. In *Status of children, youth and families*. Washington, D.C.: Administration for Children, Youth, and Families, 1980.

Gronlund, N. *Preparing criterion-referenced tests for classroom instruction*. New York: Macmillan Publishing Co., Inc., 1973.

Gross, R. From innovations to alternatives: A decade of change in education. *Phi Delta Kappan*, 1971, *53*, 22-24.

Grossman, H.J. (Ed.). *Manual on terminology and classification in mental retardation*. Washington, D.C.: American Association on Mental Deficiency, 1977.

Haggerty, D.E., Kane, L.A., & Udall, D.K. An essay on the legal rights of the mentally retarded. *Family Law Quarterly*, 1972, *6*, 59-71.

Hammill, D.D., & Bartel, N.R. (Eds.). *Teaching children with learning and behavior problems* (3d ed.). Boston: Allyn & Bacon, Inc., 1982.

Hammond, R. Context evaluation of instruction in local school districts. *Educational Technology*, 1969, *9*, 13-18.

Harris, M. *Classroom uses of behavior modification*. Columbus, Ohio: The Charles E. Merrill Publishing Co., 1972.

Harrow, A.J. *A taxonomy of the psychomotor domain: A guide for developing behavioral objectives*. New York: Longmans, Green, 1972.

Hartman, D.P., & Hall, R.V. The changing criterion design. *Journal of Applied Behavior Analysis*, 1976, *9*, 527-532.

Hartwell, L.K., Wiseman, D.E., Krus, P., & Van Reusen, T. *Child service demonstration center in secondary school age learning disabilities*. Title VI-E, End of Year Report: 1978-79 (Tech. Rep. 2). Tempe: Arizona State University, 1979.

Hartwell, L.K., Wiseman, D.E., & Van Reusen, T. Modifying course content for mildly handicapped students at the secondary level. *Teaching Exceptional Children*, *12*, 1979.

Haugh, O. The standardized test: To be or not to be. *English Journal*, 1975, *64*(3), 53-55.

Haughton, E. Counting together: Precision teaching rationale. Working paper. Eugene School District 45 and the University of Oregon, College of Education, December 1969.

Havighurst, R. *A profile of the largest city high school*. Washington, D.C.: National Association for Secondary School Principals (NAASP), 1970.

Hawkes, T. Grouping. In D.W. Allen & E. Seifman (Eds.), *The Teacher's Handbook*. Glenview, Ill.: Scott, Foresman and Co., 1971.

Hawkins, R.P., & Dobes, R.W. Behavioral definitions in applied behavior analysis: Explicit or implicit. In B.C. Etzel, J.M LeBlanc, & D.M. Baer (Eds.), *New developments in behavioral research: Theory methods and applications*. Hillsdale, N.J.: Lawrence Erlbaum Associates, Publishers, 1975.

Hayes, J. Annual goals and short-term objectives. In S. Torres (Ed.), *A primer on individualized education programs for handicapped children*. Reston, Va.: The Council for Exceptional Children, 1977.

Hayden, A.H., & Haring, N.G. Early intervention for high-risk infants and young children: Programs for Down's syndrome children. In T.D. Tjossem (Ed.), *Intervention strategies for high-risk infants and young children*. Baltimore: University Park Press, 1976.

Henrick, E., & Kriegel, L. *Experiments in survival*. New York: Association for the Aid of Crippled Children, 1961.

Hellman, H. Guiding light. *Psychology Today*, 1982, *16*(4), 22-28.

Herman, R., Gelhausen, T., & Childress, M. *Assessment of the adjudicated adolescent's self-concept: Congruity between child and parent perceptions*. Unpublished paper presented at the meeting of the Eastern Education Research Association, Norfolk, Va., March 1980.

Hersen, M., & Barlow, D.H. *Single case experimental designs: Strategies for studying behavior change*. New York: Pergamon Press, 1978.

Hewett, F. *Educating the emotionally disturbed child.* Boston: Allyn & Bacon, Inc., 1968.

Hewett, F.M. A personal perspective. In J.M. Kauffman & C.D. Lewis (Eds.), *Teaching children with behavior disorders: Personal perspectives.* Columbus, Ohio: The Charles E. Merrill Publishing Co., Inc., 1974.

Hewett, F.M., & Forness, S.R. *Education of exceptional learners.* Boston: Allyn & Bacon, Inc., 1974.

Hewett, F.M., & Taylor, F.D. *The emotionally disturbed child in the classroom: The orchestration of success.* Boston: Allyn & Bacon, Inc., 1980.

Higgins, J.P. Present level(s) of performance and assessment: Some basic considerations. In S. Torres (Ed.), *A primer on individualized education programs for handicapped children.* Reston, Va.: The Council for Exceptional Children, 1977.

Hofmeister, A. *Diagnostic math facts test.* Logan, Utah: Utah State University, Exceptional Child Center, 1972.

Hogenson, D.L. Reading failure and juvenile delinquency. *Bulletin of the Orton Society,* 1974, *24,* 164-169.

Howell, K.W., & Kaplan, J.S. *Evaluating exceptional children: A task analysis approach, Vol. II.* Columbus, Ohio: The Charles E. Merrill Publishing Company, Inc., 1980.

Howell, K.W., Kaplan, J.S., & O'Connell, C.Y. *Evaluating exceptional children: A task analysis approach.* Columbus, Ohio: The Charles E. Merrill Publishing Company, Inc., 1979.

Hoyt, K.B. *An introduction to career education: A policy paper of the U.S. Office of Education.* DHEW Publication No. (OE) 75-00504. Washington, D.C.: U.S. Government Printing Office, 1975.

Hoyt, K.B. A primer on education. *Monographs on career education.* Washington, D.C.: U.S. Office of Education, 1977.

Hoyt, K.B. Career education: Beginning of the end? Or a new beginning? *Career Development for Exceptional Individuals,* 1982, *5,* 3-12.

Hoyt, K.B., Evans, R.N., Mackin, E.F., & Mangum, G.L. *Career education and how to do it* (2nd ed.). Salt Lake City: Olympus Publishing Company, 1974.

Hoyt, K.B., & High, S.C. Career education. In H.E. Mitzel (Ed.), *Encyclopedia of educational research* (5th ed.). New York: Macmillan Publishing Company, Inc., 1982.

Hudson, F.G., & Graham, S. An approach to operationalizing the I.E.P. *Learning Disability Quarterly,* 1978, *1*(1), 13-32.

Hurlock, E. *Adolescent development.* New York: McGraw-Hill Book Company, 1973.

Isakson, R., & Ellsworth, R. The measurement of teacher attitudes toward educational research. *Educational Research Quarterly,* 1979, *4*(2), 12-18.

Jacks, K.B., & Keller, M.E. A humanistic approach to the adolescent with learning disabilities: An educational, psychological, and vocational model. *Adolescence,* 1978, *13,* 59-68.

Jensen, G.M. Year-round school: Can boards sidestep it much longer? *American School Board Journal,* 1969, *157,* 12.

Johnson, M.E.B. Teachers' attitudes to educational research. *Educational Researcher,* 1966, *9,* 74-79.

Johnson, D., Blalock, J., & Nesbitt, J. Adolescents with learning disabilities: Perspectives from an educational clinic. *Learning Disabilities Quarterly,* 1978, *1*(4), 24-36.

Jones, R.L. Labels and stigma in special education. *Exceptional Children,* 1972, *38,* 533-564.

Jones, R.L. Accountability in special education: Some problems. *Exceptional Children,* 1973, *39,* 631-642.

Jones, R.R., Reid, J.B., & Patterson, G.R. Naturalistic observation in clinical assessment. In P. McReynolds (Ed.), *Advances in psychological assessment* (Vol. 3). San Francisco: Jossey-Bass, Inc., 1975.

Jordan, J. Invisible college on mainstreaming addresses critical factors in implementing programs. *Exceptional Children,* 1974, *41,* 31-33.

Kanner, S. Emotionally disturbed children: A historical review. *Child Development,* 1962, *33,* 97-102.

Kaslow, F.W., & Cooper, B. Family therapy with the learning disabled child and his/her family. *Journal of Marriage and Family Counseling,* 1978, *4,* 41-49.

Kass, C., & Lewis, R. Favorite methods and materials of the DCLD membership. *Newsletter,* Division on Children with Learning Disabilities, 1973, *3*(winter), 1-4.

Kauffman, M., Gottlieb, J., Agard, J., & Kukic, M. Mainstreaming: Toward an explication of the construct. *Focus on Exceptional Children,* 1975, 7(3), 1-11.

Kazdin, A.E. *Behavior modification in applied settings.* Homewood, Ill: The Dorsey Press, 1980.

Kazdin, A.E. The effect of response cost and aversive stimulation in suppressing punished and nonpunished speech disfluences. *Behavior Therapy,* 1973, *4,* 73-82. (a)

Kazdin, A.E. The effect of vicarious reinforcement on attentive behavior in the classroom. *Journal of Applied Behavior Analysis,* 1973, *6,* 71-78. (b)

Kazdin, A.E. Unobtrusive measures in behavioral assessment. *Journal of Applied Behavior Analysis,* 1979, *12,* 713-724.

Keilitz, I., Zaremba, B., & Broder, P.K. *The link between learning disabilities and juvenile delinquency.* Williamsburg, Va.: National Center for State Courts, February 1979.

Kent, R.N., O'Leary, K.D., Dietz, A., & Diament, C. Comparison of observational recordings *in vivo, via* mirror, and *via* television. *Journal of Applied Behavior Analysis,* 1979, *12,* 517-522.

Kerlinger, F.P. Influence of research on education. *Educational Researcher,* 1977, 6(8), 5-12.

Kerr, C. *Giving youth a better chance: Options for education, work, and service,* Carnegie Council of Policy Studies in Higher Education. San Francisco: Jossey-Bass, Inc., 1979.

Kibler, R.J., Barker, L.L., & Miles, D.T. *Objectives for instruction and evaluation.* Boston: Allyn & Bacon, Inc., 1974.

Kiesler, D.J. Experimental designs in psychotherapy research. In A.E. Bergin & S.L. Garfield (Eds.), *Handbook of psychotherapy and behavior change: An empirical analysis.* New York: John Wiley & Sons, Inc., 1971.

Kirk, S.A. Behavioral diagnosis and remediation of learning disabilities. *Proceedings of the Annual Meeting of the Conference on Exploration into the Problems of the Perceptually Handicapped Children* (Vol. 1). Evanston, Ill.: Fund for Perceptually Handicapped Children, 1963.

Kirk, S.A. *Educating exceptional children* (2nd ed.). Boston: Houghton Mifflin Company, 1972.

Klein, R.S., Altman, S.D, Dreizen, K., Friedman, R., & Powers, L. Restructuring dysfunctional parental attitudes toward children's learning and behavior in school: Family-oriented psychoeducational therapy-Part I. *Journal of Learning Disabilities,* 1981, *14,* 15-19. (a)

Klein, R.S., Altman, S.D., Dreizen, K., Friedman, R., & Powers, L. Restructuring dysfunctional parental attitudes toward children's learning and behavior in school: Family-oriented psychoeducational therapy-Part II. *Journal of Learning Disabilities,* 1981, *14,* 99-101. (b)

Kokoszka, R., & Drye, J. Toward the least restrictive environment: High school learning disabled students. *Journal of Learning Disabilities,* 1981, *14,* 22-23.

Krathwohl, D.R. Improving educational research and development. *Educational Researcher,* 1977, 6(4), 8-14.

Krathwohl, D.R. Stating objectives appropriately for program, for curriculum, and for instructional materials development. *Journal of Teacher Education,* 1965, *12,* 83-92.

Krathwohl, D.R., Bloom, B.S., & Masia, B.B. *Taxonomy of educational objectives. Handbook II: Affective domain.* New York: Longman, Inc., 1964.

Kronick, D. *What about me? The learning disabled adolescent.* San Rafael, Calif.: Academic Therapy Publications, 1975.

Kroth, R.L. *Communicating with parents of exceptional children.* Denver: Love Publishing Company, 1975.

Kroth, R.L. Facilitating educational progress by improving parent conferences. *Focus on Exceptional Children, 4*(7), 1972.

Kroth, R.L. Involvement with parents of secondary behaviorally disordered children. In G. Brown, R. McDowell, & J. Smith (Eds.), *The emotionally disturbed adolescent: An education perspective.* Columbus, Ohio: The Charles E. Merrill Publishing Co., Inc., 1979.

Kroth, R.L., & Simpson, L. *Parent conferences as a teaching strategy.* Denver: Love Publishing Company, 1977.

Kroth, R.L., Whelan, R.J., & Stables, J.M. Teacher application of behavior principles in home and classroom environments. *Focus on Exceptional Children,* 1970, *2*(3), 1-11.

Laing, R.D. The study of family and social contexts in relation to the origin of schizophrenia. In J. Romano (Ed.), *Origins of schizophrenia.* Amsterdam: Excerpta medica, 1967.

Landis, J., Jones, R.W., & Kennedy, L.D. Curricular modification for secondary school reading. *Journal of Reading,* 1973, *16,* 374-378.

Lane, D., Pollack, C., & Sher, N. Remotivation of disruptive adolescents. *Journal of Reading,* 1972, *15,* 351-354.

Larsen, L., Goodman, L., & Glean, R. Issues in the implementation of extended school year programs for handicapped students. *Exceptional Children,* 1981, *47,* 256-263.

L'Bate, L. An input-output approach to psychodiagnosis of children. *World Journal of Psychosynthesis,* 1969, *1,* 68-73.

Leming, J.S. Cheating behavior, situational behavior, and moral development. *The Journal of Educational Research,* 1978, *71,* 214-217.

Lerner, J.W. *Children with learning disabilities: Theories, diagrams, and teaching strategies.* Boston: Houghton Mifflin Company, 1971.

Lerner, J.W. *Children with learning disabilities* (2nd ed.). Boston: Houghton Mifflin Company, 1976.

Lerner, J.W. Instructional stategies: A classification schema. In L. Mann, L. Goodman, & J.L. Wiederholt (Eds.), *Teaching the learning-disabled adolescent.* Boston: Houghton Mifflin Company, 1978.

Lerner, J.W., Evans, M.A., & Meyers, G. L.D. programs at the secondary level: A survey. *Academic Therapy,* 1977, *13,* 7-19.

Lessinger, L. Accountability: Its implications for the teacher. In D.W. Allen (Ed.), *The teacher's handbook.* Glenview, Ill: Scott, Foresman and Co., 1971.

Lillie, D.L. An overview of parent programs. In D.L. Lillie & P.L. Trohanis (Eds.), *Teaching parents to teach: A guide for working with the special child.* New York: Walker and Company, 1976.

Lillie, D.L., & Place, P.A. *Partners—A guide for working with schools for parents of children with special instructional needs.* Glenview, Ill.: Scott, Foresman & Company, 1982.

Linari, R.F. *A plan for the implementation of chapter 766 in vocational/technical school environments.* Canton, Mass: Blue Hills Regional Technical School, 1974.

Lindsley, O.R., Haughton, E., & Starlin, C. Direct measurement and prosthesis of retarded behavior. Working paper, University of Oregon, 1969.

Lindsley, O.R. Technical note: A reliable wrist counter for recording behavior rates. *Journal of Applied Behavior Analysis*, 1968, *1*, 77-78.

Lindvall, C.M., Nardozza, S., & Felton, M. The importance of specific objectives in curriculum development. In C.M. Lindvall (Ed.), *Defining educational objectives*. Pittsburgh: University of Pittsburgh Press, 1964.

Little, T.L. Training special education support personnel. *Educator*, 1977, *13*, 23-27.

Lockhead, J. An introduction to cognitive process instruction. In J. Lockhead & J. Clement (Eds.), *Cognitive process instruction*. Philadelphia: The Franklin Institute Press, 1979.

Loucks, S.F., & Hall, G.E. Assessing and facilitating the implementation of innovations: A new approach. *Educational Technology*, 1977, *17*(2), 18-21.

Love Publishing Company. *Individualized order tasks*. Denver: 1973.

Lovitt, T.C., & Curtis, K.A. Effects of manipulating an antecedent event on mathematics response rate. *Journal of Applied Behavior Analysis*, 1968, *1*, 329-334.

Mager, R.F. *Preparing instructional objectives*. Palo Alto, Calif.: Fearon Publishers, Inc., 1962.

Mager, R.F., & Pipe, P. *Analyzing performance problems, or "You really oughta wanna."* Palo Alto, Calif.: Fearon Publishers, Inc., n.d.

Mahler, C.A. *Group counseling in the schools*. Boston: Houghton Mifflin Company, 1969.

Mahoney, M.J. *Cognition and behavior modification*. Cambridge, Mass.: Ballinger Publishing Co., 1974.

Mali, P. *Managing by objectives*. New York: John Wiley & Sons, Inc., 1977.

Malouf, D., & Halpern, A. A review of secondary level special education. *Thresholds in Secondary Education*, 1976, *2*(3), 6-9, 25-29.

Mann, L., Goodman, L., & Wiederholt, J.L. (Eds.). *Teaching the learning-disabled adolescent*. Boston: Houghton Mifflin Company, 1978.

Marandola, P., & Imber, S.C. Glasser's classroom meeting: A humanistic approach to behavior change with preadolescent inner-city learning disabled children. *Journal of Learning Disabilities*, 1979, *12*, 383-387.

Marholin, D., II, & Steinman, W.M. Stimulus control in the classroom as a function of the behavior reinforced. *Journal of Applied Behavior Analysis*, 1977, *10*, 465-478.

Mark, H.J. Elementary thinking and the classification of behavior. *Science*, 1962, *135*, 75-87.

Marks, M.B. Research: The preservice missing link. *Journal of Teacher Education*, 1972, *23*, 453-456.

Marland, S.P. Career education now. *The Educational Digest*, 1971, *36*, 9-11.

Marsh, G.E., II, & Price, B.J. *Methods for teaching the mildly handicapped adolescent*. St. Louis: The C.V. Mosby Company, 1980.

Marsh, G.E., II, Gearheart, C.K., & Gearheart, B.R. *The learning disabled adolescent: Program alternatives in the secondary school*. St. Louis: The C.V. Mosby Company, 1978.

Marsh, R.L., Friel, C.M., & Eissler, V. The adult MR in the criminal justice system. *Mental Retardation*, 1975, *13*(2), 21-25.

Marshall, A.E., & Heward, W.C. Teaching self-management to incarcerated youth. *Behavioral Disorders*, 1979, *4*, 215-225.

Martin, J.H. *The education of adolescents: The final report and recommendations of the national panel on high school and adolescent education*. Washington, D.C.: U.S. Government Printing Office, 1976.

Mattina, J. New York State Supreme Court Justice, 8th Judicial District, personal communication, June 14, 1977.

Maynard, W. Basic approaches to violence and vandalism. *Phi Delta Kappan*, 1978, *59*, 359.

McAshan, H.H. *The goals approach to performance objectives*. Philadelphia: W.B. Saunders Co., 1974.

McCall, W.A. *How to experiment in education*. New York: MacMillan, 1923.

McCormack, J.E. A classroom communications system. Working paper. Manchester, Mass.: Seaside Educational Associates, 1976.

McCormack, J.E. *Proactive behavior management*. Manchester, Mass.: Seaside Educational Resources, 1978.

McCormack, J.E., Chalmers, J.A. *Early cognitive instruction for the moderately and severely handicapped*. Champaign, Ill.: Research Press Co., 1978.

McDaniels, A. The nonreading parallel alternate curriculum part III. Selected papers on learning disabilities. *Proceedings of the Eighth Annual International Conference of the Association for Children with Learning Disabilities*. San Rafael, Calif.: Academic Therapy Publications, March 1971.

McDowell, R.L., & Brown, G.B. The emotionally disturbed adolescent: Development of program alternatives in secondary education. *Focus on Exceptional Children*, 1978, *10*(4), 1-15.

McDowell, R.L. Prologue. In R.L. McDowell, G.W. Adamson, & F.H. Wood (Eds.), *Teaching emotionally disturbed children*. Boston: Little, Brown and Co., 1982.

McGrady, H.J. From diagnosis to remediation. In J.I. Arena (Ed.), *Management of the child with learning disabilities: An interdisciplinary challenge*. San Rafael, Calif.: Academic Therapy Publications, 1969.

McGrady, H.J. Communication disorders and specific learning disabilities. In R.J. Van Hattum (Ed.), *Communication disorders*. New York: Macmillan Publishing Company, Inc., 1980.

McLaughlin, T.F., & Malaby, J.E. Elementary school children as behavioral engineers. In E. Ramp & G. Semb (Eds.), *Behavior analysis: Areas of research and application*. Englewood Cliffs, N.J.: Prentice Hall, Inc., 1975.

McManman, K.M., & Cohn, M.J. A communications model for parents of adolescents with learning problems. *Journal of Clinical Child Psychology*, 1978, *7*, 151-153.

McNutt, G., & Heller, G. Services for learning disabled adolescents: A survey. *Learning Disability Quarterly*, *1*(4), 1978.

McWhirter, J.J. A parent education group in learning disabilities. *Journal of Learning Disabilities*, 1976, *9*, 16-20.

Meerbach, J. *The career resource center*. New York: Human Sciences Press, 1978.

Meers, G.D. (Ed.). *Handbook of special vocational needs education*. Rockville, Md.: Aspen Systems Corporation, 1980.

Menolascino, F.J. The mentally retarded offender. *Mental Retardation*, 1974, *12*(1), 7-11.

Mercatoris, M., & Craighead, W. Effects of nonparticipant observation on teacher and pupil classroom behavior. *Journal of Educational Psychology*, 1974, *66*, 512-519.

Mercer, J.R. *Labeling the mentally retarded*. Berkeley, Calif.: University of California Press, 1973.

Metz, A.S. *Number of pupils with handicaps in local public schools*, Bureau for Education of the Handicapped, Report No. DHEW-OE-73-11107. Washington, D.C.: U.S. Government Printing Office, 1973.

Meyen, E.L. *Instructional based appraisal system*. Bellevue, Wash.: Edmark Associates, 1976.

Michael, W.B., & Metfessel, N.S. A paradigm for developing valid, measurable objectives in the evaluation of educational programs in colleges and universities. *Educational and Psychological Measurement*, 1967, *27*, 373-383.

Miller, S.R. Secondary programming. In D.A. Sabatino (Ed.), *Learning disabilities handbook: A technical guide to program development*. DeKalb, Ill.: Northern Illinois University Press, 1975.

Miller, S.R., Sabatino, D.A., & Larsen, R.P. Issues in the professional preparation of secondary school special education. *Exceptional Children*, 1980, *46*, 344-350.

Miller, S.R., & Schloss, P.J. *Career-vocational education for handicapped youth*. Rockville, Md.: Aspen Systems Corporation, 1982.

Mills, C.M., & Walter, T.L. A behavioral employment intervention program for reducing juvenile delinquency. *Behavior Therapy*, 1977, *8*, 270-272.

Miranda v. Arizona, 384 U.S. 436 (1966).

Mitchell, A.M. Career development needs of seventeen-year-olds: How to improve career development programs. *Monograph of the National Vocational Guidance Association and the Association for Measurement and Evaluation in Guidance*. Washington, D.C.: American Personnel and Guidance Association, 1978.

Moore, A.E. *How to cut delinquency in half: The story of prevention in Oakland County, Michigan*. Washington, D.C.: U.S. Department of Health, Education, and Welfare, 1962. (ERIC Document Reproduction Service No. ED 002 168)

Morgan, D. *The individualized education program: What it is and how to do it*. Working paper, Utah State University, Department of Special Education, 1977.

Morgan, D., & Fimian, M.J. *The IEP primer: May the forms be with you*. Unpublished manuscript, Tempe: Arizona State University, 1979.

Morgan, E. State University College at Buffalo, N.Y., Department of Criminal Justice. Personal communication, June 6, 1977.

Mori, A.A. The status of career education for the handicapped. In A.A. Mori (Ed.), *Proceedings of an institute on career education for the handicapped*. Las Vegas: University of Nevada-Las Vegas, 1979.

Muehl, S., & Forrell, E.R. A follow-up study of disabled readers: Variables related to high school reading performance. *Reading Research Quarterly*, 1973, *19*, 110-123.

Murray, C.A. *The link between learning disabilities and juvenile delinquency*. Washington, D.C.: American Institute for Research, 1976.

National Assessment of Educational Progress. It's what you don't know that hurts. *NAEP Newsletter*, 1978, *11*(5), 1. (a)

National Assessment of Educational Progress. Wrap-up: Social studies/citizenship. *NAEP Newsletter*, 1978, *11*(5), 1-2. (b)

National Assessment of Educational Progress. Are 17-year-olds prepared? Doors open to real consumer work. *NAEP Newsletter*, 1979, *12*(3), 3-4.

National Association for Retarded Citizens. *An introduction to citizen advocacy*. Arlington, Texas: NARC, 1973.

National Association of State Directors of Special Education. *Guide for trainers: A resource for workshops on developing individual education programs*. Washington, D.C.: NASDSE, 1978.

National Center for Educational Statistics (NCES). *Digest of education statistics*. Washington, D.C.: U.S. Government Printing Office, 1978.

National Education Association resolution 77-33: Education for all handicapped children. *Today's Education*, 1977, *66*(4), 52.

National Education Association. *Selecting instructional materials for purchase: Procedural guidelines*. Washington, D.C.: NEA, 1972.

Neeley, E. Cars motivate nonreaders? Of course! *Teaching Exceptional Children*, 1972, *4*, 142-144.

Neisworth, J., & Smith, R. *Modifying retarded behavior*. Boston: Houghton Mifflin Company, 1973.

Nelson, R.D., Kapist, J.A., & Dorsey, B.L. Minimal reactivity of overt classroom observation on student and teacher behaviors. *Behavior Therapy*, 1978, *9*, 695-702.

Nielson, L. An in-service program for secondary learning disabilities teachers. *Journal of Learning Disabilities*, 1979, *12*, 70-74.

Nolen, P.A., Kunzelmann, H.P., & Haring, N.G. Behavioral modification in a junior high learning disabilities classroom. *Exceptional Children*, 1967, *34*, 163-168.

Ogg, E. *Securing the legal rights of retarded persons*. Public Affairs Pamphlet No. 492. New York: Public Affairs Committee, 1973.

Ohlsen, M.M. *Guidance services in the modern school*. New York: Harcourt, Brace & World, Inc., 1964.

Ohrtman, W.F. One more instant solution coming up. *The Journal of Special Education*, 1972, *6*, 377-378.

Otto, W., McMenemy, R.A., & Smith, R.J. *Corrective and remedial teaching* (2nd ed.). Boston: Houghton Mifflin Company, 1973.

Owen, R.W., Adams, P.A., Forrest, T., Stolz, L.M., & Fisher, S. Learning disorders in children: Sibling studies. *Monographs of the Society for Research in Child Development*, 1971, *36*(144).

Page, W.R., Prentice, J.J., & Thomas, D.W. Program development at the junior high school level. In J.I. Arena (Ed.), Management of the child with learning disabilities: An interdisciplinary challenge. *Proceedings of the Fourth Annual Conference of the Association for Children with Learning Disabilities*, New York, 1967.

Panushka, W. The nonreading parallel alternate curriculum, part II: Selected papers on learning disabilities. *Eighth Annual International Conference of the Association for Children with Learning Disabilities*. San Rafael, Calif.: Academic Therapy Publications, March 1971.

Pennsylvania Association for Retarded Children (PARC) v. Commonwealth of Pennsylvania, 343 F. Supp. 279 (E.D. Pa., 1972).

Perry, N. *Teaching the mentally retarded child*. New York: Columbia University Press, 1974.

Peter, L. *Prescriptive teaching*. New York: McGraw-Hill Book Company, Inc., 1965.

Phelps, L.A., & Clark, G.M. Personnel preparation for vocational programming of special needs students. *Journal of Career Education*, 1977, *3*, 35-51.

Philage, M., Kuna, D.J., & Becerril, G. A new family approach to therapy for the learning disabled child. *Journal of Learning Disabilities*, 1975, *8*, 490-499.

Phillips, E.L. Achievement place token reinforcement procedures in a home-style rehabilitation setting for predelinquent boys. *Journal of Applied Behavior Analysis*, 1968, *1*, 213-223.

Phoenix Union High School System. *Parent-teacher guide to exceptional student programs*. Phoenix Public Schools, Phoenix, Ariz., 1980.

Planned Parenthood Federation of America. *The need for planned parenthood education*. New York: Planned Parenthood, 1977.

Podboy, J.W., & Mallory, W.A. *Diagnosis of specific learning disabilities among a juvenile delinquent population*. Unpublished manuscript. Sonoma County, Calif.: Probation Department, 1977.

Popham, W.J. Normative data for criterion-referenced tests? *Phi Delta Kappan*, 1976, *57*, 593-594.

Popham, W.J. Objectives and instruction. American Educational Research Association, *Monograph Series on Curriculum Evaluation, No. 3, Instructional Objectives*. Chicago: Rand McNally Company, 1969.

Popham, W.J., & Baker, E.L. *Establishing instructional goals*. Englewood Cliffs, N.J.: Prentice-Hall, Inc., 1970.

Poremba, C. The adolescent and young adult with learning disabilities: What are his needs? What are the needs of those who deal with him? Unpublished paper presented at 3d International Conference of the Association for Children with Learning Disabilities, Pittsburgh, Penn., 1967.

Prehm, H.J., & McDonald, J.E. The yet to be served—A perspective. *Exceptional Children*, 1979, *45*, 502-507.

Preli, B.S. *Career education: Teaching/learning process*. Washington, D.C.: U.S. Government Printing Office, 1978.

President's Committee on Mental Retardation. *The mentally retarded citizen and the law*. New York: Macmillan Publishing Company, Inc., 1976.

Provus, N.W. *Teaching for relevance: An inservice training program*. Chicago: Whitehall Company, 1970.

Raymond, C.D. (Ed.) *The 1978 annual career education handbook for trainers*. Tempe, Ariz.: Palo Verde Associates, 1978.

Reckless, W.C. *The crime problem*. New York: Appleton-Century-Crofts, 1967.

Reger, R. What is a resource room? *Journal of Learning Disabilities*, 1973, *6*, 611-614.

Reynolds, M.C., & Birch, J.W. *Teaching exceptional children in all America's schools: A first course for teachers and principals*. Reston, Va.: The Council for Exceptional Children, 1977.

Richey, R.W. *Planning for teaching: An introduction to teaching* (6th ed.). New York: McGraw-Hill Book Company, 1979.

Riekes, L., Spiegel, S., & Keilitz, I. Law-related education. Mental Retardation, 1977, *15*(1), 7-9.

Riffel, R. The federal role in providing vocational education for the handicapped. *Thresholds*, 1979, *5*(4), 3-5.

Robinson, E.H., & Brosh, M.C. Communication skills training for resource teachers. *Journal of Learning Disabilities*, 1980, *13*, 55-57.

Rosenthal, R., & Jacobson, L. *Pygmalion in the classroom*. New York: Holt, Rinehart & Winston, 1968.

Ruddell, R. *Reading-language instructor: Innovative practices*. Englewood Cliffs, N.J.: Prentice-Hall, Inc., 1974.

Rusman, F.K. *A guide to the diagnostic teaching of arithmetic*. Columbus, Ohio: The Charles E. Merrill Publishing Company, 1972.

Sabatino, D.A. The information processing behaviors associated with learning disabilities. *Journal of Learning Disabilities*, 1968, *1*, 444-450.

Sabatino, D.A. Overview for the practitioner in learning disabilities. In D.A. Sabatino, T.L. Miller, & C.R. Schmidt (Eds.), *Learning disabilities: Systemizing teaching and service delivery*. Rockville, Md.: Aspen Systems Corporation, 1981.

Sabatino, D.A. Resource rooms: The renaissance in special education. *Journal of Special Education*, 1972, *6*(4), 335-347.

Sabatino, D.A., & Mauser, A.J. *Intervention strategies for specialized secondary education*. Boston: Allyn & Bacon, Inc., 1978.

Sabatino, D.A., Miller, T.L., & Schmidt, C.R. (Eds.). *Learning disabilities: Systemizing teaching and service delivery*. Rockville, Md.: Aspen Systems Corporation, 1981.

Safran, J.S. Actual and desired role competencies of secondary resource teachers. Unpublished doctoral dissertation, University of Virginia, 1980.

Sampson, E. *Contrast rendition in school lighting.* New York: Educational Facilities Laboratories, 1970.

Sanders, N.M. *Classroom questions: What kinds?* New York: Harper & Row Publishers, 1966.

Sarason, S. Mainstreaming: Dilemmas, opposition, opportunities. In M.C. Reynolds (Ed.), *Futures of education for exceptional students: Emerging structures.* Reston, Va.: The Council for Exceptional Children, 1978.

Scagers, P. *Light, vision and learning.* New York: Better Light, Better Sight Bureau, 1963.

Schilit, J. Advocacy and its relationship to the mentally retarded. *Journal for Special Education Teachers of the Mentally Retarded,* 1977, *13,* 186-190.

Schilit, J. The mentally retarded offender: A "catch 22." *The Journal for Special Educators,* 1979(a), *15,* 293-295.

Schilit, J. The mentally retarded offender and the criminal justice system. *Exceptional Children,* 1979(b), *46,* 16-22.

Schnorr, J.M. *Private schools for the learning disabled* (7th ed.). San Rafael, Calif.: Academic Therapy Publications, 1978.

Schreiber, D. 700,000 dropouts. *American Education,* 1968, *4,* 5-7.

Schultz, E.W., Hirshoren, A., Manton, A.B., & Henderson, R.A. Special education for the emotionally disturbed. *Exceptional Children,* 1971, *38,* 313-319.

Schumaker, J.B., Havell, M.F., & Sherman, J.A. An analysis of daily report cards and parent managed privileges in the improvement of adolescents' classroom performance. *Journal of Applied Behavior Analysis,* 1977, *10,* 449-464.

Schwartz, L. Opp Hall. *Mesa Magazine,* 1980, *3*(7), 37-47.

Schwartz, S.E. (Ed.). *Project retool: Institute on career education for the handicapped.* University, Ala.: University of Alabama, 1980.

Scott, O. Relative effects of four types of assignment on competence in research consumership. *The Journal of Educational Research,* 1971, *65,* 183-189.

Scranton, T.R., & Downs, M.L. Elementary and secondary programs in the U.S.: A survey. *Journal of Learning Disabilities,* 1975, *8,* 394-399.

Shanker, A. One man's view. In *Alternative schools: Pioneering districts create options for students.* Arlington, Va.: National School Public Relations Association, 1972.

Shaver, J. Randomness and replication in ten years of the American Educational Research Journal. *Educational Researcher,* 1979, *9*(1), 9-15.

Shea, T.M. *Teaching children and youth with behavior disorders.* St. Louis: The C.V. Mosby Company, 1978.

Shearer, M.S. A home-based parent training model. In D.L. Lillie & P.L. Trohanis (Eds.), *Teaching parents to teach.* New York: Walker and Company, 1976.

Shelton, M.N. Affective education and the learning disabled student. *Journal of Learning Disabilities,* 1977, *10,* 618-629.

Shore, M.F., & Massimo, J.L. The alienated adolescent: A challenge to the mental health profession. *Adolescence,* 1969, *4,* 19-34.

Siegel, E. *The exceptional child grows up.* New York: E.P. Dutton & Co., 1974.

Siegel, L.J., & Steinman, W.M. The modification of a peer-observer's classroom behavior as a function of his serving as a reinforcing agent. In E. Ramp and G. Semb (Eds.), *Behavior analysis: Areas of research and application.* Englewood Cliffs, N.J.: Prentice-Hall, Inc., 1973.

Silberberg, N., & Silberberg, M. Myths in remedial education. *Journal of Learning Disabilities*, 1969, *2*, 209-217.

Silberman, C. *Crisis in the classroom*. New York: Random House, Inc., 1970.

Sindelar, P.T., & Deno, S.L. The effectiveness of resource programming. *The Journal of Special Education*, 1978, *12*, 17-28.

Siperstein, G.N., Bopp, M.J., & Bak, J.J. Social status of learning disabled children. *Journal of Learning Disabilities*, 1978, *11*, 98-102.

Skinner, B.F. *About behaviorism*. New York: Alfred A. Knopf, Inc., 1974.

Slavin, R. Basic vs. applied research: A response. *Educational Researcher*, 1978, 7(2), 15-17.

Smith, D.D., & Snell, M.E. Classroom management and instruction of planning. In M.E. Snell (Ed.), *Systematic instruction of the moderately and severely handicapped*. Columbus, Ohio: The Charles E. Merrill Publishing Company, Inc., 1978.

Smith, R.M. *Clinical teaching: Methods of instruction for the retarded*. New York: McGraw-Hill Book Company, 1974.

Smith, R.M., & Neisworth, J.T. *The exceptional child: A functional approach*. New York: McGraw-Hill Book Company, 1975.

Snell, M.E. (Ed.). *Systematic instruction of the moderately and severely handicapped*. Columbus, Ohio: The Charles E. Merrill Publishing Company, Inc., 1978.

Spache, G.D. *Investigating the issues of reading disabilities*. Boston: Allyn & Bacon, Inc., 1976.

Splaine, J. Compulsory schooling: The legal issue. Washington, D.C.: U.S. Department of Health, Education, and Welfare, 1975. (ERIC Document Reproduction Service No. ED 117 801)

Steinitz, V. People need help, but people take advantage: The dilemma of social responsibility for upwardly mobile youth. *Youth and Society*, 1976, *7*, 399-438.

Stephens, T.M. *Directive teaching of children with learning and behavioral handicaps*. Columbus, Ohio: The Charles E. Merrill Publishing Company, Inc., 1970.

Stephens, T.M. *Teaching skills to children with learning and behavior disorders*. Columbus, Ohio: The Charles E. Merrill Publishing Company, Inc., 1977.

Stephens, T.M., Hartman, C.A., & Lucas, V.H. *Teaching children basic skills: A curriculum handbook*. Columbus, Ohio: The Charles E. Merrill Publishing Company, 1978.

Stokes, T.F., Fowler, S.A., & Baer, D.M. Training preschool children to recruit natural communities of reinforcement. *Journal of Applied Behavior Analysis*, 1978, *11*, 285-303.

Stowitschek, J.J., Gable, R.A., & Hendricksen, J.M. *Instructional materials for exceptional children: Selection, management, and adaptation*. Rockville, Md.: Aspen Systems Corporation, 1980.

Stufflebeam, D.L. *Evaluation as enlightenment for decision-making*. Proceedings of working conference on assessment theory, the Commission on Assessment of Educational Outcomes, the Association for Supervision and Curriculum Development, Sarasota, Fla., January 1969.

Stufflebeam, D.L. The relevance of the CIPP evaluation model for educational accountability. Unpublished paper, Ohio State University Evaluation Center, 1972.

Sulzer, B., & Mayer, G. *Behavior modification procedures for school personnel*. New York: Holt, Rinehart & Winston, 1972.

Sulzer-Azaroff, B., & Mayer, G.R. *Applying behavior-analysis procedures with children and youth*. New York: Holt, Rinehart and Winston, 1977.

Svoboda, W.S., & Wolfe, M.P. Looking before leaping: A basic model for planning educational change. *Educational Technology*, *14*(4), 1974, 62-63.

Szasz, T.S. Psychiatric classifications as a strategy of social constraint. In T.S. Szasz (Ed.), *Ideology and insanity*. Garden City, L.I.: Doubleday and Company, 1969.

Taplin, P.S., & Reid, J.B. Effects of instructional set and experimenter influence on observer reliability. *Child Development*, 1973, *44*, 547-554.

Taylor, S.E. Listening: What research says to the teacher. *National Education Association*, 1973, *3*, 3-7.

Terman, L.M., & Merrill, M.A. *Stanford-Binet Intelligence Scale* (1972 norms editor, Form L-M). Boston: Houghton Mifflin Company, 1973.

Thomas, J. *Learning centers: Opening up the classroom.* Boston: Holbrook Press, 1975.

Trap, J.J., Milner-Davis, P., Shirley, J., & Cooper, J.O. The effects of feedback and consequences on transitional cursive letter formation. *Journal of Applied Behavior Analysis*, 1978, *11*, 381-394.

Turnbull, A.P. Parent-professional interactions. In M.E. Snell (Ed.), *Systematic instruction of the moderately and severely handicapped.* Columbus, Ohio: The Charles E. Merrill Company, Inc., 1978.

Turnbull, A.P., & Schulz, J.B. *Mainstreaming handicapped students: A guide for the classroom teacher.* Boston: Allyn & Bacon, Inc., 1979.

Turnbull, A.P., Strickland, B.B., & Brantley, J.C. *Developing and implementing individualized education programs* (2nd ed.). Columbus, Ohio: The Charles E. Merrill Publishing Company, Inc., 1982.

Turnbull, A.P., Strickland, B., & Hammer, S.E. The I.E.P.: Guidelines for its development and implementation. *Journal of Learning Disabilities*, 1978, *11*, 40-46.

University of New Mexico/Albuquerque Public Schools Center for Parent Involvement, Albuquerque, 1979.

U.S. Bureau of the Census. *Statistical abstract of the United States: 1978* (99th ed.) Washington, D.C.: 1978.

U.S. Department of Labor. *Dictionary of occupational titles (4th ed.).* Washington, D.C.: U.S. Government Printing Office, 1977.

U.S. Government. State vocational education programs. *Title 45 a.s. Code of Federal Regulations* §*1361.* Washington, D.C.: Government Printing Office, October 1, 1979.

U.S. Office of Education. *An introduction to career education.* Office of Career Education. Washington, D.C.: U.S. Government Printing Office, 1975.

U.S. Office of Education. National Center for Educational Research and Development. The career education program status report. Washington, D.C.: U.S. Government Printing Office, 1971.

U.S. Office of Education. Occupational Clusters. Washington, D.C.: U.S. Government Printing Office, 1971.

U.S. v. Masthers, 539 F.2d 721 (D.C. Cir. 1976).

Valett, R.E. *Programming learning disabilities.* Belmont, Calif.: Fearon Publishers/Lear Siegler, Inc., 1969.

Valett, R.E. *The remediation of learning disabilities: A handbook of psychoeducational resource programs* (2nd ed.). Belmont, Calif.: Lear Siegler, Inc./Fearon Publishers, 1974.

Van Hattum, R.J. (Ed.). *Communication disorders.* New York: Macmillan Publishing Company, Inc., 1980.

Vergason, G.A. Accountability in special education. *Exceptional Children*, 1973, *39*, 367-373.

Volkmor, C., Langstaff, A., & Higgins, M. *Structuring the classroom for success.* Columbus, Ohio: The Charles E. Merrill Publishing Company, Inc., 1974.

Wagonseller, B., Burnett, A., Salzberg, B., & Burnett, J. *The art of parenting: A complete training kit.* Champaign, Ill.: Research Press Co., 1977.

Walker, H.M. *The acting-out child: Coping with classroom disruption.* Boston: Allyn & Bacon, Inc., 1979.

Walker, H.M., & Buckley, N.K. *Token reinforcement techniques.* Eugene, Oregon: E-B Press, 1974.

Wallace, G., & Kauffman, S.M. *Teaching children with learning problems.* Columbus, Ohio: The Charles E. Merrill Publishing Co., Inc., 1978.

Wallace, G., & Larsen, S.C. *Educational assessment of learning problems: Testing for teaching.* Boston: Allyn & Bacon, Inc., 1978.

Wallace, G., & McLoughlin, J.A. *Learning disabilities: Concepts and characteristics.* Columbus, Ohio: The Charles E. Merrill Publishing Co., Inc., 1975.

Walsh, J.J., Breglio, V., & Langlois, J.T. *An assessment of vocational programs for the handicapped under Part b of the 1968 amendments to the vocational education act: Executive summary.* Salt Lake City: Olympus Research Corporation, 1975.

Washington, R. A survey-analysis of problems faced by inner-city high school students who have been classified as truants. *High School Journal,* 1973, *56,* 248-257.

Waters, K., & Galloway, C. *A supplementary guide to precision teaching, planning, and charting techniques, or chart with heart.* Working paper, Eastern Nebraska Community Office of Retardation, 1972.

Watson, L.S. *Child behavior modification: A manual for teachers, nurses, and parents.* New York: Pergamon Press, 1973.

Weatherly, R., & Lipsky, M. Street-level bureaucrats and institutional innovation: Implementing special education reform. *Harvard Educational Review,* 1977, *47*(2), 171-197.

Wechsler, D. *Manual for the Wechsler Adult Intelligence Scale.* New York: Psychological Corporation, 1955.

Weinberg, W.A., & Mosby, R.J. *Developmental by-pass theory and background reading,* Vol. 1. Union Mo.: Franklin County Educational Cooperative Press, 1977.

West, F., Gobert, C.F., & LaCount, N. The ABC's of IEP's. In B. Weiner (Ed.), *Periscope: Views of the individualized education program.* Reston, Va.: The Council for Exceptional Children, 1978.

West, M., Carlin, M., Baserman, B., & Milstein, M. An intensive therapeutic program for learning disabled prepubertal children. *Journal of Learning Disabilities,* 1978, *11,* 511-514.

White, G.D. The effects of observer preferences on the activity levels of families. *Journal of Applied Behavior Analysis,* 1977, *10,* 734.

White, O.R., & Alper, T. *Precision teaching: A tool for the counselor and teacher, Working Paper No. 26* (2nd rev.). University of Oregon, College of Education, 1970.

White, O.R., & Haring, N.G. *Exceptional teaching.* Columbus, Ohio: The Charles E. Merrill Publishing Company, Inc., 1976.

Whitman, R.L., Mercurio, J.R., & Caponigri, V. Development of social responses in two severely retarded children. *Journal of Applied Behavior Analysis,* 1970, *3,* 133-138.

Wiederholt, J.L. Planning resource rooms for the mildly handicapped. *Focus on Exceptional Children,* 1974, *5*(8), 1-10.

Wiederholt, J.L, Hammill, D.D., & Brown, V. *The resource teacher: A guide to effective practices.* Boston: Allyn & Bacon, Inc., 1978.

Wiig, E.H., & Semel, E.M. *Language disabilities in children and adolescents.* Columbus, Ohio: The Charles E. Merrill Publishing Company, Inc., 1976.

Wilson, J. Selecting educational materials and resources. In D.D. Hammill & N.R. Bartel (Eds.), *Teaching children with learning and behavior problems* (3d ed.). Boston: Allyn & Bacon, Inc., 1982.

Wiseman, D.E. The non-reading parallel alternate curriculum part I, Selected papers on Learning Disabilities. *Proceedings of the Eighth Annual International Conference of the Association for Children with Learning Disabilities*. San Rafael, Calif.: Academic Therapy Publications, March 1971.

Wiseman, D.E., & Hartwell, L.K. Alternatives: Programs for secondary school age learning disabled students. *Learning Disabilities: An audio journal for continuing education*. New York: Grune Stratton, Inc., 1978.

Wiseman, D.E., Hartwell, L.K., & Krus, P. *Child service demonstration center in secondary school age learning disabilities*, Title VII-E, End of Year Report: 1977-78, Technical Report, No. 1. Tempe, Ariz.: Arizona State University, 1978.

Wolfensberger, W. The origin and nature of our institutional model. In R.B. Kugel & W. Wolfensberger (Eds.), *Changing patterns in residential services for the mentally retarded*. Washington, D.C.: President's Committee on Mental Retardation, 1969.

Woodcock, R., & Johnson, M. Woodcock-Johnson Psycho-Educational Battery. Circle Pines, Minn.: American Guidance Service, Inc., 1977.

Wrenn, C.G. *Student personnel work in college*. New York: Ronald Press, 1951.

Young, M.E. Mainstreaming and the minority child: The Philadelphia experience. In R.L. Jones (Ed.), *Mainstreaming and the minority child*. Reston, Va.: The Council for Exceptional Children, 1976.

Younie, W., & Clark, G. Personnel training needs for cooperative secondary school programs for mentally retarded. *Education and Training of the Mentally Retarded*, 1969, *4*, 186-194.

Ysseldyke, J.E., & Regan, R.R. Nondiscriminatory assessment: A formative model. *Exceptional Children*, 1980, *46*, 465-467.

Zigmond, N. A prototype of comprehensive services for secondary students with learning disabilities. *Learning Disabilities Quarterly*, 1978, *1*(1), 39-50.

Zigmond, N., & Brownlee, J. Social skills training for adolescents with learning disabilities. *Exceptional Education Quarterly*, 1980, *1*, 77-83.

Author Index

A

Abeson, A., 40, 358
Abrams, J.C., 20
Adams, P.A., 17
Agard, J., 354
Aiken, M.C., 322
Alexander, A.B., 8, 92
Alexander, R. N., 92
Algozzine R. F., 323
Allen, K.E., 164
Allen, R.C., 72, 82, 83, 87
Alley, G., 45, 58, 281
Alper, T.G., 133, 265, 292, 323
Altman, S.D., 40
Anderson, D.R., 267, 290
Arnove, R.F., 372
Ashlock, R.B., 254
Axelrod, S., 328
Ayllon, T., 149
Azrin, M., 149

B

Bachara, G.H., 347
Bachman, J.G., 13
Baer, D.N., 328
Bailey, E.J., 382
Bailey, L.J., 430, 447
Bailey, S.K., 7

Bak, J.J., 40
Baker, E.L., 136
Barlow, D.H., 339-340, 350
Barrett, J.C., 442
Bartel, N.R., 133, 140, 142
Baserman, B., 18
Bateman, B.D., 134, 136, 148, 266, 300
Bazleton, D.L., 86
Beare, D., 18, 40
Becerril, G., 18
Becker, W.C., 93, 256, 270
Behan, E.F., 349
Bendell, D., 348
Bergin, A.E., 322, 326
Berman, A., 73
Besant, L., 5
Bettencourt, B., 133, 265
Biklen, D., 71, 79
Biklen, O., 95
Birch, J.W., 354, 377
Blackhurst, A.E., 67
Blake, K.A., 141, 273
Blalock, J., 40
Bloom, B.S., 240, 254, 300
Boggs, E.M., 86
Bopp, M.J., 40
Bornstein, P.H., 328
Bracht, G.H., 321
Brantley, J.C., 158
Briard, F.K., 18

Broder, P.K., 67, 69, 76, 79
Brolin, D.E., 423-424, 427, 436,
    439-441, 447, 448, 450, 459
Brookover, W.B., 346
Brosh, M.C., 18
Brown, B.S., 67, 79, 87
Brown, S.M., 67
Brown, V., 123, 355
Browning, P.L., 11
Brownlee, J., 13
Bruininks, V.L., 40
Brutten, M., 349
Bryan, T.H., 40
Bryant, T.E., 18, 40
Buckley, N.K., 149
Budd, K., 164
Buros, O.K., 133, 273, 274
Bursuk, L.Z., 347-348
Buscaglia, L.F., 92
Buswell, G.T., 277
Buswell, J.L., 277
Butler, A.J., 11
Byrne, P., 3

C

Cahen, L.S., 320
Campbell, D.T., 320
Campbell, E.Q., 462
Cansler, O.P., 92
Canter, L., 59
Caponiger, V., 332
Carlin, M., 18
Carroll, L., 48-49
Cartwright, G.P., 271
Castor, J., 355-356
Chalmers, A., 138, 271, 304, 305
Charles, C.M., 139, 140, 143
Cheek, L.M., 192
Childress, M., 67
Clarizo, H., 233-260
Clark, G.M., 11, 21, 33, 445, 447,
    448, 451
Clifford, G.J., 319
Cob, H.V., 13

Coffey, A., 72
Cohn, M.J., 20
Cole, N., 348, 349
Colella, H.V., 349
Coleman, J.S., 462
Connolly, A.J., 254
Cook, L.D., 18, 19, 40
Cooper, B., 18, 20
Cooper, J.O., 330
Copeland, R.E., 336, 338
Courtless, T.F., 67, 79, 87
Craighead, W., 335
Crawford, D., 76-78
Cronbach, L.J., 322, 326
Cullinan, D., 381
Curtis, K.A., 328

D

D'Alonzo, B.J., 3-33, 123-151,
    153-195, 421-489
D'Alonzo, R., 59
Dauw, E.G., 322
Davis, S., 444
Deno, E., 123
Deno, S.L., 123
Deshler, D.D., 44, 45, 58, 346, 348,
    382
Devault, M.V., 318
Diament, C., 334
Dietz, A., 334
Dillner, M.H., 349
Dobes, R.W., 327
Dorsey, B.L., 335
Douglass, H.R., 5
Downs, M.L., 199, 381
Dreisen, K., 40
Drye, J., 40
DuBose, R.F., 264
Duling, F., 69
Dunn, L.M., 354, 381

E

Ebel, R.L., 281
Eddy, S., 69

Edwards, L.L., 62
Eldefonso, E., 72
Ellsworth, R., 318
Engelhart, M.D., 240, 300
Englemann, S., 256, 270
Epstein, M.H., 381
Erickson, E.L., 346
Evans, M.A., 9, 24, 59
Evans, R.N., 422, 426-427, 459
Evans, S., 21, 440

F

Faas, L.A., 94
Felton, M., 322
Filby, N.N., 362
Fimian, M.J., 123-151, 153-195,
 261-313
Fine, M., 348
Fisher, S., 17
Forrell, E.R., 347
Foster, C., 281
Fowler, S., 164, 328
Fox, R.G., 336, 338
Freeman, S.W., 19
Friedman, R., 40
Furman, W., 340, 341
Furst, B.J., 240, 300

G

Gable, R.A., 16
Gallagher, J., 318
Galloway, C., 292
Ganzer, V.J., 8
Gearhart, B.R., 8-9, 30-31, 222, 381,
 469
Gearhart, C.K., 222, 381, 409
Gelhausen, T., 67
Geller, M., 340, 341
Gilhool, T.K., 357
Glass, G.V., 321, 362
Glasser, W., 19, 59, 391

Glean, R., 466
Gobert, C.F., 166, 184
Gold, M.W., 198
Goldberg, M.F., 383
Goldfield, M.R., 327
Goldhammer, K.A., 423
Goldstein, S.A., 251-313
Good, C.V., 318
Goodman, L., 44, 57, 58, 382, 466
Gordon, T., 92
Gottlieb, J., 354
Graham, S., 137, 147
Greenlee, W.E., 18
Gregarus, F.M., 76
Gregorian, J., 138
Grinder, R.E., 14
Gronlund, N., 133, 239, 255, 269,
 274, 281, 391
Grossman, H.J., 48

H

Haggerty, D.E., 67, 71, 88
Halpern, A., 3
Hammer, S.E., 134, 147
Hammill, D.D., 123, 133, 140, 142,
 355
Hammond, R., 322
Hare, B., 18
Haring, N.G., 92, 269, 292, 293, 348
Harris, J.W., 336, 338
Harris, M., 149
Harrow, A.J., 449
Hartinger, W., 72
Hartman, C.A., 185
Hartman, D.P., 344
Hartwell, L.K., 91-120, 381-419
Hastings, J.T., 254
Haugh, O., 499
Haughton, E., 292, 330
Havighurst, R., 7
Hawks, T., 136
Hawkins, R.P., 327
Hayden, A.H., 92
Hayes, J., 184

Heller, G., 381
Heller, H.W., 33
Hellman, H., 131
Hendricksen, J.M., 16
Henrick, E., 13
Herman, R., 67
Hersen, M., 339-340, 350
Heward, W.C., 350
Hewett, F.M., 59, 126-127, 371
Higgins, J.P., 181
Higgins, M., 127
High, S.C., 459
Hill, W.H., 240, 300
Hilleboe, H.E., 86
Hobson, C.S., 462
Hofmeister, A., 278
Hogenson, D.L., 346
Howell, K.W., 133, 136, 138, 140,
    147, 265, 268-270, 273, 276, 279,
    281, 292
Hoyt, K.B., 422-423, 425-427, 435,
    459
Hudson, F. G., 134, 147
Hudson, G.D., 267, 290
Hurlock E., 40

I

Isakson, R., 318

J

Jacks, K.B., 18-19, 40
Jacobson, L., 7
Jensen, G.M., 466
Johnson, D., 40
Johnson, M.E.B., 318
Johnston, J., 13
Joiner, L.M., 346
Jones, R.L., 7, 316
Jones, R.R., 329
Jones, R.W., 349
Jones, W.G., 267, 290

K

Kane, L.A., 67, 71, 88
Kanner, S., 45
Kapist, J.A., 335
Kaplan, J.S., 133, 136-138, 140, 147,
    265, 268-270, 273, 276, 279, 281,
    292
Kaslow, F.W., 18, 20
Kass, C., 15-16
Kauffman, M., 354
Kauffman, S.M., 242
Kazdin, A.E., 329, 332, 335, 340,
    343
Keilitz, I., 67, 69, 78-79, 85
Keller, M.E., 18-19, 40
Kelley, J.A., 340-341
Kennedy, L.D., 349
Kent, R.N., 334
Kerlinger, F.P., 318
Kerr, C., 11
Kibler, R.J., 136, 239
Kiesler, D.J., 326
Kirk, S.A., 268, 468
Klein, R.S., 40
Kokaska, C.J., 423-424, 427,
    439-441, 447-448, 450
Kolstoe, O.P., 459
Krathwohl, D.R., 240, 300, 318, 322
Kreigel, L., 13
Kronick, D., 381
Kroth, R.L., 91-120
Krus, P., 382
Kukie, M., 354
Kuna D.J., 18
Kunzelmann, H.P., 348

L

LaCount, N., 166, 184
Laing, R.D., 45
Landis, J., 349
Lane, D., 349
Langley, M.B., 264
Langstaff, A., 127

Lanning-Ventura, S., 197-231
Larsen, L., 466
Larsen, R.P., 4, 9, 21
Larsen, S.C., 251
L'Bate, L., 317
Leming, J.S., 13
Lemoine, K., 133, 265
Lerner, J.W., 9, 24, 56, 59, 271, 382
Lessinger, L., 502
Lewis, R., 16
Lillie, D.L., 92-93
Linari, R.F., 444
Lindsley, O.R., 292, 330
Lindvall, C.M., 322
Lipsky, M., 316
Little, T.L., 21
Lockhead, J., 204
Loucks, S.F., 503
Lovitt, T.C., 328
Lucas, V.H., 185

M

Mackin, E.F., 422, 426-427, 459
Madaus, G.F., 254
Mager, R.F., 136
Mahler, C.A., 64
Mahoney, M.J., 330
Malaby, J.E., 270
Mali, P., 270
Mallory, W.A., 69
Malouf, D., 3
Mangum, G.L., 422, 426-427, 459
Mann, L., 44, 57-58, 382
Marandola, P., 18
Marholin, D., 331
Mark, H.J., 317
Marks, M.B., 318
Marland, S.P., 422, 424
Marsh, R.L., 503
Marshall, A.E., 350
Martin, J.H., 4, 6, 92, 382, 453-458
Masia, B.B., 240, 300
Massimo, J.L., 7
Mattina, J., 69

Mauser, A.J., 56, 58, 123-151
Mayer, G., 149, 329
Maynard, W., 367
McAshan, H.H., 136
McCall, W.A., 317
McCormack, J.E., 138, 148, 271
   287, 290, 304-305
McCoy, K.M., 233-260
McDaniels, A., 381, 385
McDartland, J., 462
McDowell, R.L., 46, 48
McGrady, H.J., 37-66
McLaughlin, T.F., 270
McLoughlin, J.A., 251
McManman, K.M., 20
McMenemy, R.A., 251
McNutt, G., 381
McWhirter, J.J., 18, 20
Meerbach, J., 127
Meers, G.D., 439
Menolascino, F.J., 504
Mecatoris, M., 335
Mercer, J.R., 504
Mercurio, J.R., 332
Metfessel, N.S., 322
Metz, A.S., 3
Meyen, E.L., 184-185
Meyers, G.L.D., 9, 24, 59
Michael, W.B., 322
Miles, D.T., 136, 239
Miller, S.R., 4, 9, 21, 439
Miller, T.L., 202
Mills, C.M., 8
Milner-Davis, P., 330
Milstein, M., 18
Mitchell, A.M., 505
Montgomery-Kasik, M., 197-232
Mood, A.M., 462
Moore, A.E., 8
Morgan, D., 155-157, 164, 183-184,
   187
Morgan. E., 78
Mori, A.A., 424
Mosby, R.J., 383
Muehl, S., 347
Murray, C.A., 67, 73-75

N

Nachtman, W., 254
Nardoza, S., 322
National Assessment of Educational
  Progress, 11-12, 14
National Association for Retarded
  Citizens, 505
National Association of State
  Directors of Special Education, 1,
  34, 147
National Center for Educational
  Statistics, 462
National Education Association,
  141, 360-361
Neeley, E., 262, 348
Neisworth, J., 149
Nelson, R.D., 335
Nesbitt, J., 40
Newlin, L., 133, 265
Nielson, L., 18
Nolen, P.A., 348

O

O'Connell, C.Y., 133, 136-138, 140,
  147, 265, 268-270, 273, 276, 279,
  281, 292
Ogg, E., 69
Ohlsen, M.M., 64
Ohrtman, W.F., 316
O'Leary, K.D., 334
Oliverson, B., 21
Otto, W., 251
Owen, R.W., 17

P

Page, W.R., 348
Palushka, J.A., 328
Panushka, J.A., 381, 385
Parsons, B.V., 8, 92
Patterson, G.R., 329

Pennsylvania Association for
  Retarded Children, 357
Perrine, M., 133, 265
Perry, N., 140-141
Peter, L., 268
Peterson, N.L., 164
Phelps, L.A., 445
Philage, M., 18
Phillips, E.L., 332
Pipe, P., 136
Place, P.A., 92
Planned Parenthood of America, 14
Podboy, J.W., 69
Pollack, C., 349
Pomerang, D.M., 327
Popham, W.J., 16, 136, 281, 322
Poppelreiter, T., 92
Poremba, C., 69
Powers, L., 40
Prehm, H.J., 507
Preli, B.S., 437
Prentice, J.J., 348
President's Committee on Mental
  Retardation, 86-88
Price, B.J., 21
Pritchett, E.M., 254
Provus, N.W., 322

Q

Querillon, R.R.., 328

R

Raymond, C.D., 436
Reckless, W.C., 7
Regen, R.R., 263, 271, 283
Reger, R., 123
Reid, J.B., 329, 334
Reynolds, M.C., 377
Richey, R.W., 136, 145
Riekes, L., 85
Rieth, H.J., 336, 338
Riffel, R., 507

Risko, V., 69
Robbins, M.J., 67
Robinson, E.H., 18
Rosenthal, R., 7
Rowbury, T.G., 164
Ruddell, R., 507
Rusman, F.K., 251

S

Sabatino, D.A., 4, 9, 21, 56, 58, 123,
    197-232, 315-350, 461-489
Safran, J.S., 21
Sampson, E., 130-131
Sanders, N.M., 240
Sarason, I.G., 8
Sarason, S., 358, 360
Scagers, P., 131
Scates, D.E., 318
Schilit, J., 67-90
Schioss, P.J., 315-350, 439
Schmidt, C.R., 202
Schnorr, J.M., 461-489
Schreiber, D., 7
Schultz, E.W., 508
Schulz, J.B., 356
Schumaker, J.B., 328, 342
Schwartz, L., 508
Schwartz, S.E., 436
Scott, O., 348
Scranton, T.R., 199, 381
Semel, E.M., 58
Shanker, A., 462
Shaver, J., 319
Shea, T.M., 40
Shearer, M.S., 92
Shelton, M.N., 18-19
Sher, N., 349
Sherman, J.A., 342
Shirley, J., 330
Shore, M.F., 7
Siegel, E., 40
Siegel, L.J., 328
Silberberg, M., 385
Silberberg, N., 385

Silberman, C., 462
Simon, S.J., 340-341
Simpson, L., 92-93
Simpson, R.L., 92
Sindelar, P.T., 123
Siperstein, G.N., 40
Skinner, B.F., 149
Slavin, R., 319
Smith, D.D., 138, 302, 309
Smith, M.L., 362
Smith, R.J., 251
Smith, R.M., 133, 149, 262, 265
Snell, M.E., 133, 137-138, 302, 309
Spache, G.D., 242
Spiegal, S., 85
Splaine, J., 7
Stables, J.M., 93
Stadt, R., 430, 447
Stagg, V., 264
Stanley, J.C., 320
Starlin, C., 292, 330
Steinitz, V., 14
Steinman, W.M., 328, 331
Stephens, T.M., 40, 185, 269
Stokes, T.F., 328
Stolz, L.M., 17
Stowitschek, J.J., 16
Strickland, B.B., 134, 147, 158
Strout, T., 372
Strupp, H.H., 326
Stufflebeam, D.L., 322
Sulzer-Azaroff, B., 149, 329
Svoboda, W.S., 421-460
Szasz, T.S., 45

T

Taplin, P.S., 334
Taylor, F.D., 59
Taylor, S.E., 15
Terman, L.M., 510
Thomas, D.R., 256, 270
Thomas, D.W., 348
Thomas, J., 126-127
Thompson, B.J., 164

Thompson, C.R., 19
Tollefson, V., 348
Trap, J.J., 330
Tudow, W.W., 86
Turnbull, A.P., 134, 147, 158, 356

U

Udall, D.K., 67, 71, 88
U.S. Bureau of the Census, 13
U.S. Government, 440
U.S. Office of Education, 425-426,
    475

V

Valana, M.C., 92
Valett, R.E., 133, 141, 145, 205
Van Hattum, R.J., 510
Van Reusen, T., 381-419
Vergason, G.A., 316
Volkmor, C., 127

W

Wagonseller, B., 510
Walker, H.M., 148-149
Wallace, G., 242, 251
Walsh, J.J., 511
Walter, T.L., 8
Ward, M., 444
Washington, R., 462
Waters, K., 292
Watson, L.S., 149

Watson, N.R., 233-260
Weatherly, R., 316
Weschler, D., 48, 69, 201
Weinberg, W.A., 383
Weinfeld, F.D., 462
Weintraub, F., 358
West, F., 166, 184
West, M., 18
Whelan, R.J., 93
White, G.D., 335
White, O.R., 269, 292-293
Whitman, R.L., 332
Wiederholt, J.L., 44, 58, 123, 355,
    383
Wiig, E.H., 58
Wilson, J., 141-142, 301
Wiseman, D.E., 21, 91-120, 381-419
Wolfe, M.P., 421-460
Wolfensberger, W., 80
Woodcock, R., 275
Wrenn, C.G., 63

Y

York, R.L., 462
Young, M.E., 373
Younie, W., 21
Yssekdyke, J.E., 263, 271, 283

Z

Zaba, J.W., 347
Zaremba, B., 67, 69, 78-79
Zigmond, N., 13, 40
Zimmerman, J., 76
Zoback, M.S., 123-151

Subject Index

A

Academic skills
  evaluation of, 172-174, 233-259,
    399-400
  and juvenile delinquents, 76-77,
    199-200
  problems on secondary level, 20,
    92, 382
  teaching basics of, 58-59, 378, 387
  tutoring in, 223
Academic success of LBP students,
  62
Accountability
  federal requirements of, 315-316,
    323
  of school principals, 377
  of teachers, 156-157
Accreditation of private schools,
  472-473, 476
Achievement tests, 273
Action plans
for parent involvement, 101-112
  prescriptive, 28
Administrators
  attitudes toward research, 316-320
  of autocratic schools, 372
  role of, 145, 375-378
Adolescents
  See also Learning Behavior
    Problem adolescents

cognitive process development of,
  205
in the criminal justice system,
  67-90
developmental characteristics of, 6,
  38, 371
in family and community systems,
  17-20
and self-image, 18, 383
sexual behavior rates of, 15
stresses of, 14
Advocacy
  checklist for legal system, 95-96
  for juvenile offenders, 68, 80-82
Affective domain and instructional
  objectives, 134-136
  and instructional objectives,
    134-136
Arizona Demonstration Resource
  Center PAC model, 387-398
Alternative Instructional
  Considerations, 406-407
Alternative programs and models for
  LBPs, 7, 97, 153-195, 384-388
Alternative public schools, 461-465
American Bar Association, 85
American Civil Liberties Union, 85
American Psychological Association,
  283
Aphasia, 39
Appeal procedures of placement, 361

Appropriate education as defined by
P.L. 94-142, 12
Arizona Child Service Demonstration
Center (CSDC), 381
Arizona Department of Education:
Career Education Matrix, 434
Arrest procedures for LBPs, 83-85
Assessment
See also Preassessment; Table of
Specifications
activity of, 146-147
of behaviors, 327-345
in case study evaluations, 168-180
definition of, 263
formative methods of, 263-299
of LBPs needs, 37-66, 131-134,
140, 166
of parents needs, 110-114
procedural analysis of, 300-312
of secondary process deficits, 202
standardized techniques of, 182,
201-202
of student's ecological system,
17-18
Association for Children with
Learning Disabilities, 76, 114
Attendance
compulsory attendance laws
and expulsion, 5, 7
and private schools
reimbursements, 472, 478
Attitudes
of criminal justice system, 68
of parents, 97
of peer tutors toward LBPs, 40,
364-366
of students toward teachers, 27,
316-320
of teachers toward LBPs, 8, 14, 39,
358-360, 363-364
about research, 315-320
Attorneys. *See* Lawyers
Audiometric screening, 182
Audiovisual materials, 144
Auditory problems and remediation,
206-213
Autocratic schools and classes,
371-373

B

Basic process problems, 252
Basic Skills. *See* Academic skills
Baseline data collection, 334-345
Behavior
appropriate for students, 148
assessment of, 326-345
causes of criminal behavior, 72-79
direct measures of, 284-292
disorders and emotional
disturbances, 3, 43, 45-46
objectives for, 237, 240-241
observational recording of, 292-299
and peer pressures, 72
sexual rates of, 14
violent, 35
Behavior management
and discipline programs, 59-61,
372
implementing programs of, 148-149
training for parents, 112
Behavior modification, 45
in the classroom, 62
and parents, 92
and reading remediation, 348-349
Behavior problems
alternative programming for,
381-419
goals for, 53
and incarceration, 7
of LBP students, 16, 379
as related to learning, 40-43
Behavior scales, 18
Billings Demonstration Program, 114
Brolin and Kokaska Model of career
education, 448-450

C

Career awareness, 429
Career development
categories of, 429-430
combined approaches of, 453-455
principles of program in, 432-439

Career education, 5
See also Vocational education
definition of, 422-424
matrix for, 434
models of, 448-452
state-of-the-art, 459-460
theories of delivery of, 425-429
Career resource center
community-based, 453-459
organization of, 127-129
Carnegie Council of Policy Studies
in Higher Education, 11
Case histories, 105
Case studies
evaluation checklist, 170-179
of LBP students, 40-42
Charts. *See* Models, and Checklists
Causes of juvenile delinquency, 72-79
Checklists. *See* Models, and
Checklists
Child abuse, 119
Child Service Demonstration Centers
(CSDC), 112-115, 387-398
Childbearing rates, 14
Children with Specific Learning
Disabilities Act, 468
Civilian Health and Medical
Program of the Uniformed
Services (CHAMPUS), 468
Clark Model of career education,
449, 451
Class. *See* Socioeconomic class
Classification systems of LBP
students, 43
Classrooms
See also Resource rooms
assessments in PAC, 396
communication systems for, 271,
305
environment of, 121, 364
learning laboratory for, 240
organization of, 123-134
size of, and individualization,
361-363, 379
Clearinghouses, in the criminal justice
system, 85-86

Clinical teaching model
of evaluation, 270
Coded Work Sheet, 250
Cognitive domain, 134, 136, 240
Cognitive process remediation, 204
Collaboration of professionals
with parents, 489
Communication
for data collection, 303-305, 316
for diagnostic teaching, 271
of parents and teachers, 91-120,
155, 374-380
in special education settings,
145-146
Community
involvement in career education,
437, 453-459
as a support system, 373
Competency-Based Infusion Model
of career education, 449-450
Competency testing, 378
Compulsory attendance law, 4, 5
Conferences
checklist for, 97-101
general strategies for, 117-119
of parent-teacher, 376-378
Confidentiality, 120, 138
Consultants as teacher, 28-29, 385
Content courses
See also Subjects
for career education, 438-439
choosing for analysis, 300
models of, 234-259
Content specialists, 233-236, 247-249,
259
Continuous recording, 294
Contracts
with private schools, 467-481
of student-teacher, 256, 258
Council for Exceptional Children,
16, 355
Division on Career Development,
422
Cost of private schools, 469, 475, 479
Cost efficiency, 315
screening and identification
programs, 387

Counseling
  with families, 7, 20, 104
  in groups, 5, 19-20, 62-64
  role in planning, 19
Courts
  and juvenile delinquents, 67-90
  right-to-education suits, 357-358
Crime
  and arrest rates, 14
  and first offenders, 8
  and LBP adolescents, 67, 72-79
Criminal justice system and LBP
  adolescents, 67-90
Crisis-resource teachers
  attitudes concerning, 28
  itinerant, 27-28
  as remedial educators, 9-10, 26-27
  training of, 10
Crisis teachers. See Crisis-resource
  teachers
Criterion-referenced tests (CRT),
  133, 166
  and evaluations, 194, 267-299, 313
  as measurement of basic skills,
    234-236, 239, 249-250, 255-256
Cross-tutorial programs, 348
Curricula
  criteria for selection of, 138-145,
    301
  functional, 12-14, 26
  implementing activities, 147-148
  infusion of career education,
    427-428, 450
  instructional materials for, 142-144
  and instructional objectives, 50-55
  laboratories, staff of, 141
  in law schools, 88
  for LBP students, 3-33, 121-151,
    462
  parallel alternative (PAC) for
    LBPs, 381-419
  in private schools, 471-472, 475,
    480-488
  and vocational education, 25,
    425-431, 442-443

D

Daily living skills, 12
D'Alonzo Model of career education,
  449-450, 452
DASIE model of formative
  evaluation, 266-267
Data-based instruction, decisions for,
  308-311
Data collection
  choosing a method of, 299-313
  and classroom organization,
    133-138
  for IEP evaluation, 191-194
  limitations in types of, 277, 316
  models of, 322-350
Data management, application to
  education, 261-313
Data sources of student
  performances, 281
Data monitoring in the classroom,
  261-313
Data recording in formative
  evaluation, 267-312
Death of a student, 119-120
Decentralization
  of career-vocational education, 453
  of handicapped students, 67
Decision-making for career
  education pupils, 434-435
Decision model for diagnostic
  teaching, 271
Deinstitutionalization of
  handicapped, 67
Delinquency
  See also Crime
  causes of, 72-79, 346-347
  and learning disabilities, 72
Democratic schools and classes,
  368-371
Department of Education. See U.S.
  Department of Education
Deprived youth and special
  education, 354, 380
Designs of research, 315-350

Development
  See also Adolescents
  of adolescents, 6, 14-15, 38, 45-46
  disorders of, 46-47
Developmental learning, 25, 317,
  345-346
Diagnosis
  instructional, 198
  of LBP pupils, 37-66
  of learning problems, 30
  of specific levels, 276
  standardized techniques of, 182
  and taxonomic systems, 45
  versus screening tests, 50, 52
Diagnostic-Prescriptive Teaching
  Model, 268
Direct Measure of Performance
  System, 286
Directive teaching, 269
Directory
  of private schools, 481-488
  of services, 116
Disabilities. *See* Learning Disabled
  (LD)
Disadvantaged youth, 354, 380
Discipline, assertive, 59
  in laissez-faire schools, 368
  problems of, 26
  programs of, 59-60
Disorders of behavior, 35, 43, 45-46
Dropouts
  and delinquency, 73-74
  and special education, 3-7
DSM-III. *See* Manual of Mental
  Disorders
Due process and student rights,
  158-159
Duration recording, 296, 332

E

Educable mentally retarded (EMR),
  43
Education for All Handicapped
  Children Act
  and alternative education, 461,
  467-468
  and evaluation, 315-316
  mandates of, 3, 12, 67, 91, 153,
  265-266, 351-381
Education programs, 29-32
  See also Programs
  individualized, 53, 57
  in private schools, 475, 480
Educational centers. *See* Learning
  centers
Educational guidance committee, 3,
  31
Educational service centers. *See*
  Learning centers
Educationally handicapped,
  identification of, 30-31
E.H. *See* Emotionally handicapped
Elementary school objectives, 10
Elementary and Secondary
  Educational Amendments of 1969,
  468
Eligibility for special education,
  153-155, 181, 466
Emotional development influences,
  45-46
Emotionally handicapped (EH), 3,
  43, 45-46
Employment programs for
  incarcerated youths, 7
EMR. *See* Educable Mentally
  Retarded
Enrollment in private schools, 471,
  482-488
Environment
  influence on behavior, 328, 349
  of private schools, 478-479
Equipment
  for basic classrooms, 125
  Form for Equipment Usage and
  Reactions, 413
Equity in education, 354
Equivalency exams, 5
Ethics of mainstreaming, 358-360
Exceptional learners
  mainstreaming of, 351-380
  models of evaluation for, 261-313

Experience-Based Model of
    vocational and career education,
    447, 453-458
Evaluation
    See also Assessment; Preassessment
    checklist for IIP, 191-193
    of IEPs, 20, 189-195
    of instruction, 136, 154-155,
        166-180, 233-259
    models of, 261-313, 315-350
    in parallel alternative curriculum,
        397-404, 407-417
    in private schools, 467-489
    reasons for, 263-265, 315-316
    of student files, 146-147
Evaluation-based instruction, 280,
    300-312
Event recording, 295, 329-331
Exams
    equivalency, 5
    using nonreading format, 389
Expulsion
    See also Attendance
    with parental involvement, 117
    of students, 5, 7

F

Faculty, 409
    See also Teachers
Failure
    of adolescents, 7, 10, 221
    and attendance, 5
    link to delinquency, 73-75, 77
    and self-image, 313
Families
    counseling with, 7, 18-20, 116-119
    as ecological system, 18-21, 91-120
    in therapy, 7, 19
Federal Bureau of Investigation
    Uniform Report of 1979, 13
Files on students, 134-138
Fine motor skills, remediation
    approaches, 216-218
First offenders, 8

Forms. See Models, and Checklists
Formative assessment, models of,
    266-267
Formative evaluation, instructional
    types and models, 265-313
Formats. See Models, and Checklists
Foundation skills and problem
    solving, 251
Frequency system of measurement,
    290
Functional skills, 12-14
    models of teaching, 25, 387
    and needs identification, 58, 182
Funding for LBP programs, 379

G

Games, as remediation approach, 203
Generic evaluation, formative model
    of, 264-271
Goals
    in career education programs,
        432-433, 459-460
    in IEPs, 154, 183, 188-189
Grading philosophy, 470-471
Graduation requirements, 195, 242
Group counseling. See Counseling
Group comparison research
    paradigm, 316, 321
Group process
    in programs, 19, 136
    for parental involvement, 95, 104
Guidance centers, 5
Guidance committee, 31
Guidance counseling, 62-64
Guidance Information System (GIS),
    129
Guidance offices, 126

H

Handicapped
    See also Mildly handicapped
    students; Public Law 94-142

applied research for, 345-350
court cases of, 82-83, 357-358
and criminal justice system, 67-90
Education for All Handicapped
    Children Act of 1975, 153-195,
    357-358
evaluation models for, 216-313
Handicapped Children Model
    Programs (HCMP), 112
identification of, 30-31
legal rights of, 67, 357-358, 466
National Center for Law and the
    Handicapped, 86
roles ascribed to, 68
secondary student data on, 9, 197
special education programs for,
    30-31, 85-90, 112
Health and first aid materials, 144
High Intensity Learning Center, 114
High schools. *See* Secondary schools
History of education, 198
Home-Based Model of career and
    vocational education, 448

I

Identification
    of educationally handicapped,
        30-32
    of LBP students, 37-66
    of offenders, 68, 86-88
Illinois Test of Psycholinguistic
    Abilities (ITPA), 268
Incarceration, 72-78
Individualized Education Program
    (IEP), 94, 97, 103, 105
    See also Handicapped
    definition of, 154
    federal regulations for, 153-155,
        315-316, 358
    IEP document development,
        180-188
    individual implementation plan
        (IIP), 175, 184
    materials for, 16-20

objectives for, 37-66, 377-378
parental involvement in, 112, 117,
    121, 130
plan checklist, 404
review and monitoring of, 180,
    190-194
team planning for, 300
use of files, 146
Individualized Instruction Program
    (IIP), 175, 184
    and criterion-referenced tests, 239
    evaluation of, 192-193
    lack of, 383-384
    standards of accuracy of, 242
Individual Performance Chart, 257
Individually Prescribed Instruction
    as evaluation system, 270
Informal Reading Inventory, 402
Inservice training, 379, 387
    for career education programs,
        435-436, 443
    in evaluation models, 316
Instructional diagnosis, 198
Instructional evaluation, 261-313
Instructional groups, 276
Instructional materials, 306
    See also Materials
Instructional objectives
    and IEP plannning, 16-20, 37-66,
        167-180
    for LBPs, 134, 197-259, 301
    for parallel alternative curriculums,
        391-394
    research on, 347-350
    short-term, 184-185
Instructional Option Form, 411-412
Instruments
    See also Models, and Checklists
    comparison of NRT and CRT,
        281-283
    kinds of, 133
Intelligence tests, 48
    use in criminal justice system,
        69-70
Integration of handicapped learners,
    351-354

Intensive level evaluation, 276-278
Interval recording, 296-299, 331-332
Intervention strategies
  with families, 7, 20, 91-120
  for LBP students, 37-66, 121-151,
    233-259
I.Q. *See* Intelligence Tests
Itinerant interventionists, 27-28
  See also Crisis-resource teachers

J

Jobs, 10-14
  See also Vocational education
Judges
  See also Criminal justice system
  education needed for, 89
  and LBP offenders, 67
Juvenile delinquency
  and achievement probelms, 382
  as LBP offenders, 67-90
  rates of, 13-14

L

Labeling
  See also Social image
  of adolescents, 7
  of LBP students, 49
  and systems of evaluation, 263,
    276
Laissez-faire schools and classes,
  367-368
Language disabilities in children and
  adolescents, 58
LBP students. See Learning Behavior
  Problem
Lasting products, number
  system of, 285-286
Laws. *See* Legislation
Law enforcement
  See also Criminal justice system
  and LBP adolescents, 67-90
Lawyers and LBP offenders, 67

Learning
  See also Learning centers
  assessment of, 182-183
  cognitive types of, 38
  developmental, 24
  goals for LBPs, 50-53, 433
  problems of, 30, 114
Learning assistance centers. *See*
  Child Service Demonstration
  Centers (CSDC); Learning centers
Learning Assistance Program for
  Educationally Handicapped
  Pupils, 30-31
Learning assistance teachers. *See*
  Learning specialists
Learning Behavior Problem (LBP)
  students
  See also Learning disabled
    students; Mildly handicapped
    students
  and academic success, 62
  alternative education for, 461-489
  applied research techniques for,
    315-350
  behavioral programs for, 148-149,
    153-155
  classification of, 4, 37-62, 351-357
  communication with parents of,
    91-120
  and criminal justice system, 67-90
  curriculum programming for, 3-33,
    133-142
  data management of, 261-313
  individualized education programs
    for, 153-195
  instructional objectives for, 37-66,
    121-151
  intervention goals for, 19-20
  labeling of, 7, 49
  learning centers for, 30-32, 112,
    115, 197
  legislation for. *See* Legislation
  mainstreaming of, 55-65, 233-259,
    351-380
  models programs for. *See*
    Programs

remediation programs for, 198-220
rights of, 157-158, 163
tutoring programs for, 220-232
vocational and career education
for, 421-460
Learning centers, 30, 32, 112-115,
141, 197
work experience at, 442, 453-459
Learning characteristics, 199
research on, 345
Learning disabilities. *See* Learning
Disabled (LD) students
Learning Disabled (LD) students
See also Learning Behavior
Problem (LBP) students;
Handicapped
alternative education for, 461-489
Association for Children with
Learning Disabilities, 76, 114
definition of, 468
diagnostic-clinical approaches,
50-53
Directory of Educational Facilities
for the Learning Disabled,
481-488
legal mandate for education of,
153, 468
reading and visual problems of, 15,
182
relationship to delinquency, 72-77,
347
strategies for, 45
U.S. v. Masthers precedent setting
case for, 83
Learning environments. *See* Resource
rooms
Learning outcomes
for career development education,
433-435
for parallel alternative curriculums,
391-394
Learning preferences, 199, 222, 389,
394-395, 401-402, 413-415
Learning problems. *See* Learning
Behavior Problem (LBP) students;
Learning disabled (LD)

Learning specialists, 31-32, 145
See also Teachers
Learning strategies, 45
LD students. *See* Learning Disabled
students
Legal advocacy, 96
Legal rights
of handicapped, 67-90
of juveniles, 153
of parents, 95
Legal system and LBP offenders,
69, 85-90
Legislation
and appropriate education, 13
Commonwealth of Massachusetts
v. Femino, 82
compulsory attendance laws, 5
Education for All Handicapped
Children Act of 1975, 3, 91
Edwards v. Arizona, 72
and funding, 422
Gideon v. Wainwright, 88
for handicapped offenders, 67
Miranda warning, 71
and parental involvement, 91-120
Rehabilitation Act of 1973, 91,
357
U.S. v. Masthers, 83
for year-round schools, 466
Listening skills, 15, 182
Log of data, 268

M

Mainstreaming
definition of, 351-357
and discipline problems, 62
of LBPs, 10, 18, 21, 24, 30, 55-65,
233-259, 351-380
and remedial education, 9
use of parallel alternative
curriculum for, 387
Management by Objectives, 270
Manual of Mental Disorders
(DSM-III), 46-48

Materials
　See also Instructional materials
　organization of, 125-126, 139,
　　142-145, 394-396
Mathematics
　instruction methods for, 251-258
　and survey level tests, 276-278
Matrix for career-vocation education,
　453-459
Measurement
　See also Evaluation
　instruments of, 132
　of learning and behaviors, 326-345
　of performance systems, 286-299
Media as teaching tool, 389
Medical history, 198
Memory, remediation approaches
　for, 206-207
Mental Retardation
　and criminal justice system, 67-90
　intelligence tests for, 48
　President's Commission on Mental
　　Retardation, 86-88
　special education for, 3, 354, 357,
　　466
Mesa Demonstration Resource
　Center, 112-114
Methodology
　of applied research, 320-350
　of instruction, 15-16
Mildly educationally handicapped.
　See Mildly handicapped students
Mildly handicapped students, 9
　alternative models for, 461-489
　career and vocational programs
　　for, 421-460
　and curriculum domains, 11-14
　identification of, 30-31, 43
　instructional approaches, 197-232
　Learning Assistance Program for
　　Educationally Handicapped
　　Pupils, 30-32
　mainstreaming of, 233-259, 351-380
　percentage in school, 197
　research designs for, 315-350

Mini PAC, 390
Minimal brain dysfunction, 468
　See also Learning Disabled (LD)
　　students
Minority youth, 12, 354-356
Miranda warning, 71-72, 86
Mirror Model for Parental
　Involvement, 101-107
Models, and Checklists
　A-B-A Design: Teacher Attention
　　and Profanity, 337
　A-B-A-B Design for Token
　　Economy in Reducing
　　Interruptive Behaviors, 338
　Addition Math Facts Probe, 275
　of advocacy methods, 95-96
　alternative instructional
　　considerations, 406-407
　of arrest procedures, 84
　for career resource centers, 127
　case study evaluation, 170-179
　classroom communication system,
　　305
　Coded Work Sheet, 250
　comparison of Two Types of
　　Evaluation Instruments, 281-283
　Competency-Based Infusion
　　Model, 449-450
　of conferences with parents,
　　98-101, 108-109, 117-119
　Continuous Recording Procedure
　　Format, 294
　Directory of Educational Facilities
　　for the Learning Disabled,
　　481-488
　Design to Validate a Positive
　　Practice Procedure, 342
　of exemplary lessons, 224-231
　Evaluation Model for Academic
　　Areas, 243
　Evaluation Model for Content
　　Areas, 234
　Form for Analyzing Use of
　　Options, 412

Form for Equipment Usage and
Reactions, 413
generic formative evaluation
model, 264
Improper Descending Baseline
Trend, 335
Individual Performance Chart, 257
Individualized Education Plan
Checklist, 404
instructional materials, 139, 142
Instructional Option Form,
411-412
Interval Recording Form, 298
Lasting Products Data, 286
Matrix of Experience-Based Learning
Situations and Structural
Components, 456-458
Multiple Baseline Across Behavior
Design, 341
Narrative Recording Procedure
Format, 295
Network Procedure for Placement of
Exceptional Students, 162
for organizing first week's
activities, 150
Points Scored Data Sheet for
Teaching Face Washing, 289
Procedural Model for IEP Use,
164-165, 168
Questions on Data Collection
Methods, 299
for recording data, 137
Recording Sheet for Rate Data,
330
Relationship of Foundation Skill
to Problem Solving, 251
rights of parents, 94
Sample Evaluation Form for
Parents, 416
Sample Evaluation Form for
Students, 414-415
Sample Evaluation Form for the
Teacher, 417
Sample Student Monitoring Form,
409-411
sample objectives, 224-231

School-Based and Experience-
Based Career and Vocational
Educational Model, 454-455
Scoring Sheet for Interval
Recording, 332
Semilogarithmic Six-Cycle Graph
for Charting Data, 293
service options for LBPs, 159-160
Simplified Evaluation Process, 323
Skills Evaluation of Student, 403
Sources of Student Performance
Data, 281
Steps in Procedural Analysis, 280
Student Learner Preference Profile
Form, 401-402
Table of Specification models, 235,
248-249, 255, 258
Ten Steps in Developing the IIP,
181
Textual Base for a Content
Outline, 245
Three Data Recording
Conventions in the Percentage
Correct System, 288
Three levels of evaluation, 272
Total Service Plan, Evaluation of
IEP, 192-193
Tuition and Fee Schedules of
Selected Private Schools, 469
Tutoring Program Management
Profile, 231
Year-end Summary Evaluation,
312
Model programs
See also Programs
as LBP alternatives, 96
for parent involvement, 112-115
for vocational and career
education, 421-460
Monitoring
See also Evaluation
of IEPs, 316
techniques of, 285-299
Multiple baseline designs for data
collection, 340-343

N

Narrative log, 268-269
Narrative Recording Procedure
Format, 295
National Assessment of Educational
Progress, 11-13
National Association of Private
Schools for Exceptional Children
(NAPSEC), 472
National Center for Educational
Statistics, 9
National Center for Law and the
Handicapped, 86
National Education Association, 141,
360-361
National Institute for Juvenile
Justice and Delinquency
Prevention, 76
National Panel on High School and
Adolescent Education, 453-459
Network Procedure for Placement of
Exceptional Students, 162
Norm-referenced tests (NRT), 133,
194, 271, 273-274, 279

O

Objectives. *See* Instructional
objectives; Task analysis
Observation
and direct evaluation methods,
284-285
recording methods of, 292-299
systems of, 299-313
Occupational development, 9,
442-443
Occupational training. *See*
Vocational education
Ombudsman for LBP offenders, 81
Open education, 465-466
Organizations of parents, 91
Orientation
for IEP planning, 164
to private schools, 481
OTTER model of formative
evaluation, 266-267

P

PAC. *See* Parallel alternative
curriculum
Parents
advocacy role of, 93-97, 120
benefits of involvement of, 107
communication and conferences
with, 91-120, 376
consent for testing, 133
and private school choice, 467
rights and responsibilities of, 120,
157-158, 166
Sample Evaluation Form for
Parents, 416
skills development training for,
112-115
strategies for involvement of,
18-19, 98-119, 373-378, 387, 437
Partial PAC, 390
Percentage correct system, 287
Peers
and criminal behavior, 72-73
perception of LBP students, 40,
364-366
as tutors, 29-30, 443
Perceptually handicapped conference,
468
Performance contracts, 256-258
Performance evaluation, 172-178,
183, 257, 267-313, 407-412
See also Evaluation
variables in, 310, 348
Periodic planning sheet, 304-305
Permission forms, 138
Personal skills, 13-14
Physical environment. *See* Resource
rooms
Placement committees, 361
Placement
justification for IEPs, 186-187
mainstreaming issues of, 354-357,
367-373
options for, 360-363
preparation for, 105, 156, 159-162,
167

in private schools, 472-488
research on, 347
vocational, 444-445
Planning
for career education, 432-433
Individualized Education Plan
Checklist, 404
with parents, 97-107
and special educators, 156
weekly plan sheets, 219
Planned Parenthood Federation of
America, 15
Points Scored Data Sheet, and
system, 286-290
Police role with LBPs, 86-87
Postsituational stage of evaluation,
322-325
Practice of learning, 16
Preassessment of entry abilities,
235-238, 247
Precision teaching evaluation model,
269
Preference PAC, 390
President's Committee on Mental
Retardation, 86-88
Presituational stage of evaluation,
322-324
Prevention
of criminal behavior, 68, 76, 82-85
role of special education in, 176
as teaching model, 27
Principal, accountability of, 377
Probation for offenders, 84-85
Problem solving
and foundation skills, 251-252
training in, 20
Procedural analysis, 280
Professions collaboration in criminal
system, 90
Profoundly Mentally Retarded
rights, 466
Program and Data File, 306
Programs
of career and vocational education,
433-460,
of instruction, 305

of mainstreaming, 351-380
options for LBPs, 96, 112-115,
421-460
trends in alternatives, 384-388
Programming
alternative models of, 351-489
for LBP students, 17-20, 38, 57,
379
Progress evaluations, 397-404
Psychological history, 198
Psychologists, 69-70
Psychology of crime and LBPs,
72-79
Psychomotor domain, 134
Puberty, 8
Public laws
P.L. 91-230, 468
P.L. 94-142. *See* Education for
All Handicapped Children Act
Public schools, alternative
models of, 461-465
Punishment of offenders, 84

Q

Questionnaire of parent needs, 107,
110-112

R

Rate system measurement of
performance, 291
Reactivity in baseline data collection,
335
Reading
and LD students, 3, 5, 382-384
and listening skills, 15, 400
research on, 347-350
standards of schools, 17
Woodcock Reading Mastery test,
275
Reality therapy, 45
Recidivism, rates of, 8
Record keeping
of instructional objectives, 411-412

or organizational information,
137-138
Recording
continuous procedure of, 294
of learner behaviors, 317, 329-345
Referral systems
of students to IEPs, 165
to teacher consultants, 28-29
Reinforcement as behavior
management, 62, 148-149, 310
Remediation, 197-220, 232
Remedial programs
for basic skills, 387
clinical approach to, 50-53
elementary model of, 421
for juvenile delinquents, 76-78
for LBP pupils, 3, 5, 15, 24-25
research on, 347
Research
applied techniques for, 315-350
trends in mainstreaming, 379
in vocational-career education, 459
Resource centers
for career education programs, 438
model programs of, 112-115
Resource rooms
history of, 385
purpose of, 23-26
organization of, 123-151, 197
Resource teachers
See also Crisis-resource teachers
methods of instruction, 233-234,
236, 259
Resource units of career education,
438-439
Response latency, 332
Response modes for testing, 238
Reversal designs, 336-339
Rights
See also Legislation
of students, 67, 69, 80, 157,
354-358
Rodman Job Corp Center, 5
Rural districts and private school
contracts, 467
Rural-residential models of career
and vocational education, 447

S

Samples
See also Models, and Checklists
of monitoring forms, 409-411
of research, 345-350
Schedules
implementation of, 146
in private schools, 475, 480
School-Based Comprehensive Model
of career and vocational education,
447, 451, 453-458
Scoring sheet for interval recording,
332
Screening checklists, 50-52
Secondary schools
objectives of, 10
and parent advocacy, 91, 93-97
and special education needs, 3-33,
123
structural climate of, 367-373
Segregation of LBP students, 123,
159-161, 359, 461
Self-image
influence on learning, 346-347, 383
and role of tutoring, 221, 349-350
Self-instruction, 328-329
Semi-logarithmic six-cycle model, 293
Service models of vocational-career
education, 446-452
Sexual behavior of adolescents, 14
Single-subject design of research,
325-345
Situational stage of evaluation,
322-325
Skills. See Academic skills;
Functional skills; Vocational
skills
Skills Evaluation of Student, 403
Social class
issues of, 5, 11, 354
and juvenile delinquency, 73
Socialization of offenders, 73
Southwest Regional Laboratory, 240
Special education
See also Legislation; Programs

and behaviorism, 21
and criminal justice system, 67,
76-77, 86-90
directors of, 315
model programs of, 30-31
philosophy of, 16
in secondary schools, 351-465
settings for, 22-23, 38
teachers of. *See* Teachers
Staff development, 373, 436
See also Inservice training
Standardized tests. *See* Norm-
referenced tests
Standards of accuracy in IIP, 242
Stanford-Binet test, 48, 69, 201
Statistics
of handicapped pupils, 9, 382
significance of, 325
Students
on handicapped pupils, 9, 382
significance of, 325
Students
attitudes of. *See* Attitudes
evaluations in PAC, 394-395, 399,
401-402, 413-415
population in private schools, 475,
479-480
Student teachers, 22, 316-318
Studies
case studies of LBPs, 40-42
conducted on youth, 11-14
methodology problems of, 78
Subjects
See also Content outlines
choices of, 139-140
evaluation of, 193-194
methods of instruction in, 225-259
Success, importance of, 221
Summary Evaluation, 312
Summative evaluation, 262, 265-266
Supervision as in loco parentis role, 6
Support services for offenders, 85-90
Surveys of student needs, 131-134
Survey level evaluation, 273, 275, 280
Survival skills. *See* Functional skills

Susceptibility rationale of
delinquency, 74
Suspension
and expulsion, 7
and juvenile crime, 74

T

Table of specifications, 235-237,
247-249, 255, 258
Tardiness, 35
Task analysis, 235-250, 270
Task Force on Law. *See* President's
Panel on Mental Retardation
Taxonomic systems, 263
Teachers
See also Crisis-resource teachers;
Learning specialists
accountability of, 156-157, 315
as advocates, 27
certification and preparation of,
9-10, 20-21
checklists for parent conferences
for, 97-101
in classroom communication
systems, 307
as consultants, 28-29
as content specialists, 383
in criminal justice system, 85-86
itinerant, 27-28
multi-disciplinary staffing model
for, 266
with PAC format, 405-407
and parental involvement, 91-120,
374-376, 489
in private schools, 472-473,
477-478
in resource rooms, 23
special education role of, 14, 20-23,
65-66, 85-86, 93-94, 376
students' perceptions of, 15
as team members, 28, 45
as vocational educators, 445-446
Teacher aides, 126-127

Teaching
of career education, 435-436
core attributes of, 148
evaluation model of, 270
of parallel alternative curriculum,
381-419
prevention model of, 28
Teacher stations, 126
Team approach in special education,
28, 45, 145, 167, 185-187, 266, 300
Truancy, 453
Tuition and fees of private schools,
469, 475, 479
Tutoring
cross-tutorial programs, 349
definition of, 199
models and approaches of, 25-26,
197, 220-232
by peers, 29-30, 443
sample objectives for, 223-231

U

Underachievers, 382-384
U.S. Bureau of Census, 4, 13
U.S. Commissioner of Education,
422
U.S. Department of Education,
Office of Special Education, 3, 386
U.S. Department of Justice, 86
U.S. Office of Education, 433

V

Vandalism, 35
Violence. *See* Behavior
Visual, Auditory, Kinesthetic, Tactile
(VAKT) system, 200
Visual problems, 203, 213, 215
Vocabulary development, 242
Vocational counseling, 5, 10, 19
Vocational education.
See also Career development
instructional objectives for, 54-55
for LBP students, 11-13, 20, 25,
92, 385-386, 439-448

W

Weschler Scales, 48
use in criminal justice system, 69
use in remediation assessment, 201
Woodcock Reading Mastery test, 275
Work sheets, 250
Workshops
See also Inservice training
for parents, 104, 112
Work-study programs, 5, 11, 112

Y

Year-round schools, 466-467

Z

Zero-reject education, 357